"For a multicultural, life-span effective therapeutic approach applied across a variety of disorders, you need to read immediately this book on the innovative application of Single Session Therapy. This practical book will cause you to think creatively about your clinical activities."

Donald Meichenbaum, *PhD, Research director of the Melissa Institute for Violence Prevention, Miami; and author of* The Evolution of Cognitive Behavior Therapy

"The editors and authors have provided a fascinating and inspiring journey of applications for single session thinking and practice. Contributors from across the world remind us that SST is real therapy. Its presence is important as a choice in the landscape of service delivery everywhere."

Karen Young, *MSW, RSW, Director, Windz Centre, Oakville, Ontario, Canada; international single-session and walk-in therapy workshop trainer and author of numerous articles and book chapters on brief narrative therapy*

"The expanding field of single session thinking and practice is one of the most exciting developments in the world of therapy and counseling today. This excellent volume makes a great contribution. The range of contexts and issues covered is extremely wide and there will be something for everyone, regardless of their chosen modality, to take away into their day-to-day practice. Highly recommended!"

Harvey Ratner, *BA, Cofounder of BRIEF, London, UK; coauthor of* Solution Focused Brief Therapy: 100 Key Points and Techniques

Single Session Thinking and Practice in Global, Cultural, and Familial Contexts

Single Session Thinking and Practice teaches readers how to implement single session approaches by encouraging practitioners and clients to collaborate in making the most of every encounter. Single session/one-at-a-time approaches are applicable in a multitude of settings, including clinics, private offices, medical centers, student counseling services – and can be used both in person and online.

Leading international figures and those practicing on the front lines provide guidance for conducting SST in a variety of contexts. Chapters feature descriptions of theoretical underpinnings, pragmatic clinical examples, cross-cultural applications, research findings, service delivery models, and implementation tips.

This text will be an instant and essential reference for anyone in the fields of brief therapy, casework, and healthcare, as well as walk-in and by-appointment single session services.

Michael F. Hoyt, PhD, is a psychologist based in Mill Valley, California. He was one of the originators (with Moshe Talmon and Robert Rosenbaum) of the Single Session Therapy approach and is the author/editor of numerous publications, including *Brief Therapy and Beyond*.

Jeff Young, PhD, is a clinical psychologist, director of The Bouverie Centre and professor of Family Therapy and Systemic Practice at La Trobe University in Melbourne, Australia. He is a coeditor of *Single-Session Therapy by Walk-In or Appointment* (with M.F. Hoyt, M. Bobele, A. Slive, & M. Talmon).

Pam Rycroft, MPsych, is a psychologist and family therapist at The Bouverie Centre in Melbourne, Australia. She has published numerous papers in the field of Single Session Therapy and was actively involved in planning the first and third international symposia on SST and walk-in services.

Single Session Thinking and Practice in Global, Cultural, and Familial Contexts

Expanding Applications

Edited by
Michael F. Hoyt, Jeff Young, and Pam Rycroft

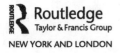

Routledge
Taylor & Francis Group

NEW YORK AND LONDON

First published 2021
by Routledge
605 Third Avenue, New York, NY 10158

and by Routledge
2 Park Square, Milton Park, Abingdon, Oxon, OX14 4RN

Routledge is an imprint of the Taylor & Francis Group, an informa business

Library of Congress Cataloging-in-Publication Data
A catalog record for this title has been requested

ISBN: 978-0-367-51468-6 (hbk)
ISBN: 978-0-367-51467-9 (pbk)
ISBN: 978-1-003-05395-8 (ebk)

Typeset in Times New Roman
by MPS Limited, Dehradun

To our clients and colleagues who have helped shape the world
of Single Session Thinking

We acknowledge the Wurundjeri People of the Greater Kulin
Nation, the traditional custodians of the land on which the third
international single session symposium was held and upon
which this book is based. We pay our respect to their Elders
past, present and emerging. We are inspired by our First
Nations' cultural heritage, traditional wisdom of
interconnectivity and relationship to the land, rivers, and sea.

"Now it appears that therapy of a single interview could become the standard for estimating how long and how successful therapy should be."
                        –Jay Haley (1993, cover endorsement of
                        Moshe Talmon's *Single Session Solutions*)

Contents

SECTION VII
Editors' Conclusion 323

Figures

Tables

About the Contributors

Editors

Michael F. Hoyt, PhD, is a psychologist based in Mill Valley, California. He was one of the originators (with Moshe Talmon and Robert Rosenbaum) of the Single Session Therapy approach. He is the author/editor of numerous publications, including *Capturing the Moment: Single-Session Therapy and Walk-In Services* (with M. Talmon); *Single-Session Therapy by Walk-In or Appointment* (with M. Bobele, A. Slive, J. Young, and M. Talmon); *Brief Therapy and Beyond: Stories, Language, Love, Hope, and Time*; and *Creative Therapy in Challenging Situations* (with M. Bobele).

Jeff Young, PhD, is a clinical psychologist and director of The Bouverie Centre at La Trobe University in Melbourne, Australia. He has published numerous papers on SST, is a past president of the *Australian and New Zealand Journal of Family Therapy*, and is a coeditor of *Single-Session Therapy by Walk-In or Appointment* (with M.F. Hoyt, M. Bobele, A. Slive, and M. Talmon). He was co-convenor of the First and Third International Symposia on Single Session Therapies and Walk-In Services, and he and his staff have been involved with training thousands of professionals in Single Session Thinking.

Pam Rycroft, MPsych, is a psychologist and family therapist at The Bouverie Centre in Melbourne, Australia. She has contributed to the training of hundreds of professionals, has published (and edited) numerous papers in the field of Single Session Therapy, and was co-convenor of the First and Third SST International Symposia.

Authors

Jorge Abia, MD, MA, is co-director of the Milton H. Erickson Institutes of Mexico City; San Juan, Puerto Rico; and Tuxtla Gutiérrez, Chiapas, Mexico. He is also co-academic chair for the Postgraduate Program in Ericksonian Hypnotherapy at the National Autonomous University of Mexico (UNAM), and secretary of the Mexican Society of Hypnosis.

Karen Alexander, ADip (Couns), BA (Visual Arts), BA (Writ), MSW, is a social worker at Metro South Addictions and Mental Health Services in an intensive community outreach team, Brisbane, Queensland, Australia.

Rachel Barbara-May, BA, BSW, is a social worker who has worked for many years in child and youth mental health and is an Open Dialogue trainer and therapist. She is currently the clinical lead at headspace Early Psychosis Program South East Melbourne; and coordinates the Eating Disorders Program at the Alfred Child and Youth Mental Health Service.

Julie Beauchamp, BAppSci (OT), MC/FTherapy, Cert IVAWT, is a family therapist, occupational therapist, and program manager for Clinical Services at The Bouverie Centre.

Rosalie Birkin, MCPP, MAN, is a child and adult psychotherapist in private practice. She established the Alfred Hospital Community Infant Mental Health Program in Melbourne which has operated for over 20 years.

Monte Bobele, PhD, ABPP, is emeritus professor of psychology at Our Lady of the Lake University in San Antonio, Texas; and faculty, Houston Galveston Institute in Houston, Texas. He is a licensed psychologist and AAMFT clinical fellow and approved supervisor. He has taught courses in walk-in/single session therapy in the U.S., Canada, Mexico, and Australia. He is the co-editor of *When One Hour is All You Have: Effective Counseling for Walk-In Clients* (with A. Slive), *Single-Session Therapy by Walk-In or Appointment* (with Hoyt, Slive, Young, and Talmon), and (with Hoyt) *Creative Therapy in Challenging Situations: Unusual Interventions to Help Clients*.

Patricia Boyhan, MCounseling, was a founding member of the Bouverie SST Team. She is a member of the Australian Psychological Society and the Australian Association of Family Therapists. Based in Melbourne, she now provides therapy and supervision in private practice.

Peter Brann, PhD, is the director of research and evaluation, and service senior psychologist, at Eastern Health Child and Youth Mental Health Service, and an adjunct lecturer with Monash University School of Clinical Sciences. Peter combines interests in routine outcome measures, health service models and diverse therapeutic approaches with the pragmatics of the service delivery world.

Flavio Cannistrà, PsyD, is a psychologist and psychotherapist. He is the founder of the Italian Center for Single Session Therapy, based in Rome, which conducts research and delivers training in SST and Brief

Therapy across Italy. He is (with Federico Piccirilli) the coeditor (in Italian) of *Terapia a Seduta Singola: Principi e Pratiche (Single Session Therapy: Principles and Practices)*.

Bonita Cohen, BSW (Hons), Grad Dip Fam Therapy, is a social worker and clinical family therapist who works at Alfred Health in the acute inpatient Mental Health Unit and in the Mental Health and Gambling Harm Service Victoria. She works with adults, older adults, families, and carers.

Kate Cordukes, MS (Arts Therapy), MS (Clinical Family Therapy), is a family therapist working at The Bouverie Centre in the clinical program and also teaches in the academic program.

Malena Cronholm-Nouicer, BS, is a psychotherapist, supervisor, and trainer with 30 years of experience in clinical work. She is a couples counselor based in Malmö, Sweden.

Gretta Daley, MSW, BS (Speech Path), is an accredited mental health social worker and couples therapist with experience working in a range of government and community sector organizations. She is a counselor at Gambler's Help Southern, a program of Connect Health and Community, Victoria, Australia.

Lars Dannerup, BS, is a couples counselor, family and solution-focused therapist, and supervisor with 25 years of experience in couples counseling. He is based in Malmö, Sweden.

James Dokona, Dip. in Counseling, Graduate Certificate in Family Therapy, is a brief solution-focused family therapist and an Indigenous counselor at The Bouverie Centre in Melbourne.

Windy Dryden, PhD, is emeritus professor of Psychotherapeutic Studies at Goldsmiths University of London, and is a fellow of the British Psychological Society. His many publications include *Single-Session Integrated CBT (SSI-CBT)*; *Single-Session Therapy: 100 Key Points and Techniques*; *Single-Session One-at-a-Time Therapy: A Rational Emotive Behavioral Approach*; and *Single-Session Counseling: Principles and Practice*.

Bronwyn Dunnachie, PhD, has a background in nursing, therapy, teaching, and clinical management and is currently a senior advisor at Werry Workforce Whāraurau, Auckland University, based in Christchurch, New Zealand. She oversees numerous portfolios of workforce development delivered across Aotearoa New Zealand, including the implementation of Supporting Parents Healthy Children (COPMIA).

Alison Elliott, BAppSc (Health Prom), M. Indigenous Studies (Wellbeing), Grad. Dip. Clin. Fam. Th., works with The Bouverie Centre's Indigenous Program as a family therapist and trainer in the Graduate Certificate in Family Therapy.

Ron Findlay, MBBS, is a medical practitioner and family therapist. He is a casual lecturer in narrative therapy at The Bouverie Centre of Latrobe University, sees families with the Elsternwick Headspace Single Session Family Team, and works in private practice doing individual, couple, and family therapy.

Carmel Fleming, MSW, is a senior social worker at Queensland Eating Disorder Service, Queensland Health, in Brisbane, QLD, Australia. She is also a PhD candidate with the School of Nursing, Midwifery and Social Work at the University of Queensland.

Denise Fry, RPN, MC FTher, is a mental health nurse and clinical family therapist working predominantly in child and youth mental health services for the last 20 years. She is currently the clinic manager at Alfred and Youth Mental Health Service.

Suzanne Fuzzard, BAppSc (OT), is a mental health occupational therapist and clinical family therapist and is the Centre Manager for headspace Murray Bridge, Mount Barker, and Victor Harbor, South Australia. As a project manager with headspace and The Bouverie Centre, she worked on increasing Family Inclusive Practice in the youth mental health setting through the use of Single Session Family Consultation (SSFC). More recently, she supported a project to embed SSFC within 50 headspace services across Australia. She is currently working to establish a walk-in service in headspace using the SST framework.

Belinda Goldsworthy, DPsych, is a senior clinical psychologist within Eastern Health Child and Youth Mental Health Service (EH CYMHS)/Deakin University Psychology Clinic, which operates using a single session framework. She also coordinates and runs an early intervention group program in schools for primary school children, 5–8 years old, and their parents.

Grace Harvey, MA, LMFT, is the clinical coordinator at the University of California–Santa Barbara Counseling and Psychological Services.

Paul Hickey, BSW (Hons), is a social work lead within the Therapies and Allied Health Team of Metro South Addictions and Mental Health Service, Brisbane, Queensland. Paul co-designed and facilitates training in Single Session Therapy within Metro South Addiction and Mental Health Service. He is also a PhD candidate at the University of Queensland.

Turi Honniger, PhD, is the clinical director of Counseling and Psychological Services at the University of California–Santa Barbara.

Lia Hunter, MPsych, is a senior clinical psychologist within Eastern Health Child and Youth Mental Health Service (EH CYMHS)/Deakin University Psychology Clinic, which operates using a single session framework. She is also a senior clinician within the EH CYMHS Access Team, which provides psychiatric triage for EH CYMHS.

Karin Isherwood, MA, is a senior consultant clinical psychologist with experience in infant, child, youth, and family mental health. Originally from the United States, Karin has been practicing in New Zealand since 1996. She currently works as a senior advisor for Werry Workforce Whāraurau, Auckland University, based in Wellington. She also has a small private practice supporting people who have experienced trauma through sexual assault, childhood sexual abuse, and homicide.

Jillian McDonald, GDipMH, RN, CMHN, is a credentialed mental health nurse working within the Therapies and Allied Health Team of Metro South Addictions and Mental Health Service, Brisbane, Queensland. Jillian is leading the implementation of Single Session Therapy across this service. She co-designed and facilitates SST training within Metro South Addictions and Mental Health Service and created the SST Practice Development Matrix.

Molly McDonald, PhD, is a staff psychologist at the University of California–Santa Barbara Counseling and Psychological Services.

Nancy McElheran, RN, MN, is a clinical nurse specialist, an AAMFT clinical fellow and approved supervisor, and a member of the Canadian Association of Marriage and Family Therapists (CAMFT). For many years she was the director and clinical coordinator of the Eastside Family Centre in Calgary, Canada, where she was involved in its development and operation. She maintains her consultation, supervisory, and teaching role at the Eastside Family Centre.

Tess McGrane, MS, MClinFamTh, is a nurse and family therapist with master's degrees in psychology and family therapy. She is coordinator and clinician for the Single Session Therapy (SST) family work at Elsternwick and Bentleigh headspace centers.

Jennifer E. McIntosh, PhD, AM, is a clinical psychologist and professor of research at The Bouverie Centre, La Trobe University, Melbourne.

Helen Mildred, DPsych (Clin), is director of the Eastern Health Child and Youth Mental Health Service/Deakin University Psychology Clinic, which operates using a single session framework. She is a senior lecturer at Deakin University with research interests in child and youth mental health, borderline personality disorder, and self-injury.

John K. Miller, PhD, LMFT, is a full professor in the school of Social Development and Public Policy at Fudan University in Shanghai, China; an adjunct professor in the Department of Psychology at the Royal University of Phnom Penh in Cambodia; and the director of the Sino-American Family Therapy Institute (SAFTI).

Myf Murphy, BApplied Science (Occupational Therapy) is an occupational therapist and has worked in Child and Adolescent Mental Health Services (CAMHS) for 18 years in Hobart and Melbourne. She was one of three principal researchers and team coordinator for a Single Session Team at the CAMHS Community Team in Hobart, Tasmania. Most recently she has started a private practice in Hobart, Tasmania.

Vicky Northe, MSW, has worked in mental health as a social worker since 1995. During her career, she has worked in maternal, child, and adolescent mental health and adult mental health. She is currently team coordinator for The Alfred Mental Health and Gambling Service, Victoria.

Rafael Núñez, MA, is the co-director of the Milton H. Erickson Institute of Mexico City; San Juan, Puerto Rico; and Tuxtla Gutiérrez, Chiapas. He is also co-academic chair for the post-graduate program in Ericksonian Hypnotherapy, the University Extension of UNAM (The National Autonomous University of Mexico); and secretary of the Mexican Society of Hypnosis.

Brendan O'Hanlon, PhD, is the Mental Health Program manager at The Bouverie Centre, La Trobe University in Melbourne. He has a strong interest in the implementation of family-based approaches in mental health services including Single Session Family Consultation and Family Psychoeducation.

Kieran O'Loughlin, PhD, is senior lecturer in counseling and psychotherapy at the Australian College of Applied Psychology (Melbourne campus). He was previously employed as a counselor, clinical supervisor, and manager at Thorne Harbour Health (previously the Victorian AIDS Council) and currently also works in private practice.

Stacey Porter draws on extensive experience in Māori mental health, Māori policy, Māori medium pedagogy and child development initiatives to support implementation of culturally responsive Single Session Family Consultation (SSFC) in Aotearoa New Zealand. Stacey descends from Ngai Takoto, Ngāti Kahu and Ngāpuhi in the far north, and Rongowhakaata, Ngāti Maru on the east coast of the North Island.

Aspasia Stacey Rabba, PhD, is a clinician-researcher and registered psychologist trained in educational and developmental psychology. She has worked in the autism field since 2008. During her PhD she developed a family support program for parents following a child's autism diagnosis. Dr. Rabba currently works as a senior psychologist within a specialist mental health and disability team in Melbourne, Australia.

Catherine Renkin, BSc, BMS, is a social worker with Metro South Addictions and Mental Health Services in Brisbane, Queensland, Australia. She is also an adjunct lecturer at the University of Queensland School of Nursing, Midwifery, and Social Work.

Alexandra ("Alix") Robinson, PhD, is a postdoctoral fellow at the University of California, Santa Barbara. She previously worked at the Eastside Family Centre in Calgary, Canada.

Robert Rosenbaum, PhD, is a psychotherapist, neuropsychologist, and international teacher of Dayan (Wild Goose) qigong and Zen meditation. He was a co-originator (with Talmon and Hoyt) of the Single Session Therapy approach. His books include *Zen and the Heart of Psychotherapy*; *Walking the Way: 81 Zen Encounters with the Tao Te Ching* (with S.M. Weitzman); and *What's Wrong with Mindfulness (and What's Not): Zen Perspectives* (edited with B. Magid). He is based in Sacramento, California.

Naomi Rottem, BSW, MClinFamTh, is a social worker and family therapist who for many years worked as Program Manager of Community Services at The Bouverie Centre. She is now Training and Consultancy Development Coordinator at Drummond Street Services in Melbourne. Her publication topics include family inclusive practice, single session work implementation, and adolescent family violence research.

Arnold Slive, PhD, is a licensed psychologist and AAMFT clinical fellow and approved supervisor. He is a visiting professor at Our Lady of the Lake University in San Antonio, Texas; and also serves as a part-time clinician and agency consultant in Austin, Texas. He founded walk-in/single session counseling services in Canada and the U.S. He is co-editor (with M. Bobele) of *When One Hour is All You Have: Effective Counseling for Walk-In Clients* and (with Hoyt, Bobele, Young, and Talmon) of *Single-Session Therapy by Walk-In or Appointment*.

Martin Söderquist, PhD, based in Malmö, Sweden, is a psychologist, and psychotherapist with 40 years of experience in clinical therapy and research – the last 12 years as a couple counselor. An important part of his work is Single Session/One-at-a-Time sessions. His most recent book (in Swedish) is *Ett Samtal i Taget: Familjerådgivning i Ny Form.* (Translation: *One Session at a Time: Couple Counseling in a New Format.*)

Sophia Sorensen, BBA, MA, RCC, is a registered clinical counselor in private practice in British Columbia, Canada, specializing in serving Indigenous and culturally diverse populations. She previously worked as a crisis outreach counselor for the First Nations Health Authority, and has also worked for government agencies, not-for-profit, and private organizations serving clients of all ages.

Moshe Talmon, PhD, is the author of the groundbreaking 1990 book, *Single Session Therapy: Maximizing the Effect of the First (and Often Only) Therapeutic Encounter*, which introduced Single Session Thinking to the world; and the author of its follow-up, *Single Session Solutions: A Guide to Practical, Effective, and Affordable Therapy*. He is also coeditor (with Hoyt) of *Capturing the Moment: Single-Session Therapy and Walk-In Services*; and coeditor (with Hoyt, Bobele, Slive, and Young) of *Single-Session Therapy by Walk-In or Appointment: Administrative, Clinical, and Supervisory Aspects of One-at-a-Time Services*. He is currently in private practice in Israel.

Kelly Tsorlinis, BSW (Hons), M (Fam Th), is a social worker and clinical family therapist and works as Intake Program Coordinator and family therapist at The Bouverie Centre in Melbourne. She also maintains a private practice.

Henry von Doussa, MA (Creative Arts), is a researcher at The Bouverie Centre in Melbourne.

Karin Wulff, MS, is a couple's counselor and solution-focused therapist based in Malmö, Sweden. She has 25 years of experience in clinical work.

Marianne Wyder, MSW, PhD, is a senior research fellow working within the Research and Learning Team of Metro South Addictions and Mental Health Service, Brisbane, Queensland. Marianne supports clinicians to conduct and facilitate practice-based research and service evaluation projects.

Dai ("Daisy") Xing, BS, is a psychotherapist and counselor at the Neiguan Counseling Center in Shanghai, China. She has worked with the Chinese Single Session Team Family Therapy project since 2016. She is an honors graduate of the Sino-American Family Therapy Institute (SAFTI) post-degree program.

Hu ("Yaoyao") Yaorui, BS, is a private practice therapist focusing on dance and movement therapy as well as family therapy in Shanghai, China. She has worked with the Chinese Single Session Family

Therapy project since 2016. She is an honors graduate of the Sino-American Family Therapy Institute (SAFTI) post-degree program.

Xu ("Eileen") Yilin, BA, is a private practice therapist focusing on family therapy in Shanghai, China. She has worked with the Chinese Single Session Family Therapy project since 2017. She is an honors graduate of the Sino-American Family Therapy Institute (SAFTI) post-degree program.

Acknowledgments

Many, many thanks:

- To the authors who wrote the chapters, the clients whose stories are told therein, and to the organizations and agencies that provided contexts for the services described; additional appreciation to Moshe Talmon for his fine Foreword
- To The Bouverie Centre: An Integrated Practice-Research Centre, La Trobe University, Melbourne. *Good on ya!* to Penny Wong and all the staff that helped make the Single Session Thinking: Going Global One Step at a Time – 3rd International Single Session Therapy and Walk-In Services Symposium so successful. Additional gratitude to headspace National Youth Mental Health Foundation for their major sponsorship; as well as the Victorian Department of Health and Human Services for their generous support
- To Nina Guttapalle, then-editor at Routledge Publishers, for embracing this project; and to Grace McDonnell, editorial assistant extraordinaire, for her excellent stewardship seeing it through to fruition. Additional thanks to Neema Sangmo Lama and MPS Limited for skillful production; to Ferenc Paczka for I.T. support; and to all those (printing, sales, delivery, and others) whose labor has made this project possible
- To our respective benefactors. For Hoyt, Kaiser Permanente, and the Stanley Garfield Memorial Award for Clinical Innovation, who granted research time for the original SST project; and to the APF Cummings Psyche Prize for its support of my writing. For Young and Rycroft, The Bouverie Centre's previous director, Dr. Colin Riess who oversaw the establishment of our original SST team, to Pat Boyhan who researched our first 50 SST families, to the staff and client families who helped us develop this way of working, and to the School of Psychology and Public Health, La Trobe University, for supporting our Centre's integration of practice and research
- To our families and friends for their love and support. For Hoyt, to my dear wife Jennifer for her endless kindness and good counsel; and

to LexiLou for her dogged perspicacity. For Young, to my wife Tric, and children Sweeney and Billie, for keeping me honest, real and compassionate. For Rycroft, to my husband and true companion, Frank, and to my adult children and my 11 glorious grandchildren for their endless encouragement, positive energy and welcome distraction
• To one another, for friendship, mutual learning, and good humor on a long and satisfying journey.

Michael F. Hoyt, Mill Valley, California, USA
Jeff Young, Melbourne, Victoria, Australia
Pam Rycroft, Melbourne, Victoria, Australia

Foreword

Moshe Talmon

It is a great honor for me to welcome you to the book, *Single Session Thinking and Practice in Global, Cultural, and Familial Contexts: Expanding Applications*, edited by my friends and colleagues Michael Hoyt, Jeff Young, and Pam Rycroft. This exciting compendium has its roots in The Third International Symposium on Single Session Therapy and Walk-In Services, which was held October 24–25, 2019, in Melbourne, Australia.

Over 30 years ago, I joined the Kaiser Permanente Medical Group in Hayward, California, as a staff psychologist on the Child and Family Team, and started seeing families and individuals. In the course of my first year at Kaiser, I stumbled upon the single session phenomenon. For the first time in my practice as a psychotherapist, about one-third of my cases did not return after the first session. I was bewildered, upset, and surprised. But soon after, I realized that this is a very wide and common phenomenon, shared by all the other members in my team.

I telephoned all of the families who chose not to return to what later I called "unplanned single session therapy" and was pleasantly surprised to know that they had realized a great deal of good after that session. So I initiated the "planned single session therapy" research project, led by Michael Hoyt and Bob Rosenbaum, both of whom worked with the Adult Team. And together, for a year, we randomly saw patients for "planned single session therapy," keeping open the possibility of additional sessions while letting families and individuals know there was a possibility that one session may be enough. Our findings were very encouraging – over one-half of patients chose to have a single session (even though more were available) and most reported benefits in both the specific problems that had brought them to therapy and in other related "ripple" issues. The book *Single-Session Therapy: Maximizing the Effect of the First (and Often Only) Therapeutic Encounter* was published in 1990; followed in 1993 by *Single Session Solutions*. Since then, all over the world, other projects and other researchers have found similar results.

With the development of walk-in clinics, single session therapy became an even more common phenomenon; in walk-in settings, about eighty percent of clients are seen for a single session with satisfying and useful outcomes.

I am glad that The Bouverie Centre in Melbourne, Australia, organized the third occasion for people all around the world to gather, share, and celebrate their experiences, and I am pleased that this book will make it possible for many readers to learn about results, ideas, and techniques for making single session therapy a common, effective, and important component within the field of psychotherapy.

Section I
Editors' Introduction

1 Single Session Thinking and Practice Going Global One Step at a Time

Michael F. Hoyt, Jeff Young, and Pam Rycroft

"A journey of a thousand miles begins with a single step."
– Lao Tzu (6th century BCE)

The essence of single session thinking is to approach the first session as if it will be the only session, while creating opportunities for further work if it is requested by the client. What emerges is a collaborative, direct, and transparent approach to providing services that puts the client in a very active role in determining the focus and length of the work. As Talmon (1993, p. 73) put it: "These concepts represent an alternative to the traditional model in psychiatry and psychotherapy: psychohealth replacing psychopathology, solutions replacing problems, and partnership replacing patronization, domination, and hierarchy."

Single session thinking is a practical and ethical response to the abundant research that shows that whether we like it or not, a significant number of therapy clients seeking help will only attend one session and will find that one session sufficient. Clinical experience shows that it is not possible to predict whether a particular client will return for further sessions. Hence, single session thinking leads to therapy and other service provision in which the practitioner and client proceed, from the beginning, with the understanding that the one meeting may be all that will occur. There might be additional sessions, or there might not be, so single session thinking leads to approaching the first session (and any subsequent session) as a one-at-a-time potentially-complete-unto-itself event. This attitude has the potential to transform healthcare service delivery.

Single session/one-at-a-time applications have expanded beyond the constraints of traditional psychotherapy. Although single session thinking emerged from therapeutic practice and clinical research – the main topic of the present volume – it should be recognized that such thinking is relevant for many types of work contexts. It can inform, for example, a collaborative, focused, efficient, and outcome-oriented approach to an ever-increasing range of services outside of the therapy room, including educational and career counseling, homeless services, hospital social work, home health agencies, and post-disaster responses.

Four common themes cut across and underlie single session thinking and practice, no matter the context:

1. *Attitude* – treating the session "as if" it might be the only one and hence making the most of every encounter, underpinned by the paramount acceptance that one session could be (and often is!) enough
2. *Accessibility* – responding in a timely manner without any unnecessary barriers to clients receiving help when they are most ready
3. *Acting Now* – accepting that the best opportunity to address change is NOW, no matter the diagnosis, severity, or complexity of the problem, and
4. *Alliance* – asking what clients want to achieve by the end of the session so that the therapist and client can work collaboratively, in the here and now, toward that goal.

Recognizing the wisdom in the old saying, "As the twig is bent, so grows the tree," various writers (e.g., Eisenthal 1976a 1976b; Haley 1977, 1989; Napier & Whitaker, 1978; Goulding, 1990; Budman, Hoyt, & Friedman, 1992) have commented on the cardinal influence of the first and sometimes only meeting. Once is often enough. As O'Hanlon and Weiner-Davis (1989, pp. 77–78) wrote: "We have observed enough 'one-session cures' to be utterly convinced that they are neither flukes, miracles, nor magic. Rather, something powerfully therapeutic occurs in the interaction between therapist and client during these sessions." Empirical support, both qualitative and quantitative, for the effectiveness of SST is substantial and keeps growing (see Mumford, Schlesinger, Glass, Parrick, & Cuerdon, 1984; Talmon, 1990, 1993; Hurn, 2005; Slive & Bobele, 2011; Campbell, 2012; Hymmen, Stalker, & Cait, 2013; Harper-Jaques & Foucault, 2014; Hoyt & Talmon, 2014; Stalker et al., 2015; Schleider & Weisz, 2017; Hoyt, Bobele, Slive, Young, & Talmon, 2018; Ewen et al., 2018; Aafjes-van Doorn & Sweeney, 2019; Cannistrà et al., 2020; Kachor & Brothwell, 2020; Schleider et al., 2021).

Single session therapy approaches are also receiving very strong endorsement by clients. A meta-review of 18 refereed journals and book chapters by Hymmen et al. (2013), for example, found client satisfaction rates of between 90–100% for both SST by walk-in (5 studies) and by appointment (13 studies). As seeking help is becoming less stigmatized, managers and policymakers are also increasingly exploring single session methods because of growing community demands for access to mental-health services at a time in which government and private funding for healthcare cannot expand to respond to this growing demand.

The History of Single Session Therapy

The field of single session therapy (SST) has grown rapidly since the 1990 publication of Moshe Talmon's groundbreaking book, *Single-Session Therapy: Maximizing the Effect of the First (and Often Only) Therapeutic Encounter* (done in collaboration with Robert Rosenbaum and Michael Hoyt at Kaiser Permanente in Northern California). Prior to the Kaiser study, there had been scattered reports of one-session therapy successes, beginning with Freud (see Sproel, 1975; Bloom, 1981/1992; Malan, Heath, Bascal, & Balfour, 1975; Rockwell & Pinkerton, 1982; O'Hanlon & Hexum, 1990; Rosenbaum, Hoyt, & Talmon, 1990; Hoyt, Rosenbaum, & Talmon, 1992), but Talmon's was the first prospective, systematic study documenting the frequency and effectiveness of planned (or intentional) single session therapies.

The basic findings of the Kaiser study were:

- Thirty-four of 58 patients (58.6%) elected to complete their therapy in one session even when more sessions were available
- More than 88% of the one-session patients reported significant improvement in their original "presenting complaint" and more than 65% also reported "ripple" improvements in related areas of functioning, and
- While not experimentally assigned to one-session or longer, on follow-up there was no difference in satisfaction and outcome scores between those who chose to stop after one visit (SST) versus those who continued for more sessions.

In 1967, walk-in psychological (and medical) services were founded at both the Los Angeles Free Clinic and at the Haight-Ashbury [San Francisco] Free Clinic, and then in 1969 the Minneapolis Walk-In Counseling Clinic opened its doors. In the early 1990s, walk-in single session services were developed by Arnie Slive, Nancy McElheran, and their colleagues at the Eastside Family Centre in Calgary, Canada (see Slive & Bobele, 2011; Slive, MacLaurin, Oakander, & Amundson, 1995; Slive, McElheran, & Lawson, 2008; McElheran, Stewart, Soenen, Newman, & MacLaurin, 2014; Miller & Slive, 2004; Stewart et al., 2018; also Chapter 11 of this volume). Walk-in SST services were subsequently taken by Monte Bobele to Our Lady of the Lake University in San Antonio, Texas, where they have been taught to graduate students, provided to the community, and promulgated in the U.S. and Mexico (see Slive & Bobele, 2011; Bobele et al., 2018; also see Chapter 4). Canada was also remarkable for its pro-liferation of walk-in SST services (see Harper-Jaques & Foucault, 2014; McElheran, Harper-Jaques, & Lawson, 2020; K. Young, 2018, 2020).

The findings of the Kaiser study and the growth of walk-in SST services set off a number of controversies. Some questioned whether a single session could even be considered therapy; others conceded "Maybe, for simple problems." There were worries about how to make a living if clients were only seen one time; some were concerned – mistakenly – that "SST" was a nefarious right-wing economic plot meant to limit clients to one visit as a way of withholding needed services. Many clinics and program managers shared these concerns, but they were also intrigued, since they had noticed that some clients were de facto electing to attend for only one session and that SST provided a way to be responsive and make the most of that time with the client. There was increasing re-cognition that single session ways of working had the potential for creating more accessible services, early intervention, and the freeing up of resources to help meet the pressing demands of other clients who wanted and truly needed more extended therapy (Hoyt, Young, & Rycroft, 2020).

By the year 1994, The Bouverie Centre of La Trobe University in Melbourne, Australia (see Young, 2018; Rycroft & Young, 2014; Young, Rycroft, & Weir, 2014; also see Chapter 3) began to offer extensive by-appointment single sessions and began training large numbers of diverse professionals, eventually assisting many organizations to implement single session practices as part of their core services. In recent years, Windy Dryden (2017, 2019, 2020; see Chapter 14 of this volume) has offered numerous SST workshops in the U.K. and internationally; Karen Young (2011, 2018, 2020) has taught single session and walk-in narrative therapy practices in Canada and internationally; and Flavio Cannistrà and Federico Piccirilli (2018; see Chapter 6) also have organized various trainings through the Italian Center for Single Session Therapy based in Rome. Recently, particularly in response to the Covid-19 pandemic, a number of organizations have begun to offer both SST client services and SST professional training online (e.g., https://www.bouverie.org.au/; www.windzcentre.com; http://ca.portal.gs/).

In the mid-2000s, in recognition of the increasing number of SST work-shop participants who found the ideas very relevant and helpful but did not identify as therapists, The Bouverie Centre broadened the terminology and began referring to *Single Session Work* (*SSW*). Continuing the theme of expanded uses for single session thinking, The Bouverie also developed an approach called *Single Session Family Consultation* (*SSFC;* see Chapters 3 and 5, plus Section VI), to assist individual treatment oriented organizations to engage families. Based on single session thinking and practice and another model called Family Consultation (Wynne & Wynne, 1986), SSFC quickly spread throughout Australia and New Zealand. In SSFC, the practitioner negotiates with their individual client regarding the potential value of in-cluding members of their family or social network for one-at-a-time meet-ings (up to three sessions) as part of the client's individual treatment. If the client agrees, the practitioner calls a key person from the client's social network to organize a single session to address the most pressing issues identified by both the client and their network.

Three International Conferences – So Far

To help herald and promote the expansion of single session therapies, The Bouverie Centre hosted the first International Symposium on Single Session Therapy and Walk-In Services on Phillip Island near Melbourne, Australia, in March 2012 – which resulted in the publication of *Capturing the Moment: Single Session Therapy and Walk-In Services* (Hoyt & Talmon, 2014). There were reports from the U.S., Canada, Australia, China, Mexico, and Israel. Chapters featured inspiring statements like these (all from authors whose latest thinking appears in the present volume):

- (from Moshe Talmon, pp. 32–33): "Some people define SST and other ultra-brief therapies as a 'psychotically optimistic' way of conducting therapy. Trusting human potential, internal and external resources, as well as the ever-surprising capabilities of the mental immune system to recover and heal is indeed relentlessly optimistic. I agree and yet I tend to see SST more as a very realistic, practical, no bullshit, and down-to-earth form of therapy."
- (from Bob Rosenbaum, pp. 48–50): "Therapy, like life, does not 'take' time because time is not a dimension we exist 'in.' We are time, and time is us [...] Nothing is ever finished, but everything is always complete."
- (from Michael Hoyt, p. 69): "Our primary therapeutic effort and expertise should be directed toward encouraging, eliciting, evoking, exploring, and elaborating whatever the client brings that can be helpful to get them to where they want to go."
- (from Monte Bobele and Arnie Slive, p. 96): "Recently a workshop participant pointed out that thinking about 'an hour being ALL we have' was inconsistent with our message. She pointed out that we should have titled the book *'When You Have a WHOLE Hour.'* And she was right! We missed the opportunity to stress that an hour was frequently more than enough time to help clients achieve some small progress toward their goals."
- (from Jeff Young, Pam Rycroft, and Shane Weir, p. 138): "We have found it a pleasure to help organizations to implement an approach that leads to accessible services for a greater range of clients."
- (from Patricia Boyhan, p. 175): "Although I originally focused on SST as a waiting list management tool, the usefulness of SST is much broader, especially in the area of engaging reluctant participants and in cross-cultural counseling [...] I now find all my sessions are informed by SST principles."
- (from Nancy McElheran, Janet Stewart, Dean Soenen, Jennifer Newman, and Bruce MacLaurin, pp. 181–182): "From the outset, the intent of the EFC [Eastside Family Centre] walk-in single session

therapy project was to provide a whole therapy in one hour. Each session was conceived as having a beginning, middle, and end [...] That rapid change is both possible and common in the human experience, and that the greatest opportunity for change comes early in the therapy process, is a basic tenet implicit in the walk-in therapy context."

- (from John Miller, p. 197): "Of all the various types of therapy services possible in the developing Chinese context, family/interpersonally-based, short-term, problem-focused, brief, and directive approaches have had the greatest appeal and acceptance among the people."

A second international symposium, called Capturing the Moment 2: Scaling New Heights in Single Session Therapy and Walk-In Services, was organized by Wood's Homes and the Eastside Family Centre and held in Banff, Canada, in September 2015. In addition to the previously mentioned countries, SST reports came from Cambodia, Haiti, Finland, and Sweden and resulted in the publication of *Single-Session Therapy by Walk-In or Appointment: Administrative, Clinical, and Supervisory Aspects of One-at-a-Time Services* (Hoyt et al., 2018). Here is a sample from contributors not previously quoted – some also appear in the present volume:

- (from Karen Young, p. 69): "Both the [brief narrative practices] approach to conversation [...] and the very existence of these [walk-in] clinics [...] have moved the field forward in ways that are congruent with our values for people to have quick access to a meaningful, collaborative and strength-oriented therapeutic encounter."
- (from Rachel Barbara-May, Paul Denborough, and Tess McGrane, p. 109): "The family felt that they had gotten what they needed from the session. No further contact was planned and the family were encouraged to contact the service should they want any further assistance in the future."
- (from Karen Story, p. 202): "The use of a single-session approach encouraged resilience and adaptation – qualities that were essential if this family was to manage the difficulties which arose as a result of the brain damage suffered by one of the parents."
- (from Sue Levin, Adriana Gil-Wilkerson, and Sylvia Rapini De Yatim, p. 258): "The success of the HGI [Houston Galveston Institute] program is due to a combination of our collaborative and dialogical therapeutic approach, the use of reflecting teams, the resourcefulness of our clients, the enthusiasm and goodwill of volunteer therapists, and the enormous need for accessible services in the community."
- (from Martin Söderquist, p. 283): "In SSCC [Single-Session Couple Counseling] you can't cover all aspects of the couple's lives. To use

the session in the most effective way for the couple, the session needs to be focused on what is most important to the couple and what they can do in the nearest future. In SSCC you narrow the focus to what is most important and achievable for the couples and go deep into (or thicken) the description of goals and signs of moving in the direction of the couple's goals."

Single session thinking and practice has continued to expand in terms of locations and venues, theories and methods, types of problems addressed, and populations served. Many more therapists and other practitioners as well as managers and policymakers – all wanting to provide readily accessible and effective client-responsive services – are seeking information and instruction. Toward this goal, the Third International Symposium on SST and Walk-In Services, *Single Session Thinking: Going Global One Step at a Time*, again organized by The Bouverie Centre, was held during October 2019 in Melbourne, Australia. The conference title, emphasizing the idea of single session thinking (or mindset), reflected the expanding range of services and systems amenable to single session approaches. The growing list of SST-reporting countries included the U.S., Canada, Australia, U.K., Israel, Mexico, Sweden, China, Cambodia, Turkey, Italy, and New Zealand.[1] Attendees also came from Norway and Singapore.

SST: By Appointment and/or by Walk-In

Although there are different single session methods that can be applied in different contexts to various problems – the subject of this book – SST can be thought of more as an affirmative mindset ("one session at a time") and as a forum or delivery system rather than as a particular theory or method (J. Young, 2018; Hoyt et al., 2018). There are two main ways to have an intentional (planned, deliberate) single session: (1) *by appointment* or (2) *by walk-in*. As Dryden (2018; Young & Dryden, 2019) has noted, these options both fall under the rubric "Help Provided at the Point of Need" (rather than "At the Point of Availability"). In addition to private offices and mental health services, single sessions also often occur in primary-care medical settings (see Martin, Rauh, Fichter, & Rief, 2007; Robinson & Reiter, 2016; Reiter, Dobmeyer, & Hunter, 2018; Luutonen, Santalahti, Makinen, Vahlberg, & Rautava, 2019); hospital and E.R.[2] meetings (e.g., Hoyt, Opsvig, & Weinstein, 1982/1995; Kosoff, 2003; Eom, Kim, Kim, Bang, & Chun, 2012; Gibbons & Plath, 2012; Rosenberg & McDaniel, 2014); college counseling centers (Center for College Mental Health, 2020; Cornish, 2020; Cornish et al., 2017; Cornish et al., 2020); inpatient psychiatric groups (Yalom & Leszcz, 2005, p. 488); second-opinion consultations; and clinical demonstration interviews (e.g., Barber, 1990; Lankton & Erickson, 1994; Keeney & Keeney, 2019; Burns, 2020[3]; Dryden, Chapter 14 of this volume).

There are also various *protocols and programs*, where people participate in some kind of structured one-session process (e.g., stress reduction, stop smoking, pain management, or improve your sleep); as well as research-validated one-session treatments for specific phobias and nightmares (Davis, Ollendick, & Öst, 2012). A single session of music therapy has been shown to improve outcomes with people who are chemically dependent (Jones, 2005) and a single session dance/movement therapy treatment protocol for people with acute schizophrenia has been described (Biondo & Gerber, 2020). Processes like guided imagery and hypnosis in palliative care (Battino, 2014, 2021), the Ericksonian mirroring hands technique (Hill & Rossi, 2017), and the use of dreamscaping for grief and loss (Gershman & Thompson, 2019) lend themselves to a one-session format. Community agencies such as homeless shelters and job counseling services may also approach issues one session at a time. We also sometimes take the session to the clients – making ourselves available at the point of need (e.g., in humanitarian disaster relief efforts) by meeting them in their home, the street, workplace, or village – rather than them coming to us. Essentially, single session thinking, making the most of the first (and any subsequent) session by treating it as if it may be the last, can be applied to many different contexts.

In the original Kaiser study (Talmon, 1990), patients/clients[4] called for an appointment and, when seen, were offered the possibility of meeting for one session of therapy (with the security of further appointments if needed). By-appointment single session approaches have also been used extensively by The Bouverie Centre and other agencies in Australia (e.g., see Carey, Tai, & Stiles, 2013; Perkins & Scarlett, 2008; Price, 1994), as well as in the U.K. (Iveson, George, & Ratner, 2014; Dryden, 2017, 2019), Italy (Cannistrà & Piccirilli, 2018), Sweden (Söderquist, 2018, 2020, also see Chapter 15), and elsewhere. The alternative main way to have an SST is by walk-in/drop-in; clients know where open-access, no-appointment-needed services are available and simply come in (usually in person, although with modern technology, possibly via computer or telephone) when wanting help. Clients can walk-in/click-in/call-in again for additional work as they did the first time. The walk-in SST approach has been featured at the Eastside Family Centre in Calgary (Stewart et al., 2018; see Chapter 11 of this volume), at Our Lady of the Lake University in San Antonio (Slive & Bobele, 2011; Bobele et al., 2018), at the Houston Galveston Institute (Levin, Gil-Wilkerson, & Rapini De Yatim, 2018), at the Walk-In Counseling Center of Minneapolis/St. Paul (Weeks & Zook-Stanley, 2018), and at clinics in Mexico City (Platt & Mondellini, 2014; Rodriguez, 2018), amongst others. Some agencies may offer both – a client can either make an appointment or simply walk-in to have a single session.

Both approaches have advantages and advocates. As Slive and Bobele (2011, 2018; also see Chapter 4) have articulated, for many clients walk-in therapy services are familiar and "user-friendly" since they are consistent with other common walk-in services (e.g., banking, haircuts); they "seize the moment," they work, and they are efficient (people come when they want, so there are no no-shows). Red tape and intake criteria can be reduced, thus making services very accessible. There is also some evidence (Stalker et al., 2015) that men are more likely to attend walk-ins than traditional appointment-based services.

On the other hand, by-appointment SSTs may be the preference of clients who want a scheduled appointment (and some clinicians may prefer to have appointments scheduled to manage their calendar); such clients can be encouraged to prepare for and thus perhaps maximize the impact of their by-appointment SST. Talmon's (1990) Kaiser study, for example, was partially inspired by the work of Steve de Shazer, who said that he approached each session as though it would be the only session and advocated a pre-session contact in which to pose the "Skeleton Key Question" that asks the client to notice what is occurring in his/her/their lives that they want to see continue and grow (see Weiner-Davis, de Shazer, & Gingrich, 1987). The approach promoted by The Bouverie Centre in Melbourne has built on this work by offering pre– and post–single session questionnaires (Young & Rycroft, 2006; also see Fry, 2012; plus Chapters 3 and 5) that have been adapted by many organizations to fit their particular context. Clients fill out a pre-session questionnaire to help begin the work before the meeting and to help maintain focus within the session itself; post-session telephone follow-ups help document change and provide an ideal time to discuss and collaboratively determine whether further work is required, needed, or wanted (see Young & Dryden, 2019). In 1995, Preston, Varzos, and Liebert published *Every Session Counts* to help clients prepare (e.g., identify specific goals, consider resources, clarify motivation) to make the most of brief therapy. Clients receiving services at "step model" college counseling services (see Cornish et al., 2017) may be asked to visit websites or otherwise read materials to cultivate their motivation and prepare for a single session. Various Indigenous[5] and shamanic practitioners may also have their clients undergo preparatory rituals in anticipation of having a single session healing encounter (see Frank & Frank, 1991; Gielen, Fish, & Draguns, 2004; Leslie, 2019). As pointed out by Moshe Talmon and Robert Rosenbaum (in a 2006 interview with Jeff Young), most healing rituals in the non-Western world are one-off events – some fascinating examples are provided in Section V of this volume.

"Could it be," as Jerome and Julia Frank wrote in *Persuasion and Healing* (1991, p. 149), "that patients wished to spend less time in therapy than therapists?" Several different ways to arrange both walk-in and by-appointment SSTs are illustrated in the chapters that follow.

A Single Session Lexicon: Terminology and Some Related Matters[6]

As the field of SST has developed and spread across the globe, a variety of terms has been used to describe aspects of single session thinking

and practice. We hope that suggesting a consistent terminology will reduce confusion and help the field to move forward.

Single Session Thinking. This umbrella term, introduced at the 2019
Melbourne symposium and highlighted in The Bouverie Centre's (2020)
online training, refers to the mindset common to all single session approaches – many of which are described below.

Single Session Therapy (SST). Talmon (1990, p. xv) originally defined
SST "as one face-to-face meeting between a therapist and a patient with no
previous or subsequent sessions within one year." Although the term
Single Session Therapy had appeared previously (e.g., Sproel, 1975; Bloom
1981; Rockwell & Pinkerton, 1982), and the definition ("one year") was
somewhat arbitrary and used for research purposes, the title of Talmon's
book brought the one-session idea to the fore. As J. Young (2018, p. 45;
also see Young & Rycroft, 2012) has noted, the term *Single Session
Therapy* represents an "in-your-face" challenge to traditional expectations
about therapy always requiring ongoing sessions and is thus "a creative
and disruptive influence on clinical practice, our theories of change, and on
service design." SST is initiated as intentionally one session at a time (see
discussion below of *OAAT* term); it is not necessarily a one-off (one and
done), but it is not therapy that might have gone on (and on...) and just
fizzled or somehow ended after one visit. SST is potentially "single" by
design, not by default (Budman & Gurman, 1988). Other related terms
include *Single Session Work* (*SSW* –Boyhan, 2006; Bouverie Centre, 2014;
Gibbons & Plath, 2012 – used to describe the application of single session
thinking outside the therapy room or when practitioners do not identify as
therapists; *Single Session Intervention* (*SSI* – see Campbell, 1999; Miller,
2011; Schleider & Weisz, 2017); *Single Session Consultation* (*SSC* –
Boyhan, 1996); and *Single Session Family Consultation* (SSFC - The
Bouverie Centre, 2014). Tess McGrane and Ron Findlay (Chapter 25) and
Myf Murphy and Denise Fry (Chapter 27) refer to their one-session
meetings with youth and families as *Single Session Family Therapy* (*SSFT*);
John Miller and his colleagues in China (Chapter 23) call their approach
with families *Single Session Team Family Therapy* (*SSTFT*). McKenzie
(2013) has also described *Single Session Peer Work* (*SSPW*). Dryden
(2017) refers to *SSI-CBT* (*Single Session Integrated CBT*). There is also the
acronym *SSS* – *Single Session Supervision* (Rycroft, 2018).

One-at-a-Time (OAAT; Hoyt, 2011; Hoyt et al., 2018), *One-Session-at-
a-Time* (Bobele & Slive, 2014; Slive & Bobele, 2018), and *One-and-Done*
(DeMelo, 2018) all synonymously refer to and emphasize the essential
single session thinking and practice idea that each meeting is approached
as a "stand alone" event (Aafjes-van Doorne & Sweeney, 2019), potentially complete unto itself. The therapist acts as if "this is it," that the one
encounter may be all that is needed (Talmon, 1990; Bobele & Slive, 2014).
Clients can return for further work, but this is usually seen as a new
"stand-alone" meeting.

Sequential Single Session Therapy (Battino, 2014, p. 405) or *Serial Single Session Therapy* (Bobele et al., 2018, p. 234) – *SSST* either way! SST/OAAT does not necessarily means "only one time"; as J. Young (2018) reports, perhaps 50% of "SST" clients eventually return for another session (or sessions). There may be intermittent or multiple SSTs; each is approached as a complete stand-alone meeting. Story (2018), for example, reports a case of "episodic long term single session therapy" in which a family coping with a parent's acquired brain injury had 32 OAAT sessions over a five-year period. Cummings and Sayama (1995; also see Budman, 1990) describe "intermittent therapy over the life cycle." Hoyt (2017, pp. 13–14) asks if the reader would consider the ten-hour-long one session reported by Berenbaum (1969) to be a prolonged brief therapy or a brief prolonged therapy?

Single Session Family Consultation (SSFC). As noted earlier, this practice involves having a one-session family meeting within the course of an individual's ongoing therapy. Hampson et al. (1999; also see Fry, 2012) at the CAMHS in Canberra also used the term *Single Session Family Consultation (SFCC)* to signify their practice of seeing the family together in family therapy, with a one-off session and then phone call to see where to next, often with a reflecting team. We would call that *Single Session Therapy (SST)* or *Single Session Family Therapy (SSFT)*, somewhat akin to what Miller et al. (Chapter 23) report doing in their *Single Session Team Family Therapy (SSTFT)* in China. SSFC as developed at The Bouverie and promoted across Australia and New Zealand is a different approach (see Chapter 5), combining Family Consultation and Single Session Thinking to create the following three-stage model:

- *Convening*: engaging with the individual client to see if they are interested in meeting with their family and, if so, calling the family to see if they are interested in a family session (based on single session practice)
- *Conducting*: having the family meeting as a single session
- *Following-Up*: making a phone call to see where to next.

Walk-in (WI) or *drop-in* refers to clients accessing services by simply arriving (usually in person, but also sometimes online or via telephone) without having pre-booked an appointment. Related terms are *open access* (see Chapter 4) and *same-day counseling* (Ewen et al., 2016).

Client/Patient/Consumer. Each term carries certain implications (see Hoyt, 2017, pp. 1–5 and 217–218). *Client* tends to emphasize a more egalitarian and less hierarchical therapeutic relationship with a subsequent de-emphasis on implications of pathology, diagnosis, and expert (top-down) strategic treatments in favor of more collaborative/facilitative/strengths-oriented approaches (see Hoyt, 1994, pp. 2–4). Indeed, for these reasons the term *consumer* is also popular in mental health services in Australia. The chapter authors herein generally prefer the use of the term *client*. As noted in Hoyt and Talmon (2014, p. 11), "What one calls the participants and the process (*therapy*? *counseling*? *treatment*? *intervention*? *consultation*? *facilitation*? *work*? *practice*? *meeting*? *encounter*? *conversation*? *coaching*?) helps to establish a meaning context (topics, roles, power relations, ideas about how change occurs), and thus, influences their work together."

Therapist/Counselor/Practitioner/Provider/Consultant/Facilitator/Worker. Paralleling the question of what to call the process and the recipient of services is the issue of what to call the person(s) offering those services. There are many possible answers (see Zeig & Munion, 1990); in the chapters that follow, the authors express their respective preferences.

Non-English Language Translations. As part of expanding globalization, single session terms are appearing in more and more languages. Writing from Mexico City, Irma Rodriguez (2018, p. 301) noted that while she understood "unique" as an invitation "to appreciate, value, and recognize what is unique, special, and different in each person and situation," her Spanish-speaking clients questioned the translation of *"single session"* as *"session unica,"* thinking it only allowed one session rather than "one-at-a-time"; so she and her colleagues decided to call their service *terapia breve sin cita" – "brief therapy without appointment."* The Italian language book edited by Cannistrà and Piccirilli (2018), called *Terapia a Seduta Singola,* translates into English as *Single Session Therapy.* (*Seduta* is the more common Italian expression for an appointment or a walk-in with a psychotherapist, but *Sessione* could also be used.) The title of Slive and Bobele's (2011) *When One Hour is All You Have: Effective Therapy for Walk-In Clients* was rendered by the publisher's Spanish translator as *Cuando Solo Tienes una Hora: Terapia Efectiva Para Clientes de Atención Inmediata* (some readers may mistake *Atención Inmediata* as meaning something like "emergency clients" even though most walk-ins are not crisis/emergency clients). The title of the book *Single-Session Therapy by Walk-In or Appointment* (Hoyt et al., 2018/2021) in Spanish is translated as *Terapia de Sesión Única, Con o Sin Cita Previa* (*Therapy of One Session, With or Without Appointment*), which correctly says that walk-ins are seen without appointment and does not suggest they are needing immediate/emergency attention. Some concepts are very hard to translate into Swedish so Swedes incorporate concepts from other languages (mostly English) and call it *Single Session Therapy* (*SST*) and *Walk-In.* (The Italian translation of "walk-in services" is also *servizi walk-in*– see Hoyt & Talmon, 2014/2018.) In Swedish, *by appointment* is *Tidsbokning.* The word-by-word Swedish translation of *One-at-a-Time* is *Ett i Taget* (*One-a-Day*) but in Malmö it is called *Ett Samtal i Taget* (*One Session a Day*).

In China, the Mandarin expression to reflect the one-time nature of the meeting is *dān cì jiǎn duǎn jiā tíng zhì liáo,* which translates as "single session family therapy." In Australia, there is no Aboriginal word for "single session" or "one-off"; *Dadirri* is a word that belongs to the language of the Ngan-gikurrungur peoples (other groups have similar concepts) that signifies a deep level of listening and engaging with what is most pressing (but without an explicit timeframe). In *Aotearoa* New Zealand, Māori consultants have indicated that SSFC would receive greater acceptance if the framework was re-named *whānau-hui* (family meeting), as the concept of *single session* may have negative connotations for families from cultures where a principle for working through family issues is "it takes as long as it takes."[7]

The Present Book

This book is a carefully curated collection selected and refined from the Third International Symposium. (Some papers from the conference are not included here.) In what follows, leading figures in the field present the latest information. There is a strong emphasis on issues of implementation, on clinical work with various problems and populations (including family and child services), and on non-Western, majority world[8] and Indigenous applications. There are many case examples and cultural nuances. Client details and circumstances have been changed throughout to protect confidentiality. This book is intended to be an essential reference for anyone working in the fields of brief therapy, healthcare, and by-appointment and/or walk-in SSTs.

In our invitation to authors, we wrote:

> We are interested in illustrating various aspects of single session thinking and practice. We would like to emphasize specific "how to" material. What principles could be garnered for use by other clinicians and managers, including cultural nuances, technical suggestions, theoretical explanations, and any cautions (including ethical considerations)? [...] The basic idea is to describe your work in an interesting way that will be helpful to readers considering expanding their usual therapeutic practice or single session thinking.

Responses were enthusiastic. Seven sections comprise this expansive volume.

Section I: Editors' Introduction (this chapter) describes the history, development, and current status of single session thinking and practice; by-appointment and walk-in SSTs; research; international terminology; and introduces the chapters that follow.

Section II: Orientations: Single Session Thinking, contains six chapters that highlight fundamental ideas about therapist mindset, sudden versus gradual change, translating single session thinking into practice, the role of family consultation, open access and service availability, and an attitude of hope and joy that promotes single sessions.

Section III: Implementation: Single Session Practice, has five chapters that highlight issues encountered when applying single session thinking and practice ideas in public mental health settings, when conducting a one-off pilot project, when the Eastside Family Centre developed its WI/SST program, and when SSFC was embedded in headspace, an Australian national youth mental health service. Two chapters describe experiences from Queensland-based Metro South Addictions and Mental Health Services (MSAMHS). In Chapter 8, Cathy Renkin, Karen Alexander, and Marianne Wyder explain how their adult services mental health team implemented Single Session Family Consultation (SSFC) as a strategy to overcome some of the fragmentation in their approaches to engaging with families; in Chapter 9, Jillian McDonald, Paul Hickey, and Marianne Wyder explain how they adapted and integrated SST to optimize the opportunity to offer families something beyond their primary assessment task.

Section IV: Single Session Thinking and Practice in Different Clinical Contexts, contains seven chapters that describe diverse situations, including a university counseling center, a CBT meet-up group, and an agency specializing in couple counseling, as well as single session work with challenging complex cases, youth mental health services, autism, infants and families, and post-HIV diagnosis counseling.

Section V: Applications in Cross-Cultural/Non-Western Contexts, has five chapters describing single session work in China, in *Aotearoa* New Zealand, with First Nations people in Western Canada, with Indigenous populations in Mexico, and with Aboriginal and Torres Strait Islander people in Australia. Ways to bring cultural humility and respect for clients' self-determination in order to avoid replicating cultural oppression are highlighted. As Alison Elliot and James Dokona note in Chapter 20, respectful listening and actually making it about what the family wants to talk about is a single session decolonizing approach; in Chapter 22, Bronwyn Dunnachie, Stacey Porter, and Karin Isherwood describe some of the processes they have undertaken to make SSFC culturally appropriate within the context of Aotearoa New Zealand. Other chapter authors also describe ways that Single Session Thinking can be applied in practice with cultural humility and competence.

Section VI: Single Session Thinking and Practice with Families, contains six chapters that illustrate ways in which a single meeting with a family can be used to augment individual treatment. Topics include ways to make the session more relaxed and "friendly," as well as the application of single session thinking to working with addictions, psychiatric crises, problem gamblers, and eating disorders.

Section VII: Editors' Conclusion – Single Session Thinking and Practice: Themes, Lessons, and a Look Toward the Future includes discussions about the importance of attitude/mindset; accessibility; working in the present, the therapeutic alliance and co-creation of single session goals;

the power of culture and family; the influence of different theories and methods; the need for additional research and training; and responses to Frequently Asked Questions.

And Now...

Single session thinking and practice offers exciting and rewarding possibilities. It is optimistic and respectful. The therapist needs to be versatile, innovative, and pragmatic, drawing on clients' hopes and resources and focusing on helping them to achieve their goals.

In what follows, readers will see how and why single session thinking and practice is continuously expanding, one step at a time.

Notes

1 In addition to these countries, Cannistrà et al. (2020) also cite SST studies from South Korea, Peru, Colombia, Finland, Norway, Switzerland, and Germany.
2 It should also be recognized that walk-in SSTs are not a form of crisis intervention, unless crisis intervention is what the client needs at the moment (Hoyt & Talmon, 2014, p. 13). Rather, walk-in/SST is a "new paradigm": "The goal of walk-in sessions is for clients to develop knowledge and skills and make use of existing resources to assist them in better managing and/or coping with their mental health-related concerns. Walk-in services, as we are describing them, are not an emergency triage service, or a way to do screening before scheduling a 'real' appointment. Walk-in services provide a form of single-session therapy" (Bobele & Slive, 2015, p. 9). For some descriptions of the use of single session principles in crisis situations, see Bisson (2003), Miller (2011), Paul & van Ommeren (2013), Akerele & Yuryev (2017), van der Veer (2017), and Guthrie (2018).
3 "Most people also know they'll just get one shot with me since I'm seeing them in the context of workshops around the country. I believe this could be a powerful factor. I let them know that I'll see them just this once and that I anticipate, but clearly cannot guarantee, complete recovery. This may function as a self-fulfilling prophecy for recovery. This is in contrast to how private practice works, where therapists are rewarded financially by a more prolonged treatment. The therapist may inform the patient that therapy will take weeks, months, or more – and that message can function as a self-fulfilling prophecy too." (Burns, 2020, p. 124)
4 See discussion of *patient/client* in Terminology section below. The Kaiser study was conducted within the context of a medical healthcare organization, so the term *patient* was used.
5 Within the Australian context, the term *Indigenous* is always capitalized (although some people prefer First Nations People, or specify Aboriginal Australian or Torres Strait Islanders); but our non-Aussie consultants indicated that the term is not necessarily capitalized elsewhere. In the chapters that follow, authors' respective preferences are used.
6 Because the co-editorship of the present volume is an American-Australian collaboration (with contributions coming from several countries in addition to the U.S. and Down Under), we generally use Americanized spelling and punctuation (e.g., *center* rather than *centre* unless a proper name or used in a

published title, *counseling* rather than *counselling*, no *u* in *behavior*) and punctuation (e.g., ending period inside quotation mark); but decided to follow Aussie practice and not hyphenate terms such as Single Session and Mental Health (but we do hyphenate Walk-In).

7 Thanks to Flavio Cannistrà for consultation regarding the Italian; to Monte Bobele and Enrique Arellano Faris for the Spanish; to Martin Söderquist for the Swedish; to John Miller, Gai Jing, and Yue Yang for the Mandarin Chinese; to Alison Elliott and Henry von Doussa for the Australian Aboriginal; and to Bronwyn Dunnachie, Karin Isherwood, and Stacey Porter regarding the Māori.

8 Miller, Platt, and Conroy (2018, p. 117) remind us that "While the Western world dominates the field of therapy, it ironically is designed to fit only for a minority of the world's population. The Western world from which most models of psychotherapy emanate represents only about 5% of the global population."

References

Aafjes-van Doorn, K., & Sweeney, K. (2019). The effectiveness of initial therapy contact: A systematic review. *Clinical Psychology Review, 74*, 101786.

Akerele, E., & Yuryev, A. (2017). Single session psychotherapy for humanitarian missions. *International Journal of Mental Health, 46*(2), 133–138.

Barber, J. (1990). Miracle cures? Therapeutic consequences of clinical demonstrations. In J.K. Zeig & S.G. Gilligan (Eds.), *Brief Therapy: Myths, Methods, and Metaphors* (pp. 437–442). New York: Brunner/Mazel.

Battino, R. (2014). Expectation: The essence of very brief therapy. In M.F. Hoyt & M. Talmon (Eds.), *Capturing the Moment: Single-Session Therapy and Walk-In Services* (pp. 393–406). Bethel, CT: Crown House Publishing.

Battino, R. (2021). *Using Guided Imagery and Hypnosis in Brief Therapy and Palliative Care.* New York: Routledge.

Berenbaum, H. (1969). Massed time-limit psychotherapy. *Psychotherapy: Theory, Research, and Practice, 6*, 54–56.

Biondo, N. Gerber, N. (2020). Single-session dance/movement therapy for people with acute schizophrenia: Development of a treatment protocol. *American Journal of Dance Therapy, 42*, 277–295.

Bisson, J.I. (2003). Single session early psychological interventions following traumatic events. *Clinical Psychology Review, 23*(3), 481–499.

Bloom, B.L. (1981). Focused single-session therapy: Initial development and evaluation. In S.H. Budman (Ed.), *Forms of Brief Therapy* (pp. 167–216). New York: Guilford Press. A revised and extended version ("Bloom's focused single-session therapy") appeared in B.L. Bloom, *Planned Short-Term Psychotherapy: A Clinical Handbook* (2nd ed., pp. 97–121). Boston: Allyn & Bacon, 1992.

Bobele, M., Fullen, C., Houston, B., Martinez, A.M., Moffat, L., & Santos, J. (2018). Westside stories: Walk-in and single-session therapy in San Antonio. In M.F. Hoyt, M. Bobele, A. Slive, J. Young, & M. Talmon (Eds.), *Single-Session Therapy by Walk-In or Appointment: Administrative, Clinical, and Supervisory Aspects of One-at-a-Time Services* (pp. 221–250). New York: Routledge.

Bobele, M., & Slive, A. (2014). One session at a time: When you have a whole hour. In M.F. Hoyt, M. Bobele, A. Slive, J. Young, & M. Talmon (Eds.), *Capturing the*

Moment: Single Session Therapy and Walk-In Services: Administrative, Clinical, and Supervisory Aspects of One-at-a-Time Services (pp. 95–121). Bethel, CT: Crown House Publishing.

Bobele, M., & Slive, A. (2015). Walk-in psychotherapy: A new paradigm. *The Milton H. Erickson Foundation Newsletter, 35*(2), 9.

Boyhan, P. (1996). Clients' perceptions of single session consultations as an option to waiting for family therapy. *Australian and New Zealand Journal of Family Therapy, 17*(2), 85–96.

Boyhan, P. (2006). Single session work (SSW): Implementation resource parcel. *Journal of Family Studies, 12*(2), 286–290.

Budman, S.H. (1990). The myth of termination in brief therapy: Or, it ain't over until it's over. In J.K. Zeig & S.G. Gilligan (Eds.), *Brief Therapy: Myths, Methods & Metaphors* (pp. 206–218). New York: Brunner/Mazel.

Budman, S.H., & Gurman, A.S. (1988). *Theory and Practice of Brief Therapy.* New York: Guilford Press.

Budman, S.H., Hoyt, M.F., & Friedman, S. (Eds.) (1992). *The First Session in Brief Therapy.* New York: Guilford Press.

Burns, D.D. (2020). *Feeling Great: The Revolutionary New Treatment for Depression and Anxiety.* Eau Claire, WI: PESI Publishing & Media.

Campbell, A. (1999). Single session interventions: An example of clinical research in practice. *Australian and New Zealand Journal of Family Therapy, 20*(4), 183–194.

Campbell, A. (2012). Single-session approaches to therapy: Time to review. *Australian and New Zealand Journal of Family Therapy, 33*(1), 15–26.

Cannistrà, F., & Piccirilli, F. (Eds.) (2018). *Terapia a Seduta Singola: Principi e Pratiche.* (Published in Italian. English translation: *Single Session Therapy: Principles and Practices.*). Firenze, Italia: Giunti.

Cannistrà, F., Piccirilli, F., Pietrabissa, G., D'Alia, P.P., Giannetti, A., Piva, L., … Ghisoni, A. (2020). Examining the clinical efficacy and clients' experiences of single session therapy in Italy: A feasibility study. *Australian and New Zealand Journal of Family Therapy, 41*(3), 271–282.

Carey, T.A., Tai, S.J., & Stiles, W.B. (2013). Effective and efficient: Using patient-led appointment scheduling in routine mental health practice in remote Australia. *Professional Psychology: Research and Practice, 44*(6), 405–414.

Center for College Mental Health (2020, January). *2019 Annual Report* (Publication No. STA 20-244).

Cornish, P.A. (2020). *Stepped Care 2.0: A Paradigm Shift in Mental Health.* Cham, Switzerland: Springer Nature.

Cornish, P.A., Berry, G., Benton, S., Barros-Gomes, P., Johnson, D., Ginsburg, R., … Romano, V. (2017). Meeting the mental health needs of today's college student: Reinventing services through Stepped Care 2.0. *Psychological services, 14*(4), 428–442.

Cornish, P.A., Churchill, A., & Hair, H.J. (2020). Open-access single-session therapy in the context of Stepped Care 2.0. *Journal of Systemic Therapies, 39*(3), 21–33.

Cummings, N.A., & Sayama, M. (1995). *Focused Psychotherapy: A Casebook of Brief, Intermittent Psychotherapy Through the Life Cycle.* New York: Brunner/Mazel.

Davis III, T.E., Ollendick, T.H., & Öst, L.-G. (Eds.). (2012). *Intensive One-Session Treatment of Specific Phobias*. New York: Springer.

Demelo, J. (2018, July). Bull's eye! One-and-done sessions give new meaning to the phrase *targeted therapy*. *O: The Oprah Magazine, 19*(63–64), 67.

Dryden, W. (2017). *Single-Session Integrated CBT (SSI-CBT)*. New York: Routledge.

Dryden, W. (2018). *Single Session Therapy*. Whiteboard video animation. London: Author.

Dryden, W. (2019). *Single-Session Therapy: 100 Key Points and Techniques*. New York: Routledge.

Dryden, W. (2020). *Single-Session Counselling: Principles and Practice*. Monmouth, U.K.: PCCS Books.

Eisenthal, S., & Lazare, A. (1976a). Specificity of patients' requests in the initial interview. *Psychological Reports, 38*, 739–748.

Eisenthal, S., & Lazare, A. (1976b). Evaluation of the initial interview in a walk-in clinic: The patient's perspective on a "customer approach." *Journal of Nervous and Mental Disease, 162*, 169–176.

Eom, S.Y., Kim, E.S., Kim, H.J., Bang, Y.O., & Chun, N. (2012). Effects of a one session spouse-support enhancement childbirth education on childbirth self-efficacy and perception of childbirth experience in women and their husbands. *Journal of the Korean Academy of Nursing, 42*(4), 599–607. doi: 10.4040/jkan.2012.42.4.599

Ewen, V., Mushquash, A.R., Bailey, K., Haggary, J.M., Dama, S., & Mushquash, C.J. (2016, January-March). Same-day counseling: Study protocol for the evaluation of a new mental health service. *JMIR Research Protocols, 5*(1), e22.

Frank, J.D., & Frank, J.B. (1991). *Persuasion and Healing: A Comparative Study of Psychotherapy* (3rd ed.). Baltimore, MD: Johns Hopkins University Press.

Fry, D. (2012). Implementing single session family consultation: A reflective team approach. *Australian and New Zealand Journal of Family Therapy, 33*(1), 54–69.

Gershman, N., & Thompson, B.E. (2019). *Prescriptive Memories in Grief and Loss: The Art of Dreamscaping*. New York: Routledge.

Gibbons, J., & Plath, D. (2012). Single session social work in hospitals. *Australian and New Zealand Journal of Family Therapy, 33*(1), 39–53.

Gielen, U.P., Fish, J.M., & Draguns, J.G. (Eds.). (2004). *Handbook of Culture, Therapy, and Healing*. Mahwah, NJ: Lawrence Erlbaum Associates.

Goulding, M.M. (1990). Getting the important work done fast: Contract plus redecision. In J.K. Zeig & S.G. Gilligan (Eds.), *Brief Therapy: Myths, Methods, and Metaphors* (pp. 303–317). New York: Brunner/Mazel.

Guthrie, B. (2018). Reflections on providing single-session therapy in post-disaster Haiti. In M.F. Hoyt, M. Bobele, A. Slive, J. Young, & M. Talmon (Eds.), *Single-Session Therapy by Walk-In or Appointment: Administrative, Clinical, and Supervisory Aspects of One-at-a-Time Services* (pp. 303–317). New York: Routledge.

Haley, J. (1977). *Problem-Solving Therapy: New Strategies for Effective Family Therapy*. San Francico: Jossey-Bass.

Haley, J. (1989). *The First Therapy Session: How to Interview Clients and Identify Problems Successfully*. Audiotape/CD. San Francisco: Jossey-Bass.

Hampson, R., O'Hanlon, J., Franklin, A., Petony, M., Fridgant, L., & Heins, T. (1999). The place of single-session family consultations: Five years' experience in Canberra. *Australian and New Zealand Journal of family Therapy, 20*(4), 195–200.

Harper-Jaques, S., & Foucault, D. (2014). Walk-in single-session therapy: Client satisfaction and clinical outcomes. *Journal of Systemic Therapies, 33*(3), 29–49.

Hill, R., & Rossi, E.L. (2017). *The Practitioner's Guide to Mirroring Hands.* Williston, VT: Crown House Publishing.

Hoyt, M.F. (1994). Introduction: Competency-based future-oriented therapy. In M.F. Hoyt (Ed.), *Constructive Therapies* (pp. 1–10). New York: Guilford Press.

Hoyt, M.F. (1995). *Brief Therapy and Managed Care.* San Francisco: Jossey-Bass.

Hoyt, M.F. (2011). Foreword. In A. Slive & M. Bobele (Eds.), *When One Hour is All You Have: Effective Therapy for Walk-In Clients* (pp. ix–xv). Phoenix, AZ: Zeig, Tucker, & Theisen.

Hoyt, M.F. (2017). *Brief Therapy and Beyond: Stories, Language, Love, Hope, and Time.* New York: Routledge.

Hoyt, M.F., Bobele, M., Slive, A., Young, J., & Talmon, M. (Eds.). (2018). *Single-Session Therapy by Walk-In or Appointment: Administrative, Clinical, and Supervisory Aspects of One-at-a-Time Services.* New York: Routledge. (Published in Spanish as *Terapia de sesión única, con o sin cita previa* (1era ed. Barcelona: Editorial Eleftheria, 2021.)

Hoyt, M.F., Opsvig, P.K., & Weinstein, N.W. (1982). Conjoint patient-staff interview in hospital case management. *International Journal of Psychiatry in Medicine, 11*, 83–87. Reprinted in M.F. Hoyt, *Brief Therapy and Managed Care* (pp. 177–181). San Francisco: Jossey-Bass, 1995.

Hoyt, M.F., Rosenbaum, R., & Talmon, M. (1992). Planned single-session therapy. In S.H. Budman, M.F. Hoyt, & S. Friedman (Eds.), *The First Session in Brief Therapy* (pp. 59–86). New York: Guilford Press.

Hoyt, M.F., & Talmon, M. (Eds.). (2014). *Capturing the Moment: Single-Session Therapy and Walk-In Services.* Bethel, CT: Crown House Publishing. (Published in Italian as: *Capturing the Moment: Terapia a Seduta Singola e Servizi Walk-In.* Roma: CISU, 2018.)

Hoyt, M.F., Young, J., & Rycroft, P. (2020). Single Session Thinking 2020. *Australian and New Zealand Journal of Family Therapy, 41*(3), 218–230.

Hurn, R. (2005). Single-session therapy: Planned success or unplanned failure? *Counseling Psychology Review, 20*(4), 33–40.

Hymmen, P., Stalker, C.A., & Cait, C. (2013). The case for single-session therapy: Does the empirical evidence support the increased prevalence of this service delivery model and walk-in services? *Journal of Mental Health, 22*(1), 60–71.

Iveson, C., George, E., & Ratner, H. (2014). Love is all around: A solution-focused single session therapy. In M.F. Hoyt & M. Talmon (Eds.), *Capturing the Moment: Single Session Therapy and Walk-In Services* (pp. 325–348). Bethel, CT: Crown House Publishing.

Jones, J.D. (2005). A comparison of songwriting and lyric analysis techniques to evoke emotional change in a single session with people who are chemically dependent. *Journal of Music Therapy, 42*(2), 94–110.

Kachor, M. & Brothwell, J. (2020). Improving youth mental health services access using a single-session therapy approach. *Journal of Systemic Therapies, 39*(3), 46–55.

Keeney, H., & Keeney, B. (2019) 120 centimeters from sainthood. In M.F. Hoyt & M. Bobele (Eds.), *Creative Therapy in Challenging Situations* (pp. 134–143). New York: Routledge.

Kosoff, S. (2003). Single session groups: Applications and areas of expertise. *Social Work with Groups, 26*(1), 29–45.

Lankton, S.R., & Erickson, K.K. (1994). The essence of a single-session success. *Ericksonian Monographs, 9*, vii–164. New York: Brunner/Mazel.

Leslie, P.J. (2019). *The Art of Creating a Magical Session: Key Elements for Transformative Psychotherapy*. New York: Routledge.

Levin, S.B., Gil-Wilkerson, A., & Rapini De Yatim, S. (2018). Single-session walk-ins as a collaborative learning community at the Houston Galveston Institute. In M.F. Hoyt, M. Bobele, A. Slive, J. Young, & M. Talmon (Eds.), *Single-Session Therapy by Walk-In or Appointment: Administrative, Clinical, and Supervisory Aspects of One-at-a-Time Services* (pp. 251–259). New York: Routledge.

Luutonen, S., Santalahti, A., Makinen, M., Vahlberg, T., & Rautava, P. (2019). One-session cognitive behavior treatment for long-term frequent attenders in primary care: Randomized controlled trial. *Scandanavian Journal of Primary Health Care, 37*(1), 98–104. doi: 10.1080/02813432.2019.1569371

Malan, D.H., Heath, E., Bascal, H., & Balfour, H. (1975). Psychodynamic changes in untreated neurotic patients. II. Apparently genuine improvements. *Archives of General Psychiatry, 32*, 110–126.

Martin, A., Rauh, E., Fichter, M., & Rief, W. (2007). A one-session treatment for patients suffering from medically unexplained symptoms in primary care: A randomized clinical trial. *Psychosomatics, 48*(4), 294–303. doi: 10.1176/appi. psy.48.4.294

McElheran, N., Harper-Jaques, S., & Lawson, A. (2020). Introduction to the special section: Walk-in single-session and booked single-session therapy in Canada. *Journal of Systemic Therapies, 39*(3), 15–20.

McElheran, N., Stewart, J., Soenen, D., Newman, J., & MacLaurin, B. (2014). Walk-in single-session therapy at the Eastside Family Centre. In M.F. Hoyt & M. Talmon (Eds.), *Capturing the Moment: Single-Session Therapy and Walk-In Services* (pp. 177–194). Bethel, CT: Crown House Publishing.

McKenzie, P. (2013). Single session peer work: A framework for peer support. In C. Chapman, K. Kellehear, M. Everett, et al., *Recovering Citizenship: Cairns Conference Proceedings 2012* (pp. 61–165). Mental Health Services Conference of Australia and New Zealand, Cairns, QLD, Australia; August *21–24.*

Miller, J.K. (2011). Single-session intervention in the wake of Hurricane Katrina: Strategies for disaster mental health counseling. In A. Slive & M. Bobele (Eds.), *When One Session Is All You Have: Effective Therapy for Walk-In Clients* (pp. 185–202). Phoenix, AZ: Zeig, Tucker, & Theisen.

Miller, J.K. (2014). Single session therapy in China. In M.F. Hoyt & M. Talmon (Eds.), *Capturing the Moment: Single Session Therapy and Walk-In Services* (pp. 195–214). Bethel, CT: Crown House Publishing.

Miller, J.K., Platt, J.J., & Conroy, K.M. (2018). Single-session therapy in the majority world: Addressing the challenge of service delivery in Cambodia and the implications for other global contexts. In M.F. Hoyt, M. Bobele, A. Slive, J.

Young, & M. Talmon (Eds.), *Single-Session Therapy by Walk-In or Appointment: Administrative, Clinical, and Supervisory Aspects of One-at-a-Time Services* (pp. 116–134). New York: Routledge.

Miller, J.K., & Slive, A. (2004). Breaking down the barriers to clinical service delivery: Walk-in family therapy. *Journal of Marital and Family Therapy, 30,* 95–105.

Mumford, E., Schlesinger, H.J., Glass, G., Parrick, C., & Cuerdon, T. (1984). A new look at evidence about reduced cost of medical utilization following mental-health treatment. *American Journal of Psychiatry, 141,* 1145–1158.

Napier, A.Y., & Whitaker, C.A. (1978). *The Family Crucible.* New York: HarperCollins.

O'Hanlon, W.H., & Hexum, A.L. (1990). *An Uncommon Casebook: The Complete Clinical Work of Milton H. Erickson, M.D.* New York: Norton.

O'Hanlon, W.H., & Weiner-Davis, M. (1989). *In Search of Solutions: A New Direction in Psychotherapy.* New York: Norton.

Paul, K.E., & van Ommeren, M. (2013). A primer on single session therapy and its potential application in humanitarian situations. *Intervention: Journal of Mental-Health and Psychosocial Support in Conflict-Affected Areas, 11*(1), 8–23.

Perkins, R., & Scarlett, G. (2008). The effectiveness of single-session therapy in child and adolescent mental health. Part 2: An 18-month follow-up study. *Psychology and Psychotherapy: Theory, Research and Practice, 81,* 143–156.

Platt, J.J., & Mondellini, D. (2014). Single session walk-in therapy for street robbery victims in Mexico City. In M.F. Hoyt & M. Talmon (Eds.), *Capturing the Moment* (pp. 215–231). Bethel, CT: Crown House.

Preston, J., Varzos, N., & Liebert, D.S. (1995). *Every Session Counts: Making the Most of Your Brief Therapy.* San Luis Obispo, CA: Impact Publishers.

Price, C. (1994). Open days: Making family therapy accessible in working class suburbs. *Australian and New Zealand Journal of Family Therapy, 15*(4), 191–196.

Reiter, J.T., Dobmeyer, A.C., & Hunter, C.L. (2018). The primary care behavioral health (PCBH) model: An overview and operational definition. *Journal of Clinical Psychology in Medical Settings, 25,* 109–126.

Robinson, P.J., & Reiter, J.T. (2016). *Behavioral Consultation and Primary Care: A Guide to Integrating Services* (2nd ed.). New York: Springer.

Rockwell, W.K., & Pinkerton, R.S. (1982). Single-session psychotherapy. *American Journal of Psychotherapy, 36,* 32–40.

Rodriguez, I.J. (2018). *Terapia breve sin cita:* Collaboration with a marginalized community in Mexico City. In M.F. Hoyt, M. Bobele, A. Slive, J. Young, & M. Talmon (Eds.), *Single-Session Therapy by Walk-In or Appointment: Administrative, Clinical, and Supervisory Aspects of One-at-a-Time Services* (pp. 291–302). New York: Routledge.

Rosenbaum, R., Hoyt, M.F., & Talmon, M. (1990). The challenge of single-session therapies: Creating pivotal moments. In R.A. Wells & V.J. Giannetti (Eds.), *Handbook of the Brief Psychotherapies* (pp. 165–189). New York: Plenum Press.

Rosenberg, T., & McDaniel, S. (2014). Single-session medical family therapy and the patient-centered medical home. In M.F. Hoyt & M. Talmon (Eds.), *Capturing the Moment* (pp. 349–362). Bethel, CT: Crown House.

Rycroft, P. (2018). Capturing the moment in supervision. In M.F. Hoyt, M. Bobele, A. Slive, J. Young, & M. Talmon (Eds.), *Single-Session Therapy by Walk-In or Appointment: Administrative, Clinical, and Supervisory Aspects of One-at-a-Time Services* (pp. 347–365). New York: Routledge.

Rycroft, P., & Young, J. (2014). SST in Australia: Learning from teaching. In M.F. Hoyt & M. Talmon (Eds.), *Capturing the Moment* (pp. 141–156). Bethel, CT: Crown House Publishing.

Schleider, J.L., Sung, J.Y., Bianco, A., Gonzalez, A., Vivian, D., & Mullarkey, M.C. (2021). Open pilot trial of single-session consultation service for clients on psychotherapy wait-lists. *The Behavior Therapist, 44*(1), 8–15.

Schleider, J.L., & Weisz, J.R. (2017). Little treatments, promising effects? Meta-analysis of single-session interventions for youth psychiatric problems. *Journal of the American Academy of Child and Adolescent Psychiatry, 56*(2), 107–115.

Slive, A., & Bobele, M. (Eds.). (2011). *When One Hour is All You Have: Effective Therapy for Walk-In Clients*. Phoenix, AZ: Zeig, Tucker, & Theisen. (Published in Spanish as *Cuando Solo Tienes una Hora: Terapia Efectiva Para Clientes de Atención Inmediata*. Mexico City: Paidós, 2013.)

Slive, A., & Bobele, M. (2018). The three top reasons why walk-in/single-sessions make perfect sense. In M.F. Hoyt, M. Bobele, A. Slive, J. Young, & M. Talmon (Eds.), *Single-Session Therapy by Walk-In or Appointment: Administrative, Clinical, and Supervisory Aspects of One-at-a-Time Services* (pp. 27–39). New York: Routledge.

Slive, A., MacLaurin, B., Oakander, M., & Amundson, J. (1995). Walk-in single-sessions: A new paradigm in clinical service delivery. *Journal of Systemic Therapies, 14*, 3–11.

Slive, A., McElheran, N., & Lawson, A. (2008). How brief does it get? Walk-in single session therapy. *Journal of Systemic Therapies, 27*, 5–22.

Söderquist, M. (2018). Coincidence favors the prepared mind: Single sessions with couples in Sweden. In M.F. Hoyt, M. Bobele, A. Slive, J. Young, & M. Talmon (Eds.), *Single-Session Therapy by Walk-In or Appointment: Administrative, Clinical, and Supervisory Aspects of One-at-a-Time Services* (pp. 270–290). New York: Routledge.

Söderquist, M. (2020). *Ett Samtal i Taget: Familjerådgivning i Ny Form*. Lund, Sweden: Studentlitteratur. (Published in Swedish. English translation: *One Session at a Time: Couple Counseling in a New Format*.)

Sproel, O.H. (1975). Single-session psychotherapy. *Diseases of the Nervous System, 36*, 283–285.

Stalker, C.A., Riemer, M., Cait, A.A., Horton, S., Booton, J., Joslig, L., & Zaczek, M. (2015). A comparison of walk-in counseling and the wait-list model for delivering counseling services. *Journal of Mental Health*. https://doi.org/10.3109/09638237.2015.1101417.

Stewart, J., McElheran, N., Park, H., Oakander, M., MacLaurin, B., Fang, C.J., & Robinson, A. (2018). Twenty-five years of walk-in single-sessions at the Eastside Family Centre: Clinical and research dimensions. In M.F. Hoyt, M. Bobele, A. Slive, J. Young, & M. Talmon (Eds.), *Single-Session Therapy by Walk-In or Appointment: Administrative, Clinical, and Supervisory Aspects of One-at-a-Time Services* (pp. 72–90). New York: Routledge.

Story, K. (2018). "Coming in for tune-ups": A family's experience of episodic long-term single session therapy at the Bouverie Centre, Melbourne. In M.F. Hoyt, M. Bobele, A. Slive, J. Young, & M. Talmon (Eds.), *Single-Session Therapy by Walk-In or Appointment: Administrative, Clinical, and Supervisory Aspects of One-at-a-Time Services* (pp. 202–220). New York: Routledge.

Talmon, M. (1990). *Single-Session Therapy: Maximizing the Effect of the First (and Often Only) Therapeutic Encounter.* San Francisco: Jossey-Bass.

Talmon, M. (1993). *Single Session Solutions: A Guide to Practical, Effective, and Affordable Therapy.* Reading, MA: Addison-Wesley.

The Bouverie Centre (2014). *Single Session Family Consultation Practice Manual.* https://www.bouverie.org.au/images/uploads/Single_Session_Family_Consultat ion_Practice_Manual_2014.pdf

van der Veer, G. (2017). Training counselors in low and middle income countries in single session counseling: Helping mental health and psychosocial workers to get on top of feelings of powerlessness. *Intervention, 15*(1), 70–75.

Weeks, M., & Zook-Stanley, L. (2018). Walk-In Counseling Center of Minneapolis/ St. Paul: The magic of our model for clients and volunteers. In M.F. Hoyt, M. Bobele, A. Slive, J. Young, & M. Talmon (Eds.), *Single-Session Therapy by Walk-In or Appointment: Administrative, Clinical, and Supervisory Aspects of One-at-a-Time Services* (pp. 135–146). New York: Routledge.

Weiner-Davis, M., de Shazer, S., & Gingrich, W.J. (1987). Using pretreatment change to construct a therapeutic solution: An exploratory study. *Journal of Marital and Family Therapy, 13*, 359–363.

Wynne, A.R., & Wynne, L.C. (1986). At the center of the cyclone: Family therapists as consultants with family and divorce courts. In L.C. Wynne, S.H. McDaniel, & T.T. Weber (Eds.), *Systems Consultation: A New Perspective for Family Therapy* (pp. 300–319). New York: Guilford Press.

Yalom, I.D., & Leszcz, M. (2005). *The Theory and Practice of Group Therapy* (5th ed.). New York: Basic Books.

Young, J. (2006). *Video Interview with Moshe Talmon and Robert Rosenbaum about Their Experiences of the Development of Single Session Therapy.* Melbourne, Australia: The Bouverie Centre.

Young, J. (2018). Single session therapy: The misunderstood gift that keeps on giving. In M.F. Hoyt, M. Bobele, A. Slive, J. Young, & M. Talmon (Eds.), *Single-Session Therapy by Walk-In or Appointment: Administrative, Clinical, and Supervisory Aspects of One-at-a-Time Services* (pp. 40–58). New York: Routledge.

Young, J., & Dryden, W. (2019). Single-session therapy – past and future: An interview. *British Journal of Guidance & Counseling, 47*(5), 645–654. Reprinted in W. Dryden, *Single Session Therapy and its Future: What SST Leaders Think* (pp. 46–63). New York: Routledge, 2021.

Young, J., & Rycroft, P. (2006). *Single Session Therapy, A Bouverie Centre Professional Development Training Workbook.* Unpublished workbook manual. Bouverie Centre: Melbourne, Australia.

Young, J., & Rycroft, P. (2012). Single session therapy: What's in a name? *Australian and New Zealand Journal of Family Therapy, 33*(1), 3–5.

Young, J., Rycroft, P., & Weir, S. (2014). Implementing single session therapy: Practical wisdoms from Down Under. In M.F. Hoyt & M. Talmon (Eds.),

Capturing the Moment: Single Session Therapy and Walk-In Services (pp. 121–140). Bethel, CT: Crown House Publishing.

Young, K. (2011). When all the time you have is NOW: Re-visiting practices and narrative therapy in a walk-in clinic. In. J. Duvall & L. Béres (Eds.), *Innovations in Narrative Therapy: Connecting Practice, Training, and Research* (pp. 147–166). New York: Norton.

Young, K. (2018). Change in the winds: The growth of walk-in therapy clinics in Ontario, Canada. In M.F. Hoyt, M. Bobele, A. Slive, J. Young, & M. Talmon (Eds.), *Single-Session Therapy by Walk-In or Appointment: Administrative, Clinical, and Supervisory Aspects of One-at-a-Time Services* (pp. 59–71). New York: Routledge.

Young, K. (2020). Multi-story listening: Using narrative practices at walk-in clinics. *Journal of Systemic Therapies, 39*(3), 34–45.

Zeig, J.K., & Munion, M. (Eds.). (1990). *What Is Psychotherapy? Contemporary Perspectives.* San Francisco: Jossey-Bass.

Section II

Orientations: Single Session Thinking

2 The Hope and Joy of Single Session Thinking and Practice

Michael F. Hoyt

In Single Session Therapy (SST), as in other therapies, we both "capture the moment" and "create the moment." As our friend and Australian colleague, the late Michael White, said (quoted in Hoyt, 1996, p. 41):

> There is a certain pleasure or joy available to us in the knowledge that we can't know beforehand what we'll be thinking at the end; in the idea that we can't know what new possibilities for action in the world might be available to us at that time.

This is what I want to talk about here: the creative SST adventure, the hope and joy of helping someone quickly. When Moshe Talmon, Bob Rosenbaum, and I collaborated in our single session therapy research project at Kaiser Permanente in Northern California in the late 1980s, who would have guessed what oaks might grow from little acorns, what "new possibilities for action" might emerge – and that 30 years later we'd be in Melbourne, Australia, gathered at the Third International Symposium on SST and Walk-In Services!

There had been other occasional reports of a one-session therapy success prior to our research, but ours was the first prospective, systematic study to demonstrate the frequency and effectiveness of SST (Talmon, 1990). There have been many studies since that have replicated and extended our results.

Opening to Single Session Possibilities

My own involvement, however, with the idea of a single session therapy being helpful existed long before our study in the late 1980s. There were key moments when someone had said something that rocked and shifted my world. My family of origin – Mom, Dad, brother Bill, and I – were an early family therapy family. I recall a time around 1964, for example, when we went to one counseling session. We knew it was only going to be for one meeting, and what the therapist said – *zing!* – really helped change things for us. There were also other instances in which a single experience, such as a comment from a friend or teacher, opened new perspectives. As Pam and Jeff (Rycroft & Young, 2014, p. 152) have written, recognizing such pivotal events in one's own life can help us to be more open to the possibilities of single session thinking and practice.

For many years I absorbed Sufi and Hasidic and Zen teaching tales, enjoying the "A-ha!" moments wherein with one stroke the listener becomes enlightened (or at least, temporarily aware). I appreciate great one-liners and other pithy statements spoken by comedians (and politicians) that cut through a lot of bullshit. I love the poets and songwriters – some famous, some not – whose eloquence opens worlds with just a few words. They get you coming, going, and where you are. And early in my training and career I was very fortunate to have a couple of mentors – Carl Whitaker and Bob Goulding – who repeatedly showed me how powerful and significant a single therapy meeting could be.

So, in 1987 when Moshe and Bob said, "It seems lots of people only come for one session. Wanna do a research project on that?" I was primed.

The Power of a Good Moment

It is good to remember that "one at a time" does not necessarily mean "only one time." A client could – and sometimes does – elect to return for another session (or sessions). We should also note that it was clients choosing to attend for one visit – not clinicians – who really "invented" single session therapy. We clinicians, recognizing that one session is *de facto* the most common length of contact, have endeavored to refine and make available for more people this naturalistically occurring phenomenon. (Actually, the most common length is ZERO sessions – people think about seeing a therapist, but never do![1] Amongst those who actually do seek counseling, ONE is the most common length of treatment ... then two, then three [Hoyt, 2018, p. 155].)

Shakespeare (*Hamlet*, Act V, Scene 2) wrote "The readiness is all," and I think that much, if not most, therapy occurs in a critical single session – we just often don't know which session it will be. The American poet Emily Dickinson (1865/1960) wrote, "Forever is composed of nows." Sometimes "moments are forever" (Talmon & Hoyt, 2014, p. 463), and various authors have described therapy models that emphasize "corrective emotional experiences," "critical moments," "good moments," "creative moments," "magical moments," "key moments," and "healing moments" occurring along an arc of preparation, change, and consolidation. Rosenbaum (2008, pp. 4–8) notes, "Psychotherapy is not short or long [....] Psychotherapy depends instead on 'good moments' where something profound shifts for a client. All the rest is preparation and consolidation." Paul Leslie (2019, p. 50) observes "Essentially, clients will feel their session is magical only if they have had a compelling new experience." Work tends to expand or contract to fit the time allotted (Appelbaum, 1973), so explicitly offering the possibility of a walk-in or by-appointment SST increases the likelihood that the first encounter may also be the only one needed.

Single session thinking and practice helps people to organize and catalyze, to integrate and motivate (Hoyt, 2018, p. 161). Most single session therapies are not particularly sensational or dramatic (but see Hoyt & Bobele, 2019). Generally speaking, we try to meet people where they are and mostly endeavor to help them to use their own resources to take the next step that works for them. To quote the psychologist Michele Ritterman (2019, p. 163):

A single stroke of the brush does not work a miracle for every client. Each person, couple, family, community is unique. As such, every case we treat requires a one-of-a-kind method of problem solving [....] As healers, we will be called upon to do what is necessary at any one moment with any given client.

Bespoke: One of a Kind, One at a Time, and Sometimes Only One Time

When we only have one meeting, therapist and client need to bring whatever is useful, so single session thinking and practice is a venue or forum for what Bob Rosenbaum (1994) has called "intrinsic integration." Outcome, not process, is most important, and numerous studies have shown a variety of theoretical orientations – solution-focused, narrative, strategic, CBT, motivational interviewing, redecision, inclusivity, Ericksonian, emotion-focused, even psychodynamic – have been used to produce positive one-session results. Although different guiding models have been articulated, SST can be thought of more as an affirmative and optimistic mindset (see Chapter 6 of this volume) and as a forum or delivery system rather than as a particular method (Young, 2018; Hoyt, Bobele, Slive, Young, & Talmon, 2018). Sometimes we help a client stop a behavior, or pivot and start something new; sometimes we help them remember to forget or forget to remember, or remember to remember or forget to forget (Rosenbaum, Hoyt, & Talmon, 1990). As Moshe (e.g., Talmon, 1990, pp. 120–123; 2014, p. 34) has emphasized, one size does not fit all.

Especially when we embrace social constructionist perspectives about knowledge, dialogue, and meanings, "Each moment, even if it is the only one, is an opportunity for hope, growth, and change" (Hair, Shortall, & Oldford, 2013, p. 20). Berg & Dolan (2001, p. 1) described their view of solution-focused brief therapy: "If we had to define the SFBT approach in one sentence without talking about philosophy or techniques, we would describe it as "the pragmatics of hope and respect." Wylie (1994) speaks of narrative therapy as "panning for gold," and Monk et al. (1997) refer to "the archeology of hope." When the focus moves from problems to solutions, good things can happen quickly. Karen Young (2018) and Alesya Courtnage (2020) elaborate how this may be accomplished in SFBT and in narrative therapy.

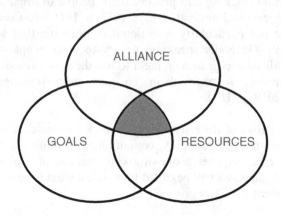

Figure 2.1 Context of Competence (from Hoyt, 2014. © M.F. Hoyt, 2014. Used with permission.)

To my mind, we seek to co-create what I have referred to as a "Context of Competence" (Hoyt, 2014, 2017; see Figure 2.1) in which, with our assistance, clients identify specific, achievable goals and bring their abilities and resources (individual, familial, social, and cultural) to bear. We welcome the deliberate, the fortuitous, and the serendipitous. Therapy, single session or otherwise, takes place where GOALS and RESOURCES intersect via the THERAPEUTIC ALLIANCE.

In SST, each session is a complete "event." There is often a temporal structure to single sessions, with different issues and tasks associated with the early, middle, and late phases of a meeting (see Figure 2.2). Clients undergo a "restoration of morale" (Frank, 1974) as they are assisted to think about positive goals and ways to achieve them.

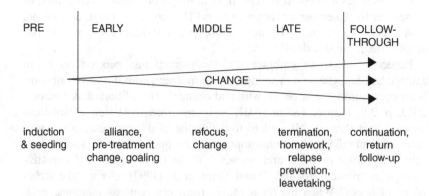

Figure 2.2 The Temporal Structure of SST (from Hoyt, 2000, p. 218. © 2000 M.F. Hoyt. Used with permission.)

Three common themes cut across and underlie effective single session thinking and practice: (1) *mindset*, which has to do with the realization that you may only have one session and hence there is a goal of making the most of every encounter; (2) *time*, which has to do with the ideas of immediate accessibility and that the best opportunity to address change is NOW; and (3) *empowerment/client activation*, which involves the assumption that clients have the wherewithal (sometimes with our facilitation) to achieve their goals (see Hoyt et al., 2018, pp. 11–15; Hoyt & Talmon, 2014, pp. 468–472). When clients are asked what they want, the therapist and client can work collaboratively to honor those hopes and intentions.

I was thinking about all of this one time while I was in Italy walking around the ancient Roman Forum. I looked up from my musings and this woman was standing in front of me! (Figure 2.3).

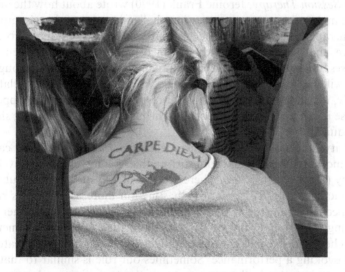

Figure 2.3 "Seize the Day" (Thank you, Horace! *Odes*, 23 BCE.)

People come to therapy, single session or otherwise, when they need help. Sometimes people change gradually, but we should also be alert to the possibility of the proverbial "bolt out of the blue." We think evolution is normally slow and incremental, but there also is the concept of "punctuated evolution" (see Alvarez, 1997; Gould, 1980; Rosenbaum et al., 1990/1995, p. 211), the phenomenon that things may go along steady state for a long time until something happens, like a meteorite strike that stirs up so much dust it blocks the sunlight and kills the vegetation and starves the dinosaurs and thus opens a niche for the mammals to flourish – or, in our field, a birth or a death, or an illness or a marriage or a divorce or a graduation or job change or a child leaving home that sets off long-term ramifications. For some, an SST is stabilizing or incremental; for others, an SST can be a watershed, a turning point. Bob Rosenbaum (2014; Rosenbaum et al., 1990/1995; see Chapter 7) has described being somewhat dubious about what could happen in a single session until he was out hiking one day and came around a curve to discover a huge avalanche changing an ancient mountain and valley in less than 30 seconds. *Both* (not either/or) sudden *and* gradual change can occur: on the mountain, wind and rain produce gradual accretion and erosion *and* an avalanche or earthquake brings more rapid alteration.

Milton Erickson (1983, p. 71) commented, "I do not think we need to presuppose or propound some long, drawn-out causation and a long, drawn-out therapeutic process. You see, if illness can occur suddenly, then therapy can occur quite as suddenly." In his Foreword to Talmon's *Single Session Therapy*, Jerome Frank (1990) wrote about how the idea of people making changes in one session challenges a lot of the assumptions that therapists have had: the beliefs that you have to gradually form an alliance, that you have to gradually uncover the underlying schemas or neuroses, that you then have to gradually work your way through or there will be too much resistance. So, when things happen relatively quickly, it's an interesting question for researchers, what really happened, because it can't be a gradual working-through process; something shifted more quickly.

Brevity does not necessarily mean superficial; the right haiku can be much more to the point and soul stirring than a long, plodding novel – or therapy (Hoyt, 2014, p. 68). There are lots of ways to think about what we clinicians do in SST. We usually function more as gardeners rather than mechanics, nurturing and bringing forth what is helpful rather than tinkering with and trying to fix something that is broken. Sometimes we're cheerleaders, or witnesses or guides, or function like a theater director evoking a performance. Sometimes our role is similar to that of a midwife, who attends the process, eases the transition, and provides a helping hand in case anything gets temporarily stuck. Ritterman (2009, pp. 129–130) reminds us that a train, taking just a slight angle onto a different track, can wind up in a brand new place. (As Gladwell, 2000, has written, little things can make a big difference.)

Therapy is a form of conversation (see Weakland, 1993; de Shazer, 1994). As Eric Berne (1966, p. 63) wrote: "The therapist does not cure anyone [...] When the patient recovers, the therapist should be able to say, 'My treatment helped nature.'" Milton Erickson (quoted in Zeig, 1980, p. 148) similarly said: "It is the patient who does the therapy. The therapist only furnishes the climate, the weather. That's all. The patient has to do all the work." In *The Gift of Therapy*, Irvin Yalom (2002,

p. 258) added: "It is a joy to see others open the taps of their own founts of wisdom."

In the novel *The Catcher in the Rye* (Salinger, 1951), the character Holden Caulfield alludes to Robert Burns' 1782 Scottish poem "Comin' Thro the Rye" as he tells his sister the story that a "catcher in the rye" was a kind of lifeguard, someone who would stand in the tall rye grass near the edge of a cliff and watch the children and make sure that none went over the edge, i.e., a protector of their innocence. In SST, we sometimes serve like that. We catch people and save them from potential hazards and we help them resolve problems without encouraging them to feel dependent or incompetent, without their needing to become "mental" or "psychiatric."

This cartoon says a lot (Figure 2.4):

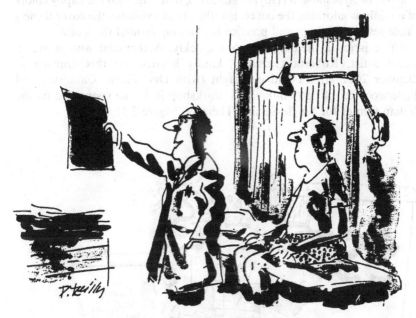

*"Basically, there's nothing wrong with you that
what's right with you can't cure."*

Figure 2.4 What's Right with You (From *The New Yorker*, February 8, 1993. © *The New Yorker*. Used with permission.) Or, as Shakespeare said in *All's Well that Ends Well*, Act I, Scene 1: "Our remedies oft in our-selves do lie."

How and where we look influences what we see and what we do. Some stories are better than others. "A 'good' story does more than merely relate 'facts': a 'good story' invigorates" (Hoyt, 2000, pp. 21–22). How we thera-pists choose to conceive and construe our clients and our work together can help enhance a sense of what the dictionary defines as *joy*: "a feeling of delight, happiness, and gladness, and a source of pleasure" (see Hoyt & Nylund, 1997/2000). This invigorating aspect of human awareness (Schutz, 1967) is especially important in the face of the problems we confront.

Images of Hope and Joy and SST

When Moshe and I edited the book *Capturing the Moment* (Hoyt & Talmon, 2014), we finished our Editors' Conclusion (p. 482) by saying: "As many clients and therapists have discovered, SST can be as up-to-date as tomorrow's sunrise." With that spirit in mind, we chose a hopeful new-day sunrise image for the cover. Then, after we had the second Capturing the Moment conference, we again produced a book, *Single-Session Therapy by Walk-In or Appointment* (Hoyt et al., 2018), that time with the happy colors of a rainbow adorning the cover. For the present volume, the cover depicts single session thinking and practice blossoming around the world.

There is joy in helping someone quickly. A therapist who is also a visual artist, Roberta Guzzardi, kindly handed me this drawing in October 2017 after I had co-taught (with Drs. Flavio Cannistrà and Federico Piccirilli) a two-day SST workshop in Rome sponsored by the Italian Center for Single-Session Therapy (Figure 2.5).

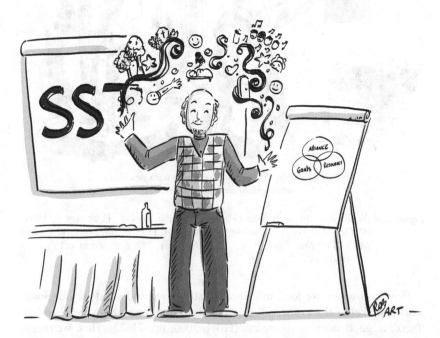

Figure 2.5 The Joy of SST (by Roberta Guzzardi. ©2020. Used by permission.)

The rainbow of figures happily floating between my hands represents some of the SST cases I had presented, in which clients in one session had overcome issues involving grief, nightmares, anxiety, depression, and relationship problems.

Will You Be Surprised by Joy, or Are You Expecting Her/Him?[2]

When Jay Haley was asked, "If you could teach students only one thing, what would it be?" Jay responded without hesitation: "Love. I'd teach them to love their clients. Everything else falls into place once a therapist loves their clients" (quoted in Davis, 2011, p. 26). At the 2nd Capturing the Moment conference, in Banff, I asked, *"Where is the magic?"* and answered, "THE MAGIC IS WITHIN, BETWEEN, and AROUND" (see Hoyt, 2017, p. 306). The Austrian philosopher Ludwig Wittgenstein (1953/1968, No. 97) and the Australian poet Gwen Harwood (2001, p. 110) both wrote: "Thought is surrounded by a halo." Call it HALO, call it LOVING-KINDNESS, call it RELATIONAL TRANCE, or call it ALLIANCE, I think it's the "BETWEEN" and "AROUND" that often brings out the "WITHIN."

And so I ask: Is your heart and soul (and mind) open and ready to help your client today? Do you really "believe in" and affirm your clients? Do you truly feel that something good will result from a one-session meeting? As Charles Snyder (2002; also see Courtnage, 2020) wrote in his paper, "Hope Theory: Rainbows of the Mind," hope is the belief that people have the agency and can see a pathway to pursue their goals. We can facilitate that, often in one visit, assisting clients to bring their goals and resources together.

Now... and Next

The fundamental idea of single session thinking and practice is that there is no time but the present (Hoyt, 1990/2017; in 2004 I edited a book called *The Present is a Gift*) and that change truly can only happen NOW. "What's past is prologue," said Shakespeare (*The Tempest*, Act II, Scene 1), meaning "Everything up to now sets the stage for what we do next." Single session therapies offer, as Michael White put it, "new possibilities for action."

I'm eager to see the next developments in SST thinking and practice.

Coda

Single session now
By walk-in or appointment
Ready when you are

In single session thinking and practice we both "capture the moment" and "create the moment." Again: Do you have hope? Are you ready for joy? In one session? Today? And tomorrow? I hope so – that's why we're here.

Notes

1 Francis and Clarkin (1981) note that "no treatment as the prescription of choice" may often be the case – people do it on their own, without professional involvement.
2 With a nod to C.S. Lewis (1956) for his book title, *Surprised by Joy*.

References

Aafjes-van Doorne, K., & Sweeney, K. (2019). The effectiveness of initial therapy contact: A systematic review. *Clinical Psychology Review, 74.* https://doi.org/10.1016/j.cpr.2019.101786

Alvarez, W. (1997). *T. Rex and the Crater of Doom.* Princeton, NJ: Princeton University Press.

Appelbaum, S.A. (1973). Parkinson's law in psychotherapy. *International Journal of Psychoanalytic Psychotherapy, 4,* 426–436.

Berg, I.K., & Dolan, Y.D. (2001). *Tales of Solution: A Collection of Hope-Inspiring Stories.* New York: Norton.

Berne, E. (1966). *Principles of Group Treatment.* New York: Oxford University Press.

Bobele, M., & Slive, A. (2014). One session at a time: When you have a whole hour. In M.F. Hoyt & M. Talmon (Eds.), *Capturing the Moment: Single Session Therapy and Walk-In Services* (pp. 95–119). Bethel, CT: Crown House Publishing.

Courtnage, A. (2020). Hoping for change: The role of hope in single-session therapy. *Journal of Systemic Therapies, 39*(1), 49–63.

Davis, S. (2011, November/December). Models or therapists? Power from a common factors perspective. *Family Therapy Magazine, 10*(6), 26–28.

DeMelo, J. (2018, July). Bull's eye! One-and-done sessions give new meaning to the phrase *targeted therapy. O: The Oprah Magazine, 19*(63–64), 67.

de Shazer, S. (1994). *Words Were Originally Magic.* New York: Norton.

Dickinson, E. (1960). *The Complete Poems of Emily Dickinson.* In T.H. Johnson (Ed.). Boston, MA: Little, Brown. (Works originally written c. 1850–1880.)

Erickson, M.H. (1983). *Healing in Hypnosis: The Seminars, Workshops, and Lectures of Milton H. Erickson (Vol. 1).* New York: Irvington.

Francis, A., & Clarkin, J.F. (1981). No treatment as the prescription of choice. *Archives of General Psychiatry, 38,* 542–545.

Frank, J.D. (1974). Psychotherapy: The restoration of morale. *American Journal of Psychiatry, 131*(3), 271–274.

Frank, J.D. (1990). Foreword. In M. Talmon (Ed.), *Single-Session Therapy* (pp. xi–xiii). San Francisco, CA: Jossey-Bass.

Gladwell, M. (2000). *The Tipping Point: How Little Things Can Make a Big Difference.* New York: Brown, Little.

Gould, S.J. (1980). *The Panda's Thumb: More Reflections on Natural History.* New York: Norton.

Hair, H.J., Shortall, R., & Oldford, J. (2013). Where's help when you need it? Developing responsive and effective brief counseling services for children, adolescents, and their families. *Social Work in Mental Health, 11,* 16–33.

Harwood, G. (2001). "Thought is Surrounded by a Halo." In G. Kratzmann (Ed.), *Selected Poems* (p. 110). Camberwell, Victoria, Australia: Penguin.

Hoyt, M.F. (1990). On time in brief therapy. In R.A. Wells & V.J. Giannetti (Eds.), *Handbook of the Brief Psychotherapies* (pp. 115–143). New York: Plenum. Expanded and reprinted in M.F. Hoyt, *Brief Therapy and Beyond* (6–32). New York: Routledge, 2017.

Hoyt, M.F. (1996). On ethics and the spiritualities of the surface: A conversation with Michael White and Gene Combs. In M.F. Hoyt (Ed.), *Constructive Therapies 2* (pp. 33–59). New York: Guilford Press. Reprinted in M.F. Hoyt, *Interviews with Brief Therapy Experts* (pp. 71–96). New York: Brunner-Routledge, 2001.

Hoyt, M.F. (2000). *Some Stories Are Better than Others: Doing What Works in Brief Therapy and Managed Care.* New York: Brunner/Mazel.

Hoyt, M.F. (2004). *The Present Is a Gift: Mo' Better Stories from the World of Brief Therapy.* New York: iUniverse.

Hoyt, M.F. (2014). Psychology and my gallbladder: An insider's account of a single-session therapy. In M.F. Hoyt & M. Talmon (Eds.), *Capturing the Moment: Single-Session Therapy and Walk-In Services* (pp. 53–72). Bethel, CT: Crown House Publishing.

Hoyt, M.F. (2017). *Brief Therapy and Beyond: Stories, Language, Love, Hope, and Time.* New York: Routledge.

Hoyt, M.F. (2018). Single-session therapy: Stories, structures, themes, cautions, and prospects. In M.F. Hoyt, M. Bobele, A. Slive, J. Young, & M. Talmon (Eds.), *Single-Session Therapy by Walk-In or Appointment: Administrative, Clinical, and Supervisory Aspects of One-at-a-Time Services* (pp. 154–174). New York: Routledge.

Hoyt, M.F., & Bobele, M. (Eds.). (2019). *Creative Therapy in Challenging Situations: Unusual Interventions to Help Clients.* New York: Routledge.

Hoyt, M.F., Bobele, M., Slive, A., Young, J., & Talmon, M. (Eds.). (2018). *Single-Session Therapy by Walk-In or Appointment: Administrative, Clinical, and Supervisory Aspects of One-at-a-Time Services.* New York: Routledge.

Hoyt, M.F., & Nylund, D. (1997). The joy of narrative: An exercise for learning from our internalized clients. *Journal of Systemic Therapies, 16*(4), 361–366. Reprinted in M.F. Hoyt, *Some Stories are Better than Others* (pp. 201–206). New York: Brunner/Mazel, 2000.

Hoyt, M.F., & Rosenbaum, R. (2018). Some ways to end an SST. In M.F. Hoyt, M. Bobele, A. Slive, J. Young, & M. Talmon (Eds.), *Single-Session Therapy by Walk-In or Appointment: Administrative, Clinical, and Supervisory Aspects of One-at-a-Time Services* (pp. 318–323). New York: Routledge.

Hoyt, M.F., & Talmon, M. (Eds.). (2014). *Capturing the Moment: Single-Session Therapy and Walk-In Services.* Bethel, CT: Crown House Publishing.

Leslie, P.J. (2019). *The Art of Creating a Magical Session: Key Elements for Transformative Psychotherapy.* New York: Routledge.

Lewis, C.S. (1956). *Surprised by Joy*. San Diego, CA: Harcourt Brace Jovanovich.

Monk, G., Winslade, J., Crocket, K., & Epston, D. (Eds.) (1997). *Narrative Therapy in Practice: The Archeology of Hope*. San Francisco: Jossey-Bass.

Ritterman, M. (2009). *The Tao of a Woman: 100 Ways to Turn*. Berkeley, CA: Skipping Stones Editions.

Ritterman, M. (2019). The single stroke: What makes "zingers" zing? In M.F. Hoyt & M. Bobele (Eds.), *Creative Therapy in Difficult Situations: Unusual Interventions to Help Clients* (pp. 163–171). New York: Routledge.

Rosenbaum, R. (1994). Single-session therapies: Intrinsic integration? *Journal of Psychotherapy Integration, 4*(3), 229–252.

Rosenbaum, R. (2008). Psychotherapy is not short or long. *APA Monitor on Psychology, 39*(7), 4, 8.

Rosenbaum, R. (2014). The time of your life. In M.F. Hoyt & M. Talmon (Eds.), *Capturing the Moment: Single-Session Therapy and Walk-In Services* (pp. 41–52). Bethel, CT: Crown House Publishing.

Rosenbaum, R., Hoyt, M.F., & Talmon, M. (1990). The challenge of single-session therapies: Creating pivotal moments. In R.A. Wells & V.J. Giannetti (Eds.), *Handbook of the Brief Psychotherapies* (pp. 165–189). New York: Plenum. Reprinted in M.F. Hoyt, *Brief Therapy and Managed Care* (pp. 105–139). San Francisco: Jossey-Bass, 1995.

Rycroft, P., & Young, J. (2014). SST in Australia: Learning from teaching. In M.F. Hoyt & M. Talmon (Eds.), *Capturing the Moment* (pp. 141–156). Bethel, CT: Crown House Publishing.

Salinger, J.D. (1951). *The Catcher in the Rye*. Boston, MA: Little, Brown.

Schutz, W.C. (1967). *Joy: Expanding Human Awareness*. New York: Grove Press.

Slive, A., & Bobele, M. (Eds.). (2011). *When One Hour is All You Have: Effective Therapy for Walk-In Clients*. Phoenix, AZ: Zeig, Tucker & Theisen.

Slive, A., & Bobele, M. (2018). The three top reasons why walk-in/single-sessions make perfect sense. In M.F. Hoyt, M. Bobele, A. Slive, J. Young, & M. Talmon (Eds.), *Single-Session Therapy by Walk-In or Appointment: Administrative, Clinical, and Supervisory Aspects of One-at-a-Time Services* (pp. 27–39). New York: Routledge.

Snyder, C.R. (2002). Hope theory: Rainbows of the mind. *Psychological Inquiry, 13*(4), 249–275.

Talmon, M. (1990). *Single-Session Therapy: Maximizing the Effect of the First (and Often Only) Therapeutic Encounter*. San Francisco: Jossey-Bass.

Talmon, M. (1993). *Single Session Solutions: A Guide to Practical, Effective, and Affordable Therapy*. Reading, MA: Addison-Wesley.

Talmon, M. (2014). When less is more: Maximizing the effect of the first (and often only) therapeutic encounter. In M.F. Hoyt & M. Talmon (Eds.), *Capturing the Moment: Single-Session Therapy and Walk-In Services* (pp. 27–40). Bethel, CT: Crown House Publishing.

Talmon, M., & Hoyt, M.F. (2014). Moments are forever: SST and walk-in services now and in the future. In M.F. Hoyt & M. Talmon (Eds.), *Capturing the Moment* (pp. 463–485). Bethel, CT: Crown House Publishing.

Weakland, J.H. (1993). Conversation – but what kind? In S.G. Gilligan & R. Price (Eds.), *Therapeutic Conversations* (pp. 136–145). New York: Norton.

Wittgenstein, L. (1968). *Philosophical Investigations* (3rd ed.; G.E.M. Anscombe, Trans.). New York: Palgrave MacMillan. (work originally published 1953).

Wylie, M.S. (1994). Panning for gold. *Family Therapy Networker, 18*(6), 40–48.

Yalom, I.D. (2002). *The Gift of Therapy: An Open Letter to a New Generation of Therapists and Their Patients.* New York: HarperCollins.

Young, J. (2018). Single-session therapy: The misunderstood gift that keeps on giving. In M.F. Hoyt, M. Bobele, A. Slive, J. Young, & M. Talmon (Eds.), *Single-Session Therapy by Walk-In or Appointment: Administrative, Clinical, and Supervisory Aspects of One-at-a-Time Services* (pp. 40–58). New York: Routledge.

Young, K. (2018). Change in the winds: The growth of walk-in therapy clinics in Ontario, Canada. In M.F. Hoyt, M. Bobele, A. Slive, J. Young, & M. Talmon (Eds.), *Single-Session Therapy by Walk-In or Appointment* (pp. 59–71). New York: Routledge.

Zeig, J.K. (1980). *A Teaching Seminar with Milton H. Erickson, M.D.* New York: Brunner/Mazel.

3 Translating Single Session Thinking into Practice

Pam Rycroft and Jeff Young

The Bouverie Centre in Melbourne, Australia, has been providing clinical single session therapy (SST), teaching it, offering implementation consultations, and hosting conferences on it since 1994.

We have pondered over those years what it is about the application of single session thinking that has appealed not only to therapists, but to a huge range of practitioners and organizations. We think we have a part answer at least: it is an accessible, timely, and responsive service which invites clients to have a voice in what they most need, and when. Clients have found it to be both respectful and practical (Hymmen, Stalker, & Cait, 2013), while managers love the fact that it is both efficient and effective.

Creating a context wherein both therapist and client approach the first session "as if" it will also be the last and inviting an overt non-judgmental discussion post session about whether further work is wanted or needed proved to be a wonderful thing for our own family therapy service. Instead of seeking equity by offering all families a pre-determined number of sessions, we realized that by making the most of the first session and then letting clients decide what they needed from us, those client families who did well with fewer sessions allowed more resources for those who needed more. This gave us the confidence to fully embrace single session thinking in practice.

In the early years, however, not all embraced the approach as we did. As we have mentioned in other places (Young, Weir, & Rycroft, 2012; Young, Rycroft, & Weir, 2014; Rycroft & Young, 2014; Young, 2018a, b) the nature of our training has changed over time. From early comments reflecting fears that this was another economic rationalist push to do more with less (or less with less?), participants' responses shifted to things like:

- "We get it that it's about making the most of the time, but how do you do that respectfully?" and
- "What makes a single session as useful as possible?"

These and many other similar questions pushed us to develop and describe our own therapeutic approach, as well as the processes we use to support this. As we moved to include work outside the therapy room (single session work rather than single session therapy), and began to consider how this approach might be (and is) adapted across very different environments, including homelessness, palliative care, disability services, online youth counseling, and emergency departments among many others, it caused us to ask ourselves:

"What are the core elements of a single session approach?"

What follows is our attempt to answer this by firstly outlining our own SST process, illustrated with a family therapy example, and secondly by naming what we see as core to our delivery of a single session approach.

Single Session Doesn't Necessarily Mean a Single Encounter: It's Often a Process

We believe that, while the therapeutic session itself is central, what happens before and after the session is also very important. In some contexts (e.g., post-disaster work – see Miller, 2011; Guthrie, 2018; Nùñez and Abia, Chapter 24 this volume), there is just the one "in the moment" opportunity. But when our clients also come along prepared to make the most of the session, so much more can be achieved, especially when they have the safeguard of knowing they can return for further work if they decide.

Our own process, as described by O'Neill and Rottem (2012) and schematically outlined below (see Figure 3.1), begins with an intake call and finishes with a follow-up phone call. We present this, as we do in our training, as one option only. Of course, folks adapt it to their own service environments.

At The Bouverie Centre, we have a *telephone intake,* conducted by a clinician, as a first response. This serves a number of purposes: it provides background to the family's current concerns, enquires about family members' hopes for the therapy, and explains Bouverie's single session approach, including our pre-session questionnaire, which is sent out to the family to be filled in and brought along to the session. (All paper work is available for download as part of our SST self-paced online training suite: https://events.bouverie.org.au/sst.) Family members choose whether to fill it in together or separately. (One very conscientious Mum brought one along which she had filled in on behalf of her three year old! She had "translated" the questions for her daughter and written down her responses.)

The column of arrowed choices on the right side of Figure 3.1 represent the various options available to clients: they may choose another single

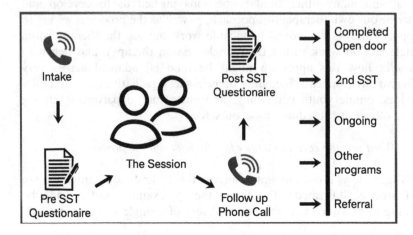

Figure 3.1 The Bouverie Centre's Single Session Therapy Process.

session, opt for ongoing regular therapy sessions, choose any other programs our service offers or in some cases consider a referral to a specialist service. Or they may choose to "go it alone," knowing that they can re-contact us at any time.

Family Therapy Example

To illustrate, we will follow Georgina, Anne, and their family through the steps of a typical Bouverie single session process.

At intake, we heard that Georgina (who preferred to be called Georgie) had partnered with Anne and brought her into the family after a number of years as a single parent, following her divorce from Ewan, and his move overseas. Georgie had four children, aged between 12 and 18. Her major concern was Liam (14), who had threatened his older brother Sean (16) with a kitchen knife following a dispute. This had scared Anne and Liam's younger sister Sophie and had caused a major upheaval in what was otherwise a relatively happy family.

Georgie and Anne had filled out the pre-session questionnaire together. When asked what they hoped to get from attending Bouverie, they had indicated that the most troubling issues for them were whether Liam needed some kind of psychiatric help and whether they as parents could or should have done more. These concerns were amplified by aspects of each woman's story: Ewan had exhibited a lot of anger while married to Georgie – in fact, it was when he "began to take this out on the kids" that she divorced him. For her part, Anne had an uncle whom she had adored as a child, but who developed a drug-related psychosis and had changed from a fun-loving young man to an angry, troubled adult.

Comment: The therapist may or may not telephone the family between the time of the intake conversation and the session itself. This is an opportunity to allay clients' anxiety and to engage with various family members (especially the more reluctant ones), answer questions, and address any concerns.

When Georgie and Anne were contacted, they both expressed grave worries about Liam's behavior. Georgie explained that, while no harm had come to anyone, she had been so concerned about Liam's rage that she had subsequently called the police, who offered to see Liam and give him an unofficial warning. Liam's behavior had triggered concerns that perhaps he had inherited his father's temper. Anne said that, on the other hand, Liam could often be thoughtful and understanding; after all, he was the one who had most welcomed her into the family. But she now wondered if he had a "split personality."

When it comes to *the session itself*, the therapist has the intake information, the family's questionnaire, and possibly information from a pre-session phone call to guide them as to the family's priorities for the session. Even so, ascertaining what each family member would like to walk away with by the end of the session provides an additional "business" engagement once the family has been settled into the room.

As a response to training participants' requests, we developed a "map" or "framework" for the session process (see Figure 3.2). It is a broad process outline rather than a specific model. The intention is to guide rather than prescribe, allowing individual practitioners to use their preferred theoretical model and personal style, given that we see single session thinking as a service delivery model rather than a therapeutic model per se (Young, 2018; Young et al., 2012). Illustrative questions are included as examples only.

While most of the above is self-evident and familiar enough to a range of therapeutic processes, the part that may or may not be so familiar is the so-called "Break." We emphasize that this may be an actual time-out or simply a punctuation in the session: a pause in the "dance," so to speak. Therapists are asked to consider what they might regret not having said, should they never get to meet this client family again. This encourages openness and directness on the part of the therapist – a "No Bullshit" approach (Young, in Findlay, 2007; also see https://events. bouverie.org.au/sst). Of course, therapists also need their clinical judgment to be on high alert – taking into consideration how individual client family members are likely to hear the reflection and feedback. Therapists may ask themselves: "What could I share that is most likely to be as helpful as possible right now to these particular folks?"

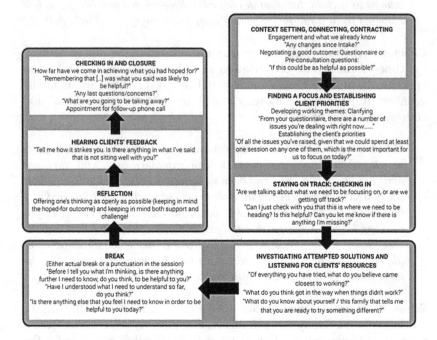

Figure 3.2 The Bouverie Centre's Single Session "Map."

What Are Our Core Elements?

In thinking about our question of what is core to our approach, there are certainly some clinical skills that we see as particularly useful for an SST approach. But beyond these, we also include some ways of thinking about how we offer the service as a whole. With our family example to illustrate, the following are what we now describe as our core elements.

1. **Negotiating a client-led outcome**
    When asked at Intake what she felt would be a good outcome for the family session, Georgie had indicated that Liam would have a better understanding of the impact of his outburst, and that she and Anne would get some advice about anything else they might have done or should do as parents. So the therapist had the Intake summary and the pre-session questionnaire as a strong starting point. But in the session itself she needed to check both Anne's and Liam's ideas about what would make this session worthwhile for them.

2. **Establishing clients' priorities**
    The therapist pointed out that she had to complete some administrative forms towards the end of the session but apart from that, the entire

session would be devoted to assisting the family get what they wanted most from the session.

Anne endorsed Georgie's hopes for the session, as well as her priorities: to establish whether Liam needed psychiatric care, and to seek advice about their parenting strategies. But Liam was reticent and had not contributed to the questionnaire, so it seemed important to get some idea of what might be an important outcome for him. "Dunno" was the answer (not unfamiliar to most practitioners working with young people). The therapist asked Liam whom he had come along to the session for. (This reframed his attendance as an act of selflessness, as he was clearly there for his Mum and for the family, not himself.) With some coaxing and encouragement from the therapist to find something that would make this worthwhile for him, he opted for "getting Mum and Anne off my back."

Comment: There may be priorities (mandatory tasks) for the therapist also, in which case time needs to be allowed for both while privileging the client or clients' needs and priorities.

3. **Finding a focus and talking about the most important things ("cutting to the chase")**
   Georgie at one stage began talking a lot about her marriage to Ewan. He had exhibited a lot of anger while married to Georgie, at times including physical abuse resulting in bruising and a huge loss in her confidence. She reiterated that it was when he "began to take things out on the kids" that she divorced him. This reminded Anne that it was her experience of her uncle's transformation from affectionate to angry and disturbed, that caused her to feel so worried about what could happen to Liam.

   Although the discussion was heartfelt and seemed to be relevant, the therapist was aware of the need to check in about the women's two major concerns, and whether the conversation was heading in the direction they felt it needed to go. It was also important to make sure that the therapist heard what was necessary to be as helpful as she could, and to capitalize on Liam's being there, because it was looking unlikely that he would engage in any ongoing therapeutic work. The therapist felt that she needed to address the issue that had led to them coming along. She looked to Liam and said: "Can I ask you something directly, Liam? It's clear that Anne and your Mum became very alarmed at the extent of your anger – threatening your brother with a knife. I'm wondering what it's like for you when you get that angry …. do you ever get worried about your own anger?"

4. **Checking in with the client(s) at regular intervals**
   As Liam acknowledged that he did get a bit worried about his own anger, Georgie began recounting in great detail the incident that had

led to the referral. The therapist became aware that, while Anne was looking at Liam and nodding her head, Liam was slowly "melting" further and further into his chair, with a look that indicated that he would rather be doing almost anything else in the world than this. The checking-in process therefore also involved asking about the experience of talking about this for each of them, particularly Liam, and more particularly after witnessing his own concern and shame in relation to his anger. The therapist also checked with Georgie and Anne whether they were getting what they were hoping from the session, and Georgie talked of wanting some advice about whether Liam needed psychiatric help. The therapist explained that she would need to explore Liam's and the family's situation in greater depth in order to respond thoughtfully, but promised she would address this question before the session ended.

5. **Interrupting respectfully when necessary, to help the client(s) get what they want.**

    The therapist became conscious very quickly that Georgie was "a talker" – and that both Anne and Liam had become accustomed to letting her talk, with Anne supporting her non-verbally with frowns and nods, while Liam "zoned out" throughout Georgie's monologues. The therapist felt a familiar tension: balancing the hearing of the distress "story" in the family members' own words while overseeing the process so that the clients get what they most want out of the session. The therapist, more than once, interrupted Georgie with comments like: "I know you are very keen to find out if Liam needs further psychiatric help, so I may have to interrupt you to get the information I need to be able to respond to this" and "Georgie – I just want to check in with Liam – what are you thinking as you hear your Mum tell us this? Is there anything you'd want to add? Disagree with?" and "Anne – I'm wondering what you might have been going through at that time?" As time went on, the therapist was able to joke with Georgie about her tendency to do all the talking.

6. **Making time your friend**

    Following on from the fact that the story itself was taking a lot of time, and the therapist was feeling pressured, she paused at one point, summed up what she had heard from each of them, and said: "Given that we have about 20 minutes left, and I want to be able to take time to think aloud in front of you before we finish, to at least provide advice about what Liam may need, I'm wondering what hasn't been said – or asked – that needs to be said or asked, at this point. Do you think I've heard what I need to hear to understand enough about what's happened and what you're all going through? Can I check in with each of you about that?" Anne said, "I think you should know that his dad had phoned to talk to the kids but had refused to talk to Liam because he hadn't acknowledged his Dad's birthday." This happened just the day before Liam had threatened his brother Sean (who happened to be Dad's favorite).

7. **Sharing your thoughts openly with clients**
   Once having established that each had said what they wanted (and were prepared) to say, the therapist went back to the family's pre-session questionnaire and quoted from their answers as to what was most troubling them, what would be a good outcome of the session and the specific questions they wanted addressed in the session. The therapist made a point of adding Liam's preferred outcome to this: to get the adults off his back. Her reflections focused on:

   - *What it meant that Liam had attended. This was something he'd much rather not have done.*
   - *How conscientious Georgie had been in involving the police, and how impressive it had been that Liam had in fact not only agreed to go along to the police station, knowing he would get a severe "talking to" – but he went along with his brother Sean who had been the target of his anger.*
   - *The concerns and questions Anne and Georgie had brought were understandable: particularly given that they each had life experiences related to the impact of anger and mental health issues. However, Liam and Sean had talked things out on the way to the police station; Liam had been remorseful and there was nothing at this point to indicate that Liam had issues that went beyond his temper.*
   - *Liam's own courage in facing up to what he had done and the fact that he had clearly known when enough was enough, and shown sufficient control to not allow his rage to dictate his behavior in using the knife.*
   - *The resources that this family brought to this problem: the adults' concern for all the children (they had talked about the different qualities of each of them, including Liam), their openness and their readiness to do things differently.*

8. **Preparing to end well (reaching closure if not solution or resolution)[1]**
   The therapist asked how far the session had come in achieving what they most wanted and needed. Georgie and Anne were very satisfied that Liam didn't need further psychiatric intervention and that they had acted with appropriate concern and care for all of the children. Liam remained reticent but said that it had made a difference hearing about how scary his Dad's anger had been for his Mum and how upsetting it would have been for Anne to have a favorite uncle become angry and

distant. He could see how his altercation with his brother would have stressed them both out.

Both Georgie and Anne felt both reassured and validated in their concern but also in their parenting.

A telephone follow-up time was arranged for 2 p.m. Thursday, two weeks after the session and written onto an appointment card for each person. Liam clearly didn't relish the idea of talking on the phone but agreed nonetheless. The therapist asked how they would communicate with the rest of the family about what had been talked about in the session – in particular with Sean. This led to a request from Georgie: sessions at this time were routinely recorded with permission from families, and she wondered if she could take the recording home to show the others. In this case, it was felt to be potentially a positive thing for this family, and they left with a copy of the DVD.[2]

9. **Leaving the door open (an "open door" policy)**
   The therapist assured the family that they could re-contact the therapist at any time prior to receiving the follow-up phone call if they needed. This appeared particularly reassuring to Georgie.

   Before the family left, the therapist reminded them that, at follow-up, together they would talk about how they found the session, "where from here," and whether they might want to request another single session, have ongoing sessions, or "go it alone," knowing that they could re-contact at any time. Georgie said that she had thought initially that, "for sure," one session wouldn't be enough and that they would need further help, but at this point she was willing to wait until the follow-up call to decide this. She and Anne were reassured that they could ring even before the follow-up call if they felt they needed to.

10. **Listening to client voices (following up, seeking feedback, and utilizing it)**
    At phone follow-up two weeks later, the therapist heard that:

    - *The family had watched the video of the session all together, more than once*
    - *Liam had commented: "Geez, I was being a bit difficult, wasn't I?"*
    - *His brother openly agreed with the therapist's comment about Liam's courage in facing up to what he had done*
    - *His sister, Sophie, talked about how Liam's temper sometimes frightens her, but how good it was to hear his own account of how it also worries – even frightens – himself*
    - *Georgie had drawn an image of a backpack (a metaphor that had come up during the session) and written down her family's thoughts*

about what resources they carried in their "backpack" as a family to get through challenging times like this.

Georgie and Anne were further commended on having listened to their kids and being open to responding in different ways.

Comment: We use a family's pre-session questionnaire as a reference point at the follow-up call. Their responses at this point (both through their descriptions and their ratings transcribed on to a post-session questionnaire during the phone call) provide a great reflection of what has changed and what hasn't, and can be compared with the pre-questionnaire ratings for evaluation purposes. Client families are also invited to give feedback about the process and the agency as a whole. Other than routine satisfaction surveys, with client consent, a researcher may contact random family members and seek their feedback.

This family used their single session to get back in touch with their own resources, and to make use of suggestions that had grown out of the therapeutic conversation. They were appreciative of the open-door policy even though they never felt the need to re-contact (other than to email a copy of the backpack image and their collected thoughts about their resources as a family).

What Is Core to a Single Session Approach?

Are all of these elements essential? The answer is – *Yes, to us.* But probably not to everyone. Walk-in services don't routinely follow up clients and they report positive outcome data[3] (see Chapters 4 and 11 of this volume). Not everyone chooses to use a reflecting process as part of a single session. Some services find that written questionnaires just don't work with their clients or service context. And those working with young clients are more likely to follow up via text messages than via formal questionnaires.

The elements we describe have developed over time because they have worked for us in applying the philosophy and values inherent in a single session approach: that clients are the heroes in their own lives (Duncan, Miller, & Sparks, 2004). Interestingly, putting the client in the driver's seat takes some of the burden from the therapist, which in turn helps the therapist to be a responsive and prudent navigator working collaboratively but actively to help get the client to where they want to go.

If we listen to what our clients want and need, when they need it, we can make the most of that first (and often only) contact – when the need is there and motivation is high – as well as using every other opportunity to help our clients get closer to their goals. We continue to experience the application of single session thinking as one of the most inspiring and rewarding ways to work with the people who seek our help.

Notes

1 The fact that these elements are numbered might suggest that they occur in a particular order. Any sequence is not "prescribed": rather it is determined by the therapist, the clients, and the nature of the conversation that occurs in any particular session. For instance, #7 and #8 could well be reversed in this example.
2 This family was seen at a time when recording (with written permission) our work was routine. On some occasions, as with this family, offering the family a copy allowed for absent family members to be informed and included in the work.
3 Whilst there is no routine follow-up for Walk-In clients, they are free to come back at any time.

References

Duncan, B.L., Miller, S.D., & Sparks, J.A. (2004). *The Heroic Client: A Revolutionary Way to Improve Effectiveness Through Client-Directed, Outcome-Informed Therapy*. San Francisco: Jossey-Bass.

Findlay, R. (2007). A mandate for honesty: Jeff Young's No Bullshit Therapy – An interview. *Australian and New Zealand Journal of Family Therapy*, *28*(3), 165–170.

Guthrie, B. (2018). Reflections on providing single-session therapy in post-disaster Haiti. In M.F. Hoyt, M. Bobele, A. Slive, A.J. Young, & M. Talmon (Eds.), *Single-Session Therapy and Walk-In Services* (pp. 303–317). New York: Routledge.

Hymmen, P., Stalker, C.A., & Cait, C. (2013). The case for single-session therapy: Does the empirical evidence support the increased prevalence of this service delivery model and walk-in services? *Journal of Mental Health*, *22*(1), 60–71.

Miller, J.K. (2011). Single-session intervention in the wake of Hurricane Katrina: Strategies for disaster mental health counseling. In A. Slive & M. Bobele ; (Eds.), *When One Hour is All You Have: Effective Therapy for Walk-In Clients* (pp. 185–202). Phoenix, AZ: Zeig, Tucker, & Theisen.

O'Neill, I., & Rottem, N. (2012). Reflections and learning from an agency-wide implementation of single session work in family therapy. *Australian and New Zealand Journal of Family Therapy*, *33*(1), 70–83.

Rycroft, P., & Young, J. (2014). Single session therapy in Australia: Learning from teaching. In M.F. Hoyt & M. Talmon (Eds.), *Capturing the Moment: Single Session Therapy and Walk-In Services* (pp. 141–156). Bethel, CT: Crown House Publishing.

Young, J. (2018a). Single session therapy: The gift that keeps on giving. In M.F. Hoyt, M. Bobele, A. Slive, J. Young, & M. Talmon (Eds.), *Single-session therapy by walk-in or appointment: Clinical, supervisory, and administrative aspects of one-at-a-time services* (pp. 40–58). New York: Routledge.

Young, J. (2018b). Putting single session therapy to work: Conceptual, training and implementation Ideas. In F. Cannistrà & F. Piccirilli (Eds.), *Terapia a*

Seduta Singola: Principi e Pratiche (pp. 169–186). Firenze, Italy: Giunti. (translated into Italian).

Young, J., Rycroft, P., & Weir, S. (2014). Implementing SST: Practical wisdoms from down under. In M.F. Hoyt & M. Talmon (Eds.), *Capturing the Moment: Single-Session Therapy and Walk-in Services: Administrative, Clinical, and Supervisory Aspects of One-at-a-Time Services* (pp. 121–140). Bethel, CT: Crown House Publishers.

Young, J., Weir, S., & Rycroft, P. (2012). Implementing single session therapy. *Australian and New Zealand Journal of Family Therapy, 34*(2), 69–74.

4 An Open Invitation to Walk-In Therapy: Opening Access to Mental Health Care[1]

Monte Bobele and Arnold Slive

The Community Counseling Service (CCS) in San Antonio, Texas, a community-based agency that trains Our Lady of the Lake University's counseling psychology graduate students, offers clients two options for psychotherapy: (1) a scheduled appointment or (2) a "no appointment necessary" walk-in session. Here is how a recent walk-in session began:

> *Therapist*: We saw that you found us online.
>
> *Jimena*: (who attended with her pre-teen daughter): I was looking for a walk-in clinic, because I've been calling other places and it was like a month to, like 3 months, to be able to get seen. I was Googling, and you were the first ones to pop out.

Another client, Geraldo, a highly anxious young man from México, walked in distraught, telling the therapists that the day before he received a text from an ex-girlfriend saying she had tested positive for HIV. The CCS is one of the few places in San Antonio where Geraldo could be seen immediately by Spanish-speaking therapists for this crisis, without a lot of red tape. It was important to us that we provide him a mental-health band-aid while helping create a plan for testing and support.[2] Geraldo decided to get tested for HIV the next day at a local resource that was discussed in the session. He was given the option of walking in again after he learned the results.[3] Geraldo arrived not having shared with anyone his distressing news; he left relieved that he had a supportive, non-judgmental conversation with the therapists.

Several times a week mental health professionals hear clients in need echoing the frustration of Jimena and Geraldo. Waiting lists, lack of accessibility, and other barriers have been identified as problems in delivery of services at the point of clients' needs (Goldner, Jones, & Fang, 2011; Possemato, Wray, Johnson, Webster, & Beehler, 2018). Barrett et al. (2008) identified obstacles that prevented prospective clients from receiving timely services including having to schedule an appointment for a first appointment and completing a time-consuming intake process before scheduling an opportunity to speak with a therapist. Their meta-analysis of 50 years of research on client attrition in a variety of settings, estimated that it took three separate contacts, often a week or more apart, with an agency before the client actually received a therapy session! Other researchers have found similar problems with the help-by-appointment model (Bebinger, 2019; Cornish, 2020; Emanuel, 2017; Possemato et al., 2018; Tatham, Stringer, Perera, & Waller, 2012). Clients already are familiar with "no appointment necessary" services such as hair stylists, medical clinics, restaurants, income tax services, church confessionals, and others (Miller, 2008; Slive & Bobele, 2012). So why haven't more mental-health service delivery systems accommodated to the world as it is lived in everyday life?

Walk-in/single session therapy[4] (WI/SST) services are based on two important ideas: first, walking in simplifies access to mental health services by eliminating the hurdle of waiting for appointments and other administrative procedures; second, single session therapy capitalizes on the well-established findings that most psychotherapy is brief. Recently, we (Slive & Bobele, 2018) highlighted three reasons that walk-in services "make perfect sense":

- **They seize the moment** by removing access hurdles and enabling clients to see a therapist at their moments of peak motivation (Slive & Bobele, 2011; Jefferies, 2003; Miller & Slive, 2004). At moments of crisis, of despair, of readiness for change, walking in provides ready access to a conversation with a mental health professional without the usual hurdles. Open access reduces frustration with the traditional appointment making processes.
- **They are effective,** as demonstrated by a growing body of research pointing to high levels of client satisfaction and positive therapeutic outcomes (Correia, 2013; Harper-Jaques & Leahey, 2011; Stalker et al., 2016). There is increasing evidence that a walk-in session reduces medical utilization, decreases stress, increases coping mechanisms, improves presenting concerns, and produces high rates of client satisfaction (Miller, 2008; Miller & Slive, 2004).
- **They are efficient** by reducing or eliminating wait lists, avoiding the use of more expensive services such as emergency rooms, and lessen overtreatment (Cornish, 2020; Emanuel, 2017: Hymmen, Stalker, & Cait, 2013; Stalker et al., 2016; Young et al., 2008).

Addressing Common Worries About WI/SST

Despite these clear advantages that WI/SST offers as a way of opening access to mental health services that are supported by increasing evidence that demonstrates effectiveness and client satisfaction, many providers worry about adding walk-in options. This chapter addresses their concerns and other potential objections that we have encountered from colleagues, students, and community members. We hope that this chapter will help facilitate the addition of walk-in services in their settings.

Will We Be Overwhelmed?

In 1990, one of us (AS) worked at Wood's Homes in Calgary, Alberta, Canada. Some of the staff members there proposed an idea to the Calgary community of offering a "no appointment necessary" walk-in counseling service. They were troubled by the growing wait list at Wood's Homes outpatient family therapy service. We had also observed the rapid emergence and utilization of walk-in medical clinics in our community. Accordingly, community members were asked for their opinions about offering walk-in mental health services. They were uniformly supportive of the idea. In fact, some were amazed that Wood's Homes (as well as other mental health professionals) wasn't already providing such easily accessible services. Still, some even wondered whether we would be overwhelmed with more than we could handle. That gave us pause for a moment, but we then realized that their unease was a sign that we were on the right track. Most walk-in clinics start out slow and find that demand increases as the word spreads. All the walk-in services that we know of have adapted creatively to increased client demand by adding hours of operation, increasing and repurposing staff, recruiting volunteer mental-health professionals, or utilizing trainees. High client demand is exactly what we are looking for.

How Do You Manage Risk When Clients Just Walk In?

What if a client comes to a walk-in service showing evidence of risk such as suicide/self-harm, threats of violence to others, or child abuse? How can we responsibly and ethically address such issues in a walk-in session? The simple answer is that in a walk-in session, these issues are handled just as they are as in "by-appointment" sessions. We assess risk. We may then work with the client to develop a safety plan. If necessary, we ensure that the person goes to a hospital emergency room for an assessment for possible admission, or we contact the relevant authorities. When possible, we may, with the client's consent, involve family members or other support persons, and arrange for a follow-up phone call. As with more traditional scheduled appointments, sometimes these measures take longer than the scheduled time.

What About Paperwork?

When clients walk in, there has been no extensive information gathering by phone or the front desk, nor are there any online forms to complete. There is no pre-assessment (see the next section). When clients arrive in a typical walk-in clinic, the receptionist gives them a short form to complete.

(See Chanut, Livingstone, and Stalker [2010] for the typical process at a walk-in clinic.) Usually, it is a one-page, two-sided form that clients can complete in five to ten minutes. Clients provide basic demographic information and indicate what they want from the session. Representative questions are:

- What is the single most important concern you would like to address today?
- Is there some background information that you would like to share about that concern?
- Some people find that one session works for them for now. At the end of your session, what will tell you that you have taken a step in the right direction?

The answers usually provide enough information for the therapist to prepare for the session. Some clients may not be able or willing to write all the requested information on the intake forms, but we learn enough through the therapeutic conversation to address what the clients want.

Following, or in some settings during, the walk-in session, the therapist completes a session note. Some clinics create a template especially for walk-in sessions that includes what the client wanted from the visit, limited background information about the problem, what was done, and future plans. When there were risk/safety issues, these are described, and details are provided about how they were addressed. The note is usually brief and can be completed in ten minutes or less. One advantage for many therapists is that once the note is completed, that's that. There are no follow-up calls to make, no appointments to book, and no future no-shows to deal with. It's one complete experience for both client and therapist.

If They Just Walk In, Is There No Pre-Assessment?

Yes, there are none of the lengthy pre-assessment procedures that are common in many clinics. Therapists working in walk-in services find that time-consuming questionnaires, psychological testing, and other speed bumps before clients and their therapists work on what is on their minds are not useful. Some clinicians and agency directors worry that by omitting a comprehensive psychosocial assessment, or a thorough risk assessment, or some other such measure they might "miss something." We have found that simply having one item in the clients' intake material is enough to alert therapists for further risk assessment when needed. An example question from a walk-in intake form might be: "Do you now, or have you had, any fears that you (or your child, or anyone with you) is at risk of harm to themselves, others, or pets?" Even when these risks are not identified on the intake form, they might arise during the session. In either case, when clients respond affirmatively to questions such as these, the clinician will assess for risk.

We cannot underestimate the issue of risk. Nor should we overestimate it. The efforts to screen for and prevent suicide have met with equivocal results over the last half century. A recent meta-analysis of such efforts to identify risk factors associated with death by suicide (Franklin et al., 2017) concluded that the current state of the research is insufficient to support common practices in predicting who is, and is not, at risk. Fifty years of researchers' efforts indicates that no currently identifiable risk factors actually predict death by suicide (see Franklin et al., 2017). Neither suicide prevention strategies (Zalsman et al., 2016), nor primary care screening have been shown to decrease deaths by suicide (Milner et al., 2017). Given that empirical support is lacking for extensive suicide assessment as a way of managing risk, perhaps a brief question on intake that is followed up by the clinician would be more efficient.

Furthermore, clients may find it intrusive when attention is directed, before a session begins, to topics such as suicide, abuse, and history of psychopathology, and before having the opportunity to talk about their immediate agendas. Such preliminaries could hinder the development of the therapeutic alliance that is a key to good outcomes. Some prospective clients will be alienated enough by this process to decide to say "no" to psychotherapy at all, thus depriving them of the care we could provide.

Is It Ethical to Not Routinely Follow-Up After Walk-In Sessions?

Typically, in our WI services at the CCS, at the Eastside Family Centre in Calgary, and many other Canadian walk-in services there is no routine follow-up contact after the session. On occasion, a session will result in the co-development of a safety plan to address a risk concern that might end with an agreement to make a call see how the plan is working. But this is a relatively rare occurrence. Apart from a prior agreement to make post-session contact for research purposes, the session ends and that's that.

We are not discouraging follow-up; in fact, we encourage it! For instance, some clients are interested in further ongoing services, and we assist by discussing options for such services. But all walk-in clients are invited to return. They can walk in again when they choose. In this way, follow-up is initiated by clients rather than by therapists. They follow up with the same ease of access as their previous session – simply by walking in. Eschewing routine follow-up is a shift from the traditional mental-health service risk-averse practice. The client oversees the process.

Can Just Anybody Walk In?

In a walk-in service, if there is no pre-screening of clients, should we be worried about risk of violence on our site or toward our staff? When this came up before we opened our center in Calgary, we consulted the police. They assured us that the threat of violence on our premises was extremely small. The greater risk would be for women at night going to their cars in the parking lot. In other words, we would have no more to worry about than any other neighborhood business. Wick (2016), in addressing general safety in walk-in medical clinics advised staff to use commonsense procedures. We have not yet heard anecdotal reports of violence at a walk-in counseling service. In our own experience, we have seen less hostility from walk-in service clients. Walk-in clients arrive less frustrated by the usual bureaucratic hurdles in getting an appointment.

What If Clients Want Something That We Don't Provide?

In many walk-in services, clients are not prescreened, so occasionally a session might not be a good fit for the client. Early in our sessions we invite clients to tell us what they want. We may ask, "What are you hoping for today?" or "When you're driving away today thinking about the session, what would tell you that it's been a good use of your time?" We then use the remainder of the session to give clients what they want. They might want increased hope, a sense of being heard, a new way of thinking about their unease, or a next small step to get back on track. For many clients, a walk-in session is their first psychotherapy experience, so we always want them to leave feeling that they've had a positive experience so that they would return or make use of other mental health services in the future if they needed (Miller, 2008).

We ask what clients want early in the session because they might be looking for something that is outside our scope of services. If desired, we give the client referral information about where those services are located. Given that there is usually time remaining, we ask if there is something else we can help with, and often there is.

What About Clients Who May Be in Therapy Elsewhere?

On occasion, clients arrive who are already in ongoing psychotherapy with another therapist. We do not send them away; we ask what they want today. We check in with them about their current therapists and whether they are planning to return to see them. If it turns out that they are discouraged about their therapy, we encourage them to bring that to their therapist's attention. We may consult with them about how to raise those matters of their care directly in the next therapy session. Some may walk in because the current therapist is unavailable. We then work with them to further the work they are doing with their ongoing therapist.

What If They Are Seeking an Ongoing Series of Sessions?

Sometimes clients walk in expecting ongoing sessions. We strongly advocate giving clients choices and respecting their decisions. One such choice is a single session or a series of sessions. If we learn that the client is primarily interested in a series of sessions, we determine, specifically, what they are hoping for and help them find a suitable service, which may include an in-house referral in our own clinic. We may then offer to use the remainder of the walk-in session as a way of getting a "head start" on their future therapy. We find that often clients are interested in having that conversation, and sometimes find that the one session had been sufficient for them at the time.

Do Clients Use a Walk-In Service as Ongoing Therapy?

Many clients return to the CCS's walk-in service. They might have come the day before, the week before, months or years before. We consider that a positive development, because we want our clients to develop a long-term alliance with the CCS (instead of specific therapists). We routinely invite clients to return for future walk-in sessions, and we treat each subsequent visit as a new single session. Some clients use our walk-in service as if it were ongoing therapy. In other words, they walk in time after time for sessions, perhaps every week. In our initial orientation to a walk-in session, we try to prevent that from occurring by using the following analogy: "As in a walk-in medical clinic, you walk in and have your session, and if you decide to walk in again at some future date you may or may not see the same therapist." Nevertheless, a few clients will return week after week. So, when we realize this, usually after just a few sessions, we work with the client to find a better fit for them at our clinic or elsewhere in the community.

However, for some clients the appeal of a walk-in service is that they can get a counseling session when it is convenient for them. Because they have an alliance with the CCS, that is more important to them than seeing the same therapist, it works for them. In fact, we have heard clients say that they find having a variety of therapists very helpful. We've come to refer to these as "serial single sessions" (Bobele et al., 2018, p. 249; Slive & Bobele, 2019) and find that this is consistent with our one-at-a-time mindset.

Are Walk-In Services Suitable for Minority and Marginalized Populations?

We believe that walk-in counseling is a move toward a more socially just way for clients to access services. We have observed that marginalized minorities who are not accustomed to therapy may be more likely to attend a walk-in service. Yet, while we have anecdotal reports, we do not have data to back up this claim. For example, at the CCS, located in a primarily Hispanic neighborhood, we provide counseling by appointment as well as walk-in in both English and Spanish (see Bobele, López,

Scamardo, & Solórzano, 2008). For more examples, see Hoyt, Bobele, Slive, Young, and Talmon (2018).

Clients find an open access service less intimidating. It follows that those trepidatious about accessing services are more likely to take a chance on a walk-in service. This seems to also be true of men, who use counseling services less often than women (Juvrud & Rennels, 2017; Liddon, Kingerlee, & Barry, 2018; Nam et al., 2010; Susukida, Mojtabai, & Mendelson, 2015). However, more men seem to utilize walk-in counseling than we usually see in other services. Recently in studying client satisfaction and outcomes, Harper-Jaques and Foucault (2014) recruited the first 100 individual adult walk-in clients who agreed to participate in the research project. It turned out that exactly 50% were male and 50% were female. We are not sure what accounted for such an unusually high percentage of men. Perhaps a walk-in service is a way for some men, undecided about psychotherapy, to test the waters.

What About Structure, Training, and Support for New Walk-In Services?

We agree with our Australian colleagues (Young, Rycroft, & Weir, 2014) that walk-in/single session therapy, like by-appointment/single session therapy services, need strong organizational support. That means administrative support from the top, training for staff that focuses on (1) the single session mindset (Talmon, 1990), (2) addressing the fears about walk-in services described in this chapter, and (3) a support group of like-minded colleagues. Also helpful is what Young et al. (2014) called a "clinical champion" who is passionate about this work and is respected by colleagues as a go-to person for clinical consultations. In addition, walk-in services require a supportive "front end," someone who greets clients, informs them about the process, collects brief intake documents, and answers questions about fees or other matters. It is common that when walk-in services first open their doors, there is some down time for staff members. As word spreads in the community about this easy-access option, there is typically consistent high utilization. Even when occasional less busy periods occur, staff members can use that time in the same way as when "no shows" and late cancellations occur for scheduled appointments: catching up with record keeping or consulting with colleagues about ongoing cases.

It is important to note that walk-in/single session services are implemented with a variety of staffing and administrative schemes (see Hoyt et al., 2018; Slive & Bobele, 2014). Some offer a walk-in option during all the hours the agency is open, some are open for walk-ins one day a week, and some only a half-day per week. Length of sessions range from half-hour to 1½ hours. Some utilize all their staff members and others only those that are interested in this form of service. Others have trainees and/or volunteer mental health professionals who provide some of the services. Some operate with teams of therapists working together and others with each therapist working independently (though perhaps with a consultant available as needed). Many clinics in the U.S. and Canada that offer WI/SST also offer single session therapy by appointment and have on-going therapy options. Where walk-in has been added to already existing services, inevitable by-appointment no-shows and cancellations create opportunities to handle walk-in clients without adding staff. Australia, in considering adding walk-in services, has the advantage of already having many experienced single session therapists in the workforce. We recommend, though, that when walk-in services are introduced, a system of support be built in for the less experienced single session therapist.

Conclusion

Walking in is one way to facilitate access to mental health services by enabling therapeutic conversations at a client's moment of high need and eliminating frustrating, intrusive, unreliable, and discouraging intake processes. In this chapter, we have addressed common worries and fears about walk-in services, which are understandable given that they are new concepts for many therapists and administrators. We hope that by putting these "on the table" we have provided food for thought that will assist mental health professionals evaluating the goodness of fit of walk-in services. Across Canada and in places in the U.S. and Mexico, walk-in SST has been embraced and has flourished. Indeed, provincial governments in Canada are moving toward even wider applications of open access to mental health (Cornish, 2020). We invite single session thinkers, in Australia and around the globe, to an ongoing conversation about whether walk-in single session services make sense as a component of a mental health continuum of services.

Notes

1 Portions of this chapter appeared in A. Slive and M. Bobele (2019). Ideas for addressing doubts about walk-in-single-session therapy. *Journal of Systemic Therapies, 38*(4), 17–30. ©JST Institute 2019. Used with permission.
2 The term *band-aid* is sometimes used dismissively. In this context, we see it differently. Sometimes a bandage is all that is needed; it promotes healing and prevents the spread of infection; at other times, it is an important starting point for additional treatment (see Slive & Bobele, 2014, p. 85).
3 *Editors' note*: For a discussion of single session counseling post-HIV testing, see O'Loughlin, Chapter 19 of this volume.
4 We will use the terms *counseling*, *therapy*, and *psychotherapy* interchangeably in this paper to refer to the practice of providing mental health services to individuals, couples, and families.

References

Barrett, M.S., Chua, W.-J., Crits-Christoph, P., Gibbons, M.B., Casiano, D., & Thompson, D. (2008). Early withdrawal from mental health treatment: Implications for psychotherapy practice. *Psychotherapy*, *45*(2), 247–267. http://doi.org/10.1037/0033-3204.45.2.247

Bebinger, M. (2019). Urgent care on demand, except this time for mental health. https://www.wbur.org/commonhealth/2019/04/19/urgent-care-on-demand-except-this-time-for-mental-health.

Bobele, M., Fullen, C., Houston, B., MartinezA.M., Moffat, L., & Santos, J. (2018). Westside stories: Walk-in and single-session therapy in San Antonio. In M.F. Hoyt, M. Bobele, A. Slive, J. Young, & M. Talmon (Eds.), *Single-Session Therapy by Walk-In or Appointment: Administrative, Clinical, and Supervisory Aspects of One-at-a-Time Services* (pp. 221–250). New York: Routledge.

Bobele, M., López, S., Scamardo, M., & Solórzano, B. (2008). Single-session/walk-In therapy with Mexican-American Clients. *Journal of Systemic Therapies*, *27*(4), 75–89.

Chanut, S., Livingstone, S., & Stalker, C. (2010). An inventory of walk-in therapy clinics in Southern Ontario. Unpublished paper, available at http://www.childrenscentre.ca/resources/research_and_eval/Research%20Reports/Walk%20In%20Inventory-%20June%206%20final_3.pdf.

Cornish, P.M. (2020). *Stepped Care 2.0: A Paradigm Shift in Mental Health*. Cham, Switzerland: Springer Nature.

Correia, T.D. (2013). *Once was Enough: A Phenomenological Inquiry into Clients' Experiences with Single Session Therapy* (Doctoral dissertation). Retrieved from ProQuest Dissertations & Theses Global database. (UMI No. 1287127968).

Emanuel, E.J. (2017). *Prescription for the Future: The Twelve Transformational Practices of Highly Effective Medical Organizations*. New York: PublicAffairs.

Franklin, J.C., Ribeiro, J.D., Fox, K.R., Bentley, K.H., Kleiman, E.M., Huang, X., ... Nock, M.K. (2017). Risk factors for suicidal thoughts and behaviors: A meta-analysis of 50 years of research. *Psychological Bulletin*, *143*(2), 187–232.

Goldner, E.M., Jones, W., & Fang, M.L. (2011). Access to and waiting time for psychiatrist services in a Canadian urban area: A study in real time. *Canadian Journal of Psychiatry*, *56*(8), 474–480. http://doi.org/10.1177/070674371105600805

Harper-Jaques, S. & Foucault, D. (2014). Walk-in single session therapy: Client satisfaction and clinical outcomes. *Journal of Systemic Therapies*, *33*(3), 29–49.

Harper-Jaques, S., & Leahey, M. (2011). From imagination to reality: Mental health walk-in at South Calgary Health Centre. In A. Slive & M. Bobele (Eds.), *When One Hour is All You Have: Effective Therapy for Walk-In Clients* (pp. 167–183). Phoenix, AZ: Zeig, Tucker, & Theisen.

Hoyt, M.F., Bobele, M., Slive, A., Young, J., & Talmon, M. (Eds.). (2018). *Single-Session Therapy by Walk-In or Appointment: Administrative, Clinical, and Supervisory Aspects of One-at-a-Time Services*. New York: Routledge.

Hymmen, P., Stalker, C.A., & Cait, C.A. (2013). The case for single-session therapy: Does the empirical evidence support the increased prevalence of this service delivery model? *Journal of Mental Health*, *22*(1), 60–71. doi:10.3109/09638237.2012.670880

Jefferies, A. (2003). Dropping-in: The unexamined encounter. *Psychodynamic Practice*, *9*(2), 173–186. Retrieved from http://search.ebscohost.com/login. aspx?direct=true&db=a9h&AN=9780245&site=ehost-live

Juvrud, J., & Rennels, J. (2017). "I don't need help": Gender differences in how gender stereotypes predict help-seeking. *Sex Roles*, *76*(1-2), 27–39. https://doi. org/10.1007/s11199-016-0653-7

Liddon, L., Kingerlee, R., & Barry, J.A. (2018). Gender differences in preferences for psychological treatment, coping strategies, and triggers to help-seeking. *British Journal of Clinical Psychology*, *57*(1), 42–58.

Miller, J.K. (2008). Walk-in single session team therapy: A study of client satisfaction. *Journal of Systemic Therapies*, *27*(3), 78–94. https://doi.org/10.1521/jsyt.2008.27.3.78

Miller, J.K., & Slive, A. (2004). Breaking down the barriers to clinical service delivery: Walk-in family therapy. *Journal of Marital and Family Therapy*, *30*(1), 95–103.

Milner, A., Witt, K., Pirkis, J., Hetrick, S., Robinson, J., Currier, D., Spittal, M.J., Page, A., & Carter, G.L. (2017). The effectiveness of suicide prevention delivered by GPs: A systematic review and meta-analysis. *Journal of Affective Disorders*, *210*, 294–302.

Nam, S., Chu, H., Lee, M., Lee, J., Kim, N., & Lee, S. (2010). A meta-analysis of gender differences in attitudes toward seeking professional psychological help. *Journal of American College Health*, *59*(2), 110–116. https://doi-org.ezproxy. ollusa.edu/10.1080/07448481.2010.483714

Possemato, K., Wray, L.O., Johnson, E., Webster, B., & Beehler, G.P. (2018). Facilitators and barriers to seeking mental health care among primary care veterans with posttraumatic stress disorder. *Journal of Traumatic Stress*, *31*(5), 742–752. https://doi-org.ezproxy.ollusa.edu/10.1002/jts.22327

Slive A., & Bobele, M. (2011). *When One Hour is All You Have: Effective Therapy for Walk-In Clients*. Phoenix, AZ: Zeig, Tucker, & Theisen.

Slive, A., & Bobele, M. (2012). Walk-in counselling services: Making the most of one hour. *Australian and New Zealand Journal of Family Therapy*, *33*(1), 27–38.

Slive, A., & Bobele, M. (2014). Walk-in single session therapy: Accessible mental health services. In M.F. Hoyt & M. Talmon (Eds.), *Capturing the Moment: Single Session Therapy and Walk-In Services* (pp. 73–94). Bethel CT: Crown House Publishing.

Slive, A., & Bobele, M. (2018). The three top reasons why walk-in/single-sessions make perfect sense. In M.F. Hoyt, M. Bobele, A. Slive, J. Young, & M. Talmon (Eds.), *Single-Session Therapy by Walk-In or Appointment: Administrative, Clinical, and Supervisory Aspects of One-at-a-Time Services* (pp. 27–39). New York: Routledge.

Slive, A., & Bobele, M. (2019). Ideas for addressing doubts about walk-in-single-session therapy. *Journal of Systemic Therapies*, *38*(4), 17–30.

Stalker C.A., Horton S., & Cait C.-A. (2012). Single-session therapy in a walk-in counseling clinic: A pilot study. *Journal of Systemic Therapies*, *31*, 38–52.

Stalker, C.A., Riemer, M., Cait, C.-A., Horton, S., Booton, J., Josling, L. … Zaczek M. (2016). A comparison of walk-in counseling and the wait list model for delivering counselling services. *Journal of Mental Health*, *25*(5), 403–409. http://doi.org/10.3109/09638237.2015.1101417

Susukida, R., Mojtabai, R., & Mendelson, T. (2015). Sex differences in help seeking for mood and anxiety disorders in the national comorbidity survey-replication. *Depression & Anxiety, 32*(11), 853–860. https://doi-org.ezproxy.ollusa.edu/10.1002/da.22366

Talmon, M. (1990). *Single-Session Therapy: Maximizing the Effect of the First (and Often Only) Therapeutic Encounter.* San Francisco: Jossey-Bass.

Tatham, M., Stringer, H., Perera, S., & Waller, G. (2012). 'Do you still want to be seen?' The pros and cons of active waiting list management. *International Journal of Eating Disorders, 45*(1), 57–62. doi:10.1002/eat.20920

Wick, J.Y. (2016). Safety in the walk-in clinic: Consistent consciousness. *Contemporary Clinic.* Retrieved from https://contemporaryclinic.pharmacytimes.com/news-views/safety-in-the-walk-in-clinic-consistent-consciousness

Young, K., Dick, M., Herring, K., & Lee, J. (2008). From waiting lists to walk-in: Stories from a walk-in therapy clinic. *Journal of Systemic Therapies, 27*(4), 23–39.

Young, J., Rycroft, P., & Weir, S. (2014). Implementing single-session therapy: Practical wisdoms from down under. In M.F. Hoyt & M. Talmon (Eds.), *Capturing the Moment: Single-Session Therapy and Walk-In Services* (pp. 121–140). Bethel, CT: Crown House Publishing

Zalsman, G., Hawton, K., Wasserman, D., van Heeringen, K., Arensman, E., Sarchiapone, M., & Purebl, G. (2016). Suicide prevention strategies revisited: 10-year systematic review. *The Lancet Psychiatry, 3*(7), 646–659.

5 Single Session Family Consultation (SSFC)

Brendan O'Hanlon and Naomi Rottem

SSFC is a model of brief family engagement and inclusion in the care of an individual client, typically involving between one and three sessions, and then as needed. It includes a meeting organized by a practitioner with their client (a service user) and their family to collaboratively respond to family-identified needs and clarify how the family will be involved in the individual's ongoing care.

How SSFC Developed

The Bouverie Centre at La Trobe University is an integrated practice-research service in Melbourne, Australia. It has a government-funded role in building the capability of mental health and alcohol and other drugs (AOD) services to include families in treatment and care. The Centre has adopted a range of models of practice and the methods to promote implementation of these models over the past 30 years. This includes conducting statewide training in Family Sensitive Practice (Furlong, 2001) and implementation of evidence-based family psycho-educational interventions (McFarlane, 2016). SSFC has been an important development in our approach to improving family inclusiveness in these sectors.

In 2016, The Bouverie Centre articulated its vision for family involvement in mental health and AOD services through a document titled *From Individual to Families: A Client Centred Framework for Family Involvement*. A "Pyramid of Family Involvement," described within that document, is shown in Figure 5.1. This paralleled similar frameworks, particularly in the U.S., where the concept of offering a range of services to families had been articulated (Cohen et al., 2008; Dausch et al., 2012). SSFC could respond directly to family needs and link them to more intensive interventions and other services as required. Thus, SSFC became part of an integrated response, complementing rather than competing with existing approaches and services for families (Figure 5.2).

As its name suggests, Single Session Family Consultation essentially brings together concepts and practices from two models, Single Session

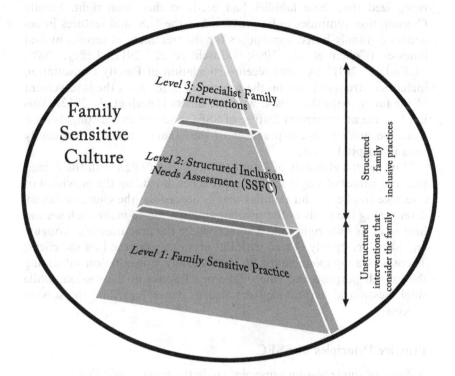

Figure 5.1 The Bouverie Pyramid of Family Involvement (based on a framework developed by Mottaghipour & Bickerton, 2005) ©2016 The Bouverie Centre; used by agreement.

Therapy (SST) and Family Consultation (FC – discussed below), as well as drawing on ideas from family therapy and family meetings in health care.

The Bouverie Centre has been an active proponent of single session ideas and practices for many years (Young & Rycroft, 2012; Young, Weir, & Rycroft, 2012). In terms of its role in the development of SSFC, single session family therapy was conducted as part of the Centre's clinical program. Training in SST was also a popular offering as part of the Centre's external workforce development activity.

Family Consultation was first proposed by a key figure in the development of family therapy, Lyman Wynne (Wynne & Wynne, 1986), who articulated a rationale for practitioners adopting a consultative position that responded to families' expressed needs. This contrasted with the prevailing practices at the time of assuming that all families wanted or needed family therapy. Wynne's notion of consultation with families marked an important shift away from families being co-opted into a treatment modality designed to treat their relative to an approach that recognized that these families had needs in their own right. Family Consultation continues to be promoted in the U.S. and features in accounts of family-based approaches for the treatment of serious mental illnesses (Cohen et al., 2008; Dausch et al., 2012; Lefley, 2009; McFarlane, 2016). A more recent articulation of Family Consultation includes a stronger focus on the process of negotiating the involvement of the family with the person with the illness (Jewell et al., 2012). This has become an important feature of SSFC and one that distinguishes it from the more common practices of the "family meeting" frequently used in hospital settings.

Many of the elements of Family Consultation align with the principles and values of single session approaches, including the provision of a service to clients and families that is accessible; the client or family determining the goals of the session; an intention to make each session helpful in its own right; and a stance where the practitioner's thoughts and ideas are openly shared with but in no way imposed on the client. There was a complementary fit, with Family Consultation informing the overall purpose and role of the practitioner in the session, while single session ideas provided detailed guidance regarding the session process.

Practice Principles of SSFC

A series of single session principles guide the practice of SFCC:

1. A process of active invitation is needed to engage service clients and their families. The practitioner offers SSFC as a positive service response

2. The client's preferences inform the convening and conducting of sessions (discussed below). The client can decide who will be invited to the consultation session and what will and will not be discussed

3. The client is supported to be an active participant. The SSFC practitioner assists the family to appreciate what might be helpful (and unhelpful) in supporting recovery

4. A needs orientation is adopted. It is not an assessment of family functioning nor is it family therapy where the explicit aim is to change relationships. The practitioner is interested to acknowledge what is working well in the family and supports the family in identifying their needs in the session

5. Consultation sessions promote a reciprocal process involving exchange between the service user, family members, and the practitioner – providing an opportunity for all participants to hear and learn from each other

6. Each consultation session should be helpful in its own right and may have a range of outcomes including no further sessions, a decision to meet again, or referral to other services.

The Model in Practice

SSFC is a process involving three stages: *Convening, Conducting,* and *Following-Up.* The term *Single Session Family Consultation* refers to all these three stages rather than just the session involving the meeting with the family (which is usually referred to as the "consultation session"). In what follows it is assumed that the practitioner who sees the individual client (service user) also conducts the consultation session. Notice that much of the process of the consultation session is informed by single session thinking:

- Family members are invited to prioritize issues that they want to address
- The practitioner checks in during the session about whether the current focus or the experience of the session is helpful
- An awareness of available time is encouraged to maximize the value of the session
- The practitioner is transparent in their process of conducting the session and in sharing reflections on the family's issues and dilemmas.

Case Vignette

Let's consider the *Convening, Conducting,* and *Following-Up* steps in turn; we will illustrate each with an unfolding case example.

Part I: Convening

The convening stage refers to the key tasks and activities associated with setting up the session with the family. The process generally involves the following sequence:

- The idea of a meeting with the family is explored by the practitioner with their individual client. The client's desired outcomes for the session are clarified along with their preferences regarding what will be discussed – and importantly, what will not be discussed – and who will attend
- The practitioner may at this point also flag what they would like to discuss at the consultation session
- If "the *who,* the *what,* and the *how*" of the consultation sessions are agreed, the client is invited to nominate a family member to be contacted by the practitioner so they can be invited to the session

- The practitioner then contacts the family members to invite them to the session, explains briefly the proposed agenda, and then asks the family members to identify what they would like to discuss at the consultation session. If there are conflicting preferences, such as the family wanting to talk about the service user's drug use when the service user has indicated this will not be discussed, the practitioner explains this limitation to the family
- These discussions provide a tentative mapping of the issues to be discussed in the consultation session, not a fixed agenda.

Noel is a 57-year-old married man who lives with his wife, Annette (56), and Sarah (23), the youngest of their three children. Noel works as an assistant manager in a large transport and distribution business. Noel is on sick leave following a recent episode of bipolar affective disorder during which he became disinhibited and aggressive towards his work colleagues. At an appointment with his mental health practitioner, Ronan, Noel talks about the impact of his recent episode on his family and his work situation. Ronan identifies the opportunity to bring the family together in an SSFC session. He reflects that given they "have all been through a lot" it might be good to meet with the family. Ronan suggests to Noel that a meeting might help family members to know how to best support him. Ronan talks with Noel about who should attend the meeting and what might be discussed. Noel says his wife and daughter could attend. Noel feels Annette doesn't understand how hard it is for him to go back to work. He knows Sarah is worried about him but doesn't know what she has been told. He is happy for Annette and Sarah to come to the session but doesn't want to be "interrogated" by Annette about what he did or said at his workplace when he was unwell.

With Noel's agreement, Ronan calls Annette and invites both Annette and Sarah to the session. Annette says she is concerned about Noel getting back to work. She wants to support him but feels like she just upsets him. Annette says that they have tended to keep Sarah "out of the picture" as she is already quite an anxious person and she and Noel don't want to stress her any further. Ronan encourages Annette to invite Sarah to the session, reflecting that Sarah obviously knows "something is wrong" and might feel less anxious if she understands more about what is happening with her Dad.

Part II: Conducting

The conducting stage of SSFC refers to the session with the client and their family that was convened during the previous stage. The conducting stage typically takes an hour and can be in an interview room or at the family home. The session is divided into five steps; here is a schematic:

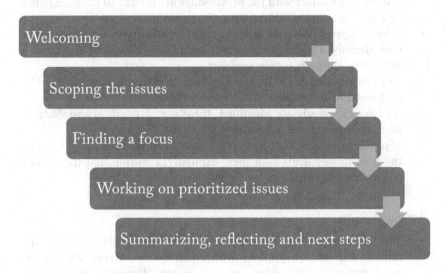

Figure 5.2 A Session "Map."

Let's take a closer look at the key tasks, then see how they occur in our illustration.

Welcoming

- The practitioner introduces themself to the family and provides an explanation of the practitioner's role in relation to the client
- The practitioner connects with each individual family member
- The practitioner explains that the purposes of the session are to assist the family in their role of supporting their relative who is experiencing mental health difficulties, and to identify and respond to their own needs, concerns, or questions
- The practitioner then outlines the session structure, its duration, process (e.g., hearing from everyone, being practically useful), and possible outcomes (e.g., information, problem solving, referral).

Scoping the Issues

- The practitioner summarizes the issues that were identified in the convening stage as being those that the client wants to discuss, and also confirms the issues identified by other family members
- There is also an opportunity for family members to raise additional issues at this point, which may be important if new priorities have emerged since the convening stage, or for those present who have not previously spoken to the practitioner. Family members for whom this

is their first contact with the practitioner are invited to propose issues or topics they want addressed in the session

- Where appropriate, and with the client's permission, the practitioner may directly ask family members about the impact of the client's difficulties on each family member
- The practitioner can also raise any issue that they believe needs to be addressed in the session
- As issues or needs are identified, these are clarified, acknowledged, and (as appropriate) normalized
- If topics are raised that have previously been identified as off limits, the practitioner deals with these explicitly, ensuring that the client's wishes are respected.

Finding a Focus

- The practitioner briefly summarizes the issues identified by the family, and then negotiates which one or two issues will be the most important to address in the session. Typically, more issues are raised than can be usefully addressed in the session, so prioritizing a focus is explained to the family in terms of wanting them to experience the session as helpful. A number of strategies can be utilized separately or in combination. These include:

  o Inviting the family to nominate a priority
  o Selecting issues that are relevant to most of those present in the session rather than an issue relating exclusively to one family member
  o Working on a problem that has the best prospect of a productive outcome
  o Considering the time available and the relative complexity of the issue
  o Taking into account the scope and limits of the practitioner's expertise or role.

- Issues or concerns that are not the focus of a particular session can be deferred, if necessary, either through the options of a subsequent session, directing people to relevant resources, or referral to other services.

Working on Prioritized Issues

- The practitioner decides the approach that they will adopt in responding to the prioritized issues and lets the family know, checking that this is acceptable to them. The response should be commensurate with the practitioner's role, knowledge, and skills, and may include:

o   Sharing information about a condition
o   Facilitating a conversation in which family members can share their lived experience of the difficulty
o   Gathering more information to make an informed referral or to undertake advocacy
o   Collaborating to address day-to-day problems
o   Including an individual practitioner with specialized knowledge to address a particular issue (e.g., a psychiatrist to answer questions about medication or a rehabilitation worker to talk about employment options).

Summarizing Progress, Sharing Reflections, and Agreeing on Next Steps

•   The practitioner summarizes progress in the session and offers reflections about what has been discussed or achieved during the session. Family members are invited to briefly respond to these reflections or to the session in general
•   The practitioner clarifies and confirms with the family any actions that were agreed upon in the consultation to address their needs
•   Next steps are confirmed, including scheduling a follow-up phone call to the family, or another session as appropriate
•   A plan for how further communication will occur between the practitioner and the family can be made as appropriate.

Ronan meets with the family using the SSFC session structure. After describing his role as Noel's treating clinician, he summarizes what each family member wants from the session and checks that he has understood their concerns and needs. He makes a point of acknowledging that he is meeting Sarah for the first time and that she has not had an opportunity until now to say what she hopes for in the session. Sarah says she feels like she has been kept in the dark about her dad's condition and hearing anything would be an improvement. Annette says there is a lot on her mind, the most immediate issue being that she is not sure whether she should be pushing Noel, given he is spending most of his time sitting in his armchair. Noel reports that he finds it hard to even think about work, wondering given his age whether he will work again. Ronan suggests that he wants to make the most of the time they have together by having a focus for the session. The family agrees that it would be good to be "all on the same page" regarding Noel's condition including how they can best support Noel at the moment. Ronan proposes that getting a better understanding of Noel's condition might help address all family members' concerns. He facilitates a discussion where Noel shares his experience of being unwell, though is mindful of Noel's request not to go into detail about what has happened at

Noel's workplace. Ronan provides relevant information about bipolar disorder, its treatment, and what helps with recovery. He also asks Annette and Sarah about their experience of Noel's condition, normalizing their concern and fears about a further manic episode. In appreciating how embarrassed Noel feels about his behavior towards his work colleagues, Annette agrees that she will stop asking Noel about work for the time being. Noel in turn offers to do a few small jobs around the house to help out and to get himself up and going again. Sarah says she has found the information helpful but would like to find out more. Ronan suggests websites for Sarah about bipolar disorder and particularly the experience of children whose parent has a mental illness. Ronan concludes the session by acknowledging that Noel's manic episode has rocked the whole family and yet, perhaps in contrast to past episodes, they have opted to address the impact of Noel's condition more directly. He is impressed with Annette's and Sarah's support for Noel and with Noel's willingness to share more about his experience of bipolar disorder. While all family members respond by thanking Ronan for being the first person to involve the family and for the session, they opt to "see how things go" rather than schedule a further session. Ronan makes a time in three weeks to call Annette and Sarah separately while he continues to see Noel on a weekly basis.

Part III: Following-Up

An appointment for a phone call follow-up is made during the consultation session with the time period varying from a few days to three weeks, dependent on the service setting. (Note: This step does not occur if the family has opted to return for a further session.)

- The follow-up call can involve one or multiple family members who can be contacted separately or together
- The practitioner contacts the family at the scheduled time for the following purposes:
  - Checking in to see how the service-user/family members are doing in relation to issues addressed in session
  - Following up any actions/decisions/referrals decided upon at the meeting
  - Deciding next steps - including any ongoing arrangements for contact between the family and the practitioner, and if available and desired by the service user and family, the option of a further consultation session or referral to another service.

- The practitioner can also seek feedback from the family about the experience of the session to help inform future sessions with the family and for the practitioner's ongoing efforts to improve their practice of SSFC.

Ronan calls Annette and Sarah, as planned, as part of the SSFC follow-up stage. Annette reports that Noel is still not talking about going back to work and that she for the most part has kept to her commitment to not ask him about work. She feels reassured after the session, knowing more about Noel's condition and having Ronan as a point of contact if she becomes increasingly worried about Noel. Ronan wonders whether Annette might appreciate talking to other families who have had similar experiences, but Annette says that she doesn't feel like she needs that at the moment. Sarah reports that she found the session helpful and has been reading a lot of information on the websites that Ronan provided. She feels the session raised a number of issues for her and she would like to see a counselor who understands mental illness but is not connected with her dad's care. Ronan agrees to send Sarah some affordable referral options. At his next session with Ronan, Noel said he was pleased with the way the session went and wondered whether they could have another SSFC in a few months.

Toward the Future

The limited published research in relation to SSFC indicates that service users and their families in a youth mental health service rated sessions highly. At follow-up, practitioners also have reported improved familiarity with approaches to working with families and confidence in using family interventions (Poon, Harvey, Fuzzard, & O'Hanlon, 2017). These findings are consistent with The Bouverie Centre's own evaluation of SSFC in adult mental health and AOD services (O'Hanlon, Rottem, Bamberg, & Wills, 2017; The Bouverie Centre, 2015). More research is needed to understand how SSFC may improve important outcomes such as family member distress or service user well-being.

Nonetheless SSFC has made family work "do-able" and has been widely accepted by practitioners, service managers, and funding bodies. This has created a supportive context for the further development of SSFC. Comprehensive self-paced online training has been developed at The Bouverie Centre (https://events.bouverie.org.au/ssfc) and plans are underway to develop specialist modules around particular contexts (e.g., AOD, disability, health care in the military) as well as in relation to particular challenges such as working with conflict, the inclusion of children in sessions, and working cross culturally. Single session thinking and practice will inform all of these developments and ultimately benefit more service users and their families.

References

Cohen, A.N., Glynn, S.M., Murray-Swank, A.B., Barrio, C., Fischer, E.P., McCutcheon, S.J., … Dixon, L.B. (2008). The family forum: Directions for the implementation of family psychoeducation for severe mental illness. *Psychiatric Services, 59*(1), 40–48. doi:10.1176/ps.2008.59.1.40

Dausch, B.M., Cohen, A.N., Glynn, S., McCutcheon, S.J., Perlick, D.A., Rotondi, A.J., ... Dixon, L.B. (2012). An intervention framework for family involvement in the care of persons with psychiatric illness: Further guidance from Family Forum II. *American Journal of Psychiatric Rehabilitation, 15*(1), 5–25. doi:10.1080/15487768.2012.655223

Furlong, M. (2001). Constraints on family-sensitive mental health practices. *Journal of Family Studies, 7*(2), 217–231. Retrieved from http://dx.doi.org/10.5172/jfs.7.2.217

Jewell, T., Smith, A., Hoh, B., Ladd, S., Evinger, J., Lamberti, J.S., ... Salerno, A.J. (2012). Consumer centered family consultation: New York State's recent efforts to include families and consumers as partners in recovery. *American Journal of Psychiatric Rehabilitation, 15*(1), 44–60. Retrieved from http://dx.doi.org/10.1080/15487768.2012.655230

Lefley, H. (2009). *Family Psychoeducation for Serious Mental Illness.* New York: Oxford University Press.

McFarlane, W.R. (2016). Family interventions for schizophrenia and the psychoses: A review. *Family Process, 55*(3), 460–482. doi:10.1111/famp.12235

Mottaghipour, Y., & Bickerton, A. (2005). The pyramid of family care: A framework for family involvement with adult mental health services. *Australian e-Journal for the Advancement of Mental Health, 4*(3), 210–217.

O'Hanlon, B., Rottem, N., Bamberg, J., & Wills, M. (2017). *The Catchment Beacon Project Report.* Unpublished paper. Melbourne, Australia: The Bouverie Centre, La Trobe University.

Poon, A.W.C., Harvey, C., Fuzzard, S., & O'Hanlon, B. (2017). Implementing a family inclusive practice model in youth mental health services in Australia. *Early Intervention in Psychiatry,* 1–8. 10.1111/eip.12505

The Bouverie Centre (2015). *Mental Health Beacon: Implementing Family Inclusive Practices in Victorian Mental Health Services.* Retrieved from http://www.bouverie.org.au/images/uploads/MH_Beacon_Project_Report_March_2015.pdf

Wynne, A.R. & Wynne, L.C. (1986). At the center of the cyclone: Family therapists as consultants with family and divorce courts. In L.C. Wynne, S.H. McDaniel, & T.T. Weber (Eds.), *Systems Consultation: A New Perspective for Family Therapy* (pp. 300–319). NewYork: Guilford Press.

Young, J., & Rycroft, P. (2012). Single session therapy: What's in a name? *Australian and New Zealand Journal of Family Therapy, 33*(1), 3–5. doi:10.1017/aft.2012.1

Young, J., Weir, S., & Rycroft, P. (2012). Implementing single session therapy. *Australian and New Zealand Journal of Family Therapy, 33*(1), 84–97. doi:10.1017/aft.2012.8

6 The Vital Role of the Therapist's Mindset

Flavio Cannistrà

How we look – which is directed by our mindset – influences what we see, and what we see influences how we proceed. This chapter is about mindset, but also about epistemological and trans-theoretical matters.

My meta-intention is that the reader becomes more aware of how our mindset shapes clinical reasoning processes, the logic within how we listen and how we speak, the choice and clarification of the words we use, and thus, how we work with our clients – and how we may help them in a single session.

1. **According to many studies, all the main approaches in psychotherapy seem to be effective.**

    1.1 For example, the American Psychological Association (APA, 2012) says that "most valid and structured psychotherapies are roughly equivalent in effectiveness." And even if some authors claim the opposite (e.g., Westmacott & Hunsley, 2007), still others defend the first position (e.g., Wampold & Imel, 2015).

      At this moment, the decision seems to fall in a not well-defined "future" and hence into the present readers' hands.

    1.2 There's not a dominant point of view about which approach to psychotherapy is most effective. Also this sentence ("There's not a dominant point of view") can be supported by quoting some authors (Laudan, 1977) and probably questioned by quoting other authors.

      1.2.1 Writing articles in psychology seems largely a matter of quoting authors who support the writer's point.

      1.2.2 The consequence for this chapter will be that every paragraph could be supported or questioned without reaching an ultimate point.

2. **There is a thing about which every study seems implicitly to agree: even if the effectiveness is the same, the duration is not.**

2.1 For example, Solution Focused Brief Therapy (SFBT) typically lasts around 3 to 7 sessions (see Macdonald, 2011; McKergow & Korman, 2009). Cognitive Behavioral Therapy generally lasts around 5 to 20 sessions (NHS, n.d.). In treating unipolar depression, psychodynamic therapy lasts an average of 88 sessions and psychoanalytic therapy an average of 234 sessions (Huber, Henrich, Clarkin, & Klug, 2013). And according to Single Session Therapy studies, often one session is all that is needed (e.g., see Talmon, 1990; Hoyt & Talmon, 2014; Hoyt, Bobele, Slive, Young, & Talmon, 2018).

We can go over and over research of this kind.

2.2 Let's say that: it seems that different approaches and models need different numbers of sessions to get the desired result.

2.2.1 "Result" is another hard matter. "What a result is" seems strongly related to the therapist's theoretical and epistemological position. In this case, we can use the vague definition of "result" as "the end of the therapy with the accomplishment of the client's goals."

2.2.2 "Client" is a not easy matter, again. Who is the client? What if a child is in therapy? Is he/she the client or are his/her parents? Who decides what the result is? And if the person is sent by a court?

Those questions are extremely important to define the duration of a therapy – and its effectiveness.

2.3 Again, it seems impossible to have a unique definition of who is the client and what is the result of the therapy.

3. **So, some interventions seem to take (significantly) less time than others. Why?**

We can't give an ultimate answer, but we can give some kind of explanation that can be useful for clinicians who want to understand the implications for how to reduce the duration of therapy.

3.1 Actually, according to a postmodern view (Gergen, 2006), I don't even think it is possible for an ultimate answer to be given. I will simply try to give one of the possible answers, with (I hope) some useful practical consequences.

3.2 Before I give mine, I will explore some other answers to the question "Why do some interventions take less time than others?"

3.2.1 In our professional practice there is a widespread idea that techniques are what can make therapy briefer – and what can make therapy work. This is seen in the literature's ubiquitous emphasis on old and new kinds of techniques as the best way to solve contemporary problems.

3.2.1.1 Here, by "technique" I mean "behavioral prescriptions" in or between sessions.

3.2.1.2 But what is "a technique"?

Is the Miracle Question a technique? Yes, but it is also a question. So is a question a technique?

And a *double-bind question* – is that a technique? The technique is the question or is it the double-bind? The double-bind is the effect of the question, isn't it? But according to the definition of "therapeutic double-bind" (Watzlawick, Bavelas, & Jackson, 1967), it needs a specific relationship – and a specific context, the therapy context – or it simply can't be a "*therapeutic* double-bind." So "technique" is composed of a question asked in a particular context with two (or more) persons in a particular relationship.

3.2.1.3 So, when someone says that "techniques make therapy briefer" (meaning that some techniques are better than others to shorten the number of sessions), we could ask: "What do you mean by 'techniques'?"

3.2.2 The idea about the central role of techniques in reducing the number of sessions needed is common in the brief therapy field.

3.2.2.1 After all, at the beginning of brief therapy's history some authors gave (both directly and indirectly) considerable importance to behavioral prescriptions (e.g., Levy & Shelton, 1990; de Shazer, 1985; Watzlawick, Weakland, & Fisch, 1974).

However, subsequently others reconsidered that role.

Actually, it seems that even Milton Erickson said that psychotherapy is mostly a matter of commonsense (Zeig, 1985).

de Shazer and other SFBT therapists, after giving great emphasis to behavioral prescriptions, then changed the model to an increasingly question-centered one (de Shazer, 1994; Iveson, George, & Ratner, 2012).

Hoyt (2009, 2017) considers that the most important things in (brief) therapy are Alliance, Goals, and Clients' Resources (which he calls *The Context of Competence* – see Chapter 2), not behavioral prescriptions.

Much of the recent Single Session Therapy literature seems to be strongly focused on clients' resources and strengths, rather than techniques (Cannistrà, 2020; Hoyt & Cannistrà, 2019; Hoyt & Talmon, 2014; Talmon & Hoyt, 2014; Hoyt et al., 2018).

3.2.2.2 This also can be recognized by our common-day experiences.

As Hoyt (2017, p. 294; also see Chapter 2) has noted, the most common number of sessions in psychotherapy is 0. People (we) can solve most problems by themselves, without techniques prescribed by an "expert."

3.2.2.3 Migone (2014, p. 632), close to a psychoanalytic mindset, did a critique of the concept of "brief therapy" and landed on the premise that "The only way to operationalize the definition of 'brief therapy' as 'brief' is by making reference to a set time limit decided a priori as a ground rule laid out before the beginning of treatment."

Brief therapy authors seem to disagree with this view.

For example, Zeig (2007, p. 6) said that "The term 'brief therapy' was probably coined in the work of David Malan and James Mann, but their approaches were narrowly defined within psychoanalytic parameters. Haley brought into the mainstream of psychotherapy a robust and generic brief therapy."

Haley (1990, p. 3) also said that "long-term therapists are made, not born. Therapists do not have innate skills in committing clients to long-term contracts. Without training, they must learn by trial and error to do interminable therapy when they get into practice."

So, "making reference to a set time limit decided a priori as a ground rule laid out before the beginning of treatment" (Migone, 2014, quoted above) is *not* "the only way to operationalize the definition of 'brief therapy' as 'brief.'"

Rosenbaum (2008 p. 8) noted: "Psychotherapy is not long or short; to view it this way sets up a false dichotomy." Rather, he said (in Hoyt, Rosenbaum, & Talmon, 1992, p. 81), "my desire is to see everyone for one full moment, as long as that takes."

3.2.3 Away from a brief therapy context, other studies also reduce the importance of techniques in therapy.

For example, Asay and Lambert (1999, p. 32) say that: "Although some practitioners [...] imagine that they or their techniques are the most important factor contributing to outcome, the research literature does not support this contention" (p. 30). Instead, "the difference in outcome could be attributed to patient factors, such as the nature of the patient's personality makeup, including ego organization, maturity, motivation, and ability to become productively involved in therapy."

Ahn and Wampold (2001) showed that if you remove the main technique from a therapy (i.e., the behavioral prescription that is supposed to produce the main therapeutic effect) the result is the same – there's no significant difference.

3.3 Thus, despite the large amount of research, it seems that there is not an approach with "better techniques" versus others with "poorer techniques."

So, you can learn different techniques and still have difficulty making therapy brief or single session.

4. **My thesis is that the therapist's mindset plays a vital role in ensuring that the result can be reached in few sessions – often even one.**

4.1 By "mindset" I mean "the established set of attitudes held by someone" (Lexico 2020), where "attitudes" are "a feeling or *opinion* about something or someone, or a *way of behaving* that is caused by this" (Cambridge Dictionary, 2020. italics added).

4.1.1 My thesis is that the therapist's opinions and resulting behaviors – verbal and non-verbal interventions – are what most influence the length of therapy.

This has been summarized by Hoyt (2017, p. 230): "How we look influences what we see, and what we see influences what we do, 'round and 'round."

Let me give some examples.

4.1.1.1 The International Psychoanalytical Association (2020) says that, even if the time frame for doing an analysis is hard to predict, "an average of three to five years can be expected."

4.1.1.1.1 With those mindsets it can be expected that a therapy can't last only one or a few sessions.

The therapist will be influenced by the *opinion* that the work with that client will be expected to last about "three to five years."

And he/she/they will choose and use a series of other theoretical constructs that will support and form this *opinion*.

4.1.1.1.2. A mindset creates (and comes out of) constructs.

For example, in a psychoanalytic mindset there is the construct of "flight into health." As Frick (1999, p. 63) explains, "reports to the therapist of rapid improvement and a return to feelings of well-being are viewed with suspicion. Such positive patient reports, sometimes accompanied by early termination, are considered to be 'self-deceptive' [...], are 'fraught with inherent dangers' [...], are 'not trustworthy' [...], and are 'pseudo-successes.'"

How can therapy be brief or single session with a mindset based on these kind of *opinions*?

But the most interesting thing is that Frick proposes a new way to conceptualize "flight into health." At first Frick uses a psychoanalytic mindset to explain that "these regressions have been interpreted to mean that the changes were not authentic, that insight has not been achieved, or that the patient's neurotic 'core' has not been touched. This was *the psychoanalytic flight into health perspective*" (p. 75, emphasis added). Then, once he embraced a different psychotherapeutic approach, he changed the mindset and so the same event is different: "From *the perspective of the ambiguous Gestalt*, however, the shift into the healthy mode [...] is substantial and real, and a shift back into the neurotic pattern does not invalidate the previous emergence of the patient's healthy organization. [...] We can anticipate, therefore, that such shifts will occur and welcome them as opportunities to further strengthen the healthy organization as we help weaken the neurotic one" (p. 76, italics added).

With a change of mind(set) the client's behavior goes from being problematic to being healthy.

4.1.1.1.3 So, there are epistemological and theoretical knowledges that the therapist will embrace to construct and support his/her observations and ideas. In psychoanalysis these will often work as a theoretical and practical confirmation that it takes a long time to solve problems.

4.1.1.2 Switching to brief therapies, it seems that the brief therapist's mindset often comes from observations of what works briefly in common life (see 3.2.2.2) and in therapeutic settings, with the idea that if something works for one person it could work again for someone else.

According with this (see also 3.2.2.3) we can also say that "brief therapy" is a label that identifies a heterogeneous group of therapies whose authors operate from *opinions* and resulting methods that help to keep the number of sessions low.

4.1.1.2.1 There is not one "International Association" of Brief Therapy, so we don't have a unique or "official" way to define brief therapy.

4.1.1.2.2 Anyway, we can say that historically many brief therapy ideas were born from observations of common-day behaviors with common people (Bateson, 1972; Milton Erickson's life and work are another masterful example) and through unidirectional mirrors and videotapes of patients (de Shazer, 1982; Watzlawick & Weakland, 1977), consultation of clinical records (Talmon, 1990), and as the necessity to give an effective and quick response to problems generated by war and social-economical issues (Hoyt, 2009, pp. 13–17; Megglé, 2011).

4.2 Of course, there are also epistemological and theoretical knowledges that the therapist will study to construct and support his/her observations and ideas. And those will support the *opinion* – and the resulting behaviors – that few sessions are necessary to get the result. Basically, we could say that the idea that the therapy can be brief or long is based on opinions that it can be so. And the practice will produce results that will confirm them.

4.2.1 If the result will disconfirm those *opinions*, the clinician could probably:

1. *change his/her mind*: consider that his/her theory is wrong and change his/her mind.
2. *integrate the new results*: modify his/her theory in the face of the disconfirmations
3. *deny the new results*: like saying that results are wrong, born from a misinterpretation of what has been observed, etc.

4.2.2 So, to make therapy more efficient, one option seems to be to adopt a mindset which leads to the result in a lesser number of sessions than other mindsets.

Or simply adopt *opinions* that lead to behaviors which lead to the result in a lesser number of sessions than other opinions/behaviors.

4.2.2.1 To adopt one or another kind of mindset is exactly what clinicians do. The question is if they are aware that the mindset is a choice.

There doesn't seem to exist an ultimate reason (different from the choice of greater brevity) to choose one approach or another. The reason can't be that one approach is more effective, because of what was said in 1.1. And yet that argumentation is based on specific opinions – that is, on a specific mindset.

One can think that *the* choice is "follow the science." But science has many different voices, mindsets, theories, epistemologies (Gergen, 2006; Laudan, 1977). And, again, this is a point of view.

It's a loop and we simply can't exit from it. We just can decide to adopt one mindset rather than another. But, again, this sentence is another expression of a specific mindset. Other mindsets simply can't imagine the idea of "decide to adopt a mindset rather than another"; or they see that idea as less useful than to adopt a specific kind of mindset (itself).

4.3 The clinician who wants to be briefer should decide what kind of mindset he/she/they want to adopt.

And yet "brief" is not an empty condition. It's replete with theoretical issues.

Every clinician has his idea of what "brief" brings with itself. Even the well-known brief therapist de Shazer (1991, pp. ix–x), to the question "How brief is brief?" answered "Not even one more than is necessary," without explaining what "necessary" is – or who decides how much is "necessary," or when "what's necessary" is accomplished.

Nor can "Ask the client" be an ultimate answer – because it still depends on a specific mindset.

4.4 In the end, we can only say that the clinician who wants to be briefer should study how to do that. But since it is impossible to decide if a particular mindset is better than another, what he/she/they will decide to study and the results he/she/they will accomplish will depend on them.

5. A choice must be made.
   Actually, a choice is always made.
   Here, I present my choices to be briefer in therapy.

5.1 *The first choice is to be pragmatic.*

   5.1.1 Since *pragmatism* has a long history, let's synthesize it saying that with "to be pragmatic" we mostly mean "to consider the effects of interventions." Or, as Scott Miller put it (in Hoyt, Miller, Held, & Matthews, 2001, p. 218): "Ultimately, the meaning of an idea is in its use."

   5.1.2 A pragmatic intervention is one that produces an effect which leads to the desired *result* (see 2.2.1).

   5.1.3 Since we can have different kinds of mindsets, which lead to many different interventions, the best are those which lead us to the best result. But who defines the best result?

5.2 *The second choice is to be efficient.*

   5.2.1 Efficient means to reach the result in the least amount of time. Since there can be many different mindsets, so many different interventions to get the result, choose those which help you achieve it most quickly.

   According to 4.3, the question is: less than what? Less time taken compared to other interventions.

   Surprisingly, this can be achieved within every mindset or approach.

5.3 *The third choice is to avoid theory reification.*

   5.3.1 Theories and constructs are tools. You need them to find the best ways to help your client. They are not things or truths. This also means that you don't have to be a slave to your constructs. Put constructs at your service.

   5.3.2 Choose theories and constructs that help you to choose interventions which help to get the result in a lesser amount of time compared to other interventions – and to other theories/constructs.

5.4 *The fourth choice is to adopt a multi-theoretical mindset.*

   5.4.1 Considering that theories and constructs have to help you to get the result in a lesser amount of time compared to others, a multi-theoretical mindset can give you more options.

   Our attitude (see 4) should be to not fall in love with a unique approach and to adopt different approaches as long as they help us to reach the result in a lesser amount of time compared to other theories/constructs.

5.4.2 We suppose that it is more useful to choose different tools depending on the person, the problem, and/or the moment of the therapy.

Conclusion

I conclude with a question for you, dear reader: *What choices in thinking and practice will you make to increase the likelihood that fewer sessions (even one) will produce the result?*

References

Ahn, H., & Wampold, B. (2001). Where oh where are the specific ingredients? A meta-analysis of component studies in counseling and psychotherapy. *Journal of Counseling Psychology*, *48*(3), 251–257.

APA. (2012, August). *Recognition of Psychotherapy Effectiveness*. American Psychological Association. www.apa.org/about/policy/resolution-psychotherapy.

Asay, T.P. & Lambert, M.J. (1999). The empirical case for the common factors in therapy: Quantitative findings. in M.A. Hubble, B.L. Duncan, & S.D. Miller (Eds.), *The Heart and Soul of Change: What Works in Therapy* (pp. 23–55). Washington, DC: APA Books.

Bateson, G. (1972). *Steps to an Ecology of Mind*. Chicago, IL: University of Chicago Press.

Cambridge Dictionary (2020). Attitude. Retrieved March 14, 2020, from dictionary.cambridge.org/dictionary/english/attitude

Cambridge Dictionary (2020). Efficient. Retrieved March 14, 2020, from dictionary.cambridge.org/it/dizionario/inglese/efficient

Cannistrà, F. (2020). Single session therapy: The Italian method. *The Science of Psychotherapy*, May, pp. 20–39. Retrieved from https://www.thescienceofpsychotherapy.com/the-science-of-psychotherapy-may-2020/

de Shazer, S. (1982). *Patterns of Brief Family Therapy: An Ecosystemic Approach*. New York: Guilford Press.

de Shazer, S. (1985). *Keys to Solution in Brief Therapy*. New York: Norton.

de Shazer, S. (1991). Foreword. In Y.D. Dolan (Ed.), *Resolving Sexual Abuse* (pp. ix–x). New York: Norton.

de Shazer, S. (1994). *Words Were Originally Magic*. New York: Norton.

Frick, W.B. (1999). Flight into health: A new interpretation. *Journal of Humanistic Psychology*, *39*(4), 58–81.

Gergen, K.J. (2006). *Therapeutic Realities: Collaboration, Oppression and Relational Flow*. Chagrin Falls, OH: Taos Institute.

Haley, J. (1990). Why not long-term therapy? In J.K. Zeig & S.G. Gilligan (Eds.), *Brief Therapy: Myths, Methods, and Metaphors* (pp. 3–17). New York: Brunner/Mazel.

Hoyt, M.F. (2009). *Brief Psychotherapies: Principles & Practice*. Phoenix, AZ: Zeig, Tucker & Theisen.

Hoyt, M.F. (2017). *Brief Therapy and Beyond: Stories, Language, Love, Hope and Time*. New York: Routledge.

Hoyt, M.F., Bobele, M., Slive, A., Young, J., & Talmon, M. (Eds.). (2018). *Single-Session Therapy by Walk-In or Appointment: Administrative, Clinical, and Supervisor Aspects of One-at-a-Time Services*. New York: Routledge.

Hoyt, M.F. & Cannistrà, F. (2019). Single-session therapy: A healthful approach to effectively and efficiently solve client problems. *Italian Journal of Mental Health (Revista Sperimentale di Freniatria)*, *143*(1), 73–85. (In English and Italian). doi: 10.3280/RSF2019-001005

Hoyt, M.F., Miller, S.D., Held, B., & Matthews, W. (2001). About constructivism (or, if four colleagues talked in New York, would anyone hear it?): A conversation with Scott Miller, Barbara Held, and William Matthews. In M.F. Hoyt, *Interviews with Brief Therapy Experts* (pp. 206–225). New York: Brunner-Routledge.

Hoyt, M.F., Rosenbaum, R., & Talmon, M. (1992). Planned single-session psychotherapy. In S.H. Budman, M.F. Hoyt, & S. Friedman (Eds.), *The First Session in Brief Therapy* (pp. 59–86). New York: Guilford Press.

Hoyt, M.F., & Talmon, M. (2014). Editors' introduction: Single session therapy and walk-in services. In M.F. Hoyt & M. Talmon (Eds.), *Capturing the Moment: Single Session Therapy and Walk-In Services* (pp. 1–26). Bethel, CT: Crown House Publishing.

Huber, D., Henrich, G., Clarkin, J., & Klug, G. (2013). Psychoanalytic versus psychodynamic therapy for depression: A three-year follow-up study. *Psychiatry: Interpersonal and Biological Processes*, *76*, 132–149.

International Psychoanalytical Association. (2020). *About Psychoanalysis – The Core Psychoanalytic Method and Setting*. Retrieved on March 16, 2020, from www.ipa.world/en/Psychoanalytic_Treatment/About__Psychoanalysis.aspx

Iveson, C., George, E., & Ratner, H. (2012). *Brief Coaching: A Solution Focused Approach*. New York: Routledge.

Laudan, L. (1977). *Progress and Its Problems. Towards a Theory of Scientific Growth*. London: Routledge & Kegan Paul.

Levy, R.L., & Shelton, J.L. (1990). Tasks in brief therapy. In R.A. Wells & V.J. Giannetti (Eds.), *Handbook of the Brief Psychotherapies* (pp. 145–164). New York: Plenum Press.

Lexico (2020). Mindset. Retrieved March 16, 2020, from www.lexico.com/en/definition/mindset.

Macdonald, A. (2011). *Solution-Focused Therapy: Theory, Research and Practice* (2nd ed.). London: SAGE.

McKergow, M., & Korman, H. (2009). In between – neither inside nor outside: The radical simplicity of Solution-Focused Brief Therapy. *Journal of Systemic Therapies*, *28*(2), 34–39.

Megglé, D. (2011). *Les Therapies Breves* (2nd ed.). Molenbeek-Saint-Jean, France: Satas.

Migone, P. (2014). What does "brief" mean? A theoretical critique of the concept of brief therapy from a psychoanalytic viewpoint. *Journal of the American Psychoanalytic Association*, *62*(4), 631–656.

NHS. (2020). *Overview: Cognitive Behavioural Therapy (CBT)*. National Health System. Retrieved March 14, 2020, from www.nhs.uk/conditions/cognitive-behavioural-therapy-cbt/

Rosenbaum R. (2008). Psychotherapy is not short or long. *APA Monitor on Psychology, 39*(7), 4, 8.

Talmon, M. (1990). *Single Session Therapy: Maximizing the Effect of the First (and Often Only) Therapeutic Encounter.* San Francisco: Jossey-Bass.

Talmon, M., & Hoyt, M.F. (2014). Moments are forever: SST and walk-in services now and in the future. In M.F. Hoyt & M. Talmon (Eds.), *Capturing the Moment. Single Session Therapy and Walk-In Services* (pp. 463–486). Bethel, CT: Crown House Publishing.

Wampold, B.E., & Imel, Z.E. (2015). *Counseling and Psychotherapy. The Great Psychotherapy Debate: The Evidence for What Makes Psychotherapy Work* (2nd ed.). New York: Routledge.

Watzlawick, P., Bavelas, J.B., & Jackson, D.D. (1967). *Pragmatics of Human Communication: A Study of Interactional Patterns, Pathologies, and Paradoxes.* New York: Norton.

Watzlawick, P., & Weakland, J.H. (Eds.). (1977). *The Interactional View: Studies at the Mental Research Institute, Palo Alto, 1965–1974.* New York: Norton.

Watzlawick, P., Weakland, J.H., & Fisch, R. (1974). *Change: Principles of Problem Formation and Problem Resolution.* New York: Norton.

Westmacott, R., & Hunsley, J. (2007). Weighing the evidence for psychotherapy equivalence: Implications for research and practice. *The Behavior Analyst Today, 8*(2), 210–225.

Zeig, J.K. (1985). *Experiencing Erickson: An Introduction to the Man and His Work.* New York: Brunner/Mazel.

Zeig, J.K. (2007). A tribute to Jay Haley, 1923–2007. *American Journal of Clinical Hypnosis, 50*(1), 5–9.

7 Gradually and Suddenly: What Zen Teaches Us About Change in SST

Robert Rosenbaum

Psychotherapists disagree about whether change occurs suddenly, in leaps of insight and abrupt shifts of behavior, or whether it takes place progressively, bit by bit. This underlies the dispute between those convinced therapy intrinsically requires multiple sessions and those who have witnessed clients realize significant benefits in brief therapies, even in a single session. Zen Buddhists have been arguing a similar question for over a thousand years: is the realization of enlightenment sudden or gradual? The story of Zen's doctrinal dispute provides some lessons for present-day meditation practitioners, and for psychotherapists too.

The *Platform Sutra* (Yampolsky, 1967) was written in China toward the end of the 8th century. It describes how Zen master Hongren, to determine who would succeed him as the temple's abbot, instructed his monks to compose a poem demonstrating their level of understanding The head monk, Shenxiu, wrote:

> Our body is the bodhi tree
> Our mind a mirror bright
> Carefully we wipe them hour by hour
> And let no dust alight.

Publicly Hongren praised the poem, but privately told Shenxiu to try again.

Huineng was an illiterate layperson who had never received any Buddhist teaching. One day while walking through the town square he heard a monk recite the Diamond Sutra: in a sudden flash Huineng realized *annutara samyak sambodhi* ("complete perfect enlightenment"). Huineng did not tell anyone about this, but travelled to Hongren's monastery where instead of becoming a monk, he obtained work as a humble laborer in the temple's kitchens. Hearing of the poem contest, Huineng composed his own verse and asked a monk to write it on the monastery's wall:

> There is no Bodhi tree,
> No stand of a mirror bright.

Originally there is not a single thing:
Where can dust alight?

When Hongren discovered Huineng was the author of the verse, he invited Huineng to come to his rooms in secret. He certified Huineng's understanding and made him his official successor but, knowing the monks would be furious he'd given his imprimatur to an illiterate lay-person, he told Huineng to flee the monastery, lest he be killed. It wasn't until 10 years later that Huineng became abbot of a monastery, where he was recognized as the head of the Southern school of Zen.

Here is an account of a client who, instead of hearing a sutra during a walk, resolved an important life issue one day on a department store's escalator.

Erica was a 34-year-old woman who came to psychotherapy feeling depressed at a life impasse. Four years ago her mother was diagnosed with dementia; with nobody else in the family available, Erica arranged for her mother to move in with her. Erica had a good relationship with her mother and during the early stages of her mother's illness all went well. As her mother's condition worsened and Erica's caregiver responsibilities increased, more and more of Erica's energy was spent tending to her mother's needs. Erica's social life dwindled to nothing and her professional career suffered. For the past year, Erica had felt increasingly torn between taking care of her mother and taking more care of herself. She would take steps to place her mother in residential care, but whenever a spot opened up in a facility she'd feel too guilty to act on it.

Psychotherapy focused on resolving this conflict. Erica was able to express both her love for her mother and how draining it was to tend to her needs. She was frustrated and resentful about putting her life on hold, but also felt a strong need to keep her mother with her at home – "not only for my mother's sake, but so I feel I've done all I could." She would tell herself dementia had already taken away the woman who used to be her mother, but then think of all the ways her mother had cared for her, feel overwhelmed with tenderness and guilt, and decide anew her mother ought to stay with her.

During four sessions of therapy, Erica went back-and-forth on the topic without any resolution. I asked her if she felt therapy was helping, and Erica said she felt she was going around in circles. I agreed with her, and proposed an intervention:

Rather than keeping on going around in circles, how about this? When you're ready – but not before – to make a firm decision and stick to it, devote a whole day to the process. On that day go to downtown San Francisco first thing in the morning; go to the Nordstrom's department store; start at the circular escalator on the bottom floor. Get on the escalator, circle round and round without getting off at any of the intervening floors all the way to the top floor. Then get back on and go round and round until you reach the bottom. Keep doing that until, at some point, you feel you know what to do.

Erica felt this could be helpful. She and I agreed it didn't make sense to meet again until she'd done the task, so she said she would call me to schedule another appointment after she had gone 'round and 'round in Nordstrom's.

Three months later Erica returned. She described how, going 'round and 'round on the escalator, it became clear to her: it was time to move on. She made her decision and placed her mother in a good care facility where she visited her once a week. Erica said she was coping with some feelings of loss and sadness but also felt excited about advancing in her professional work. She had resumed dating, and was enjoying socializing. She felt the therapy had been successful and she did not need any more sessions.

Both the Zen and clinical stories are examples where a discrete incident led to a leap of insight and significant practical consequences. These appear as sudden changes, but when we examine them in more detail we find the situation less clear.

It turns out the account in Zen's Platform Sutra is probably apocryphal – is a piece of propaganda written by a later Zen teacher, Shen-hui, a fervent proponent of the Southern school of sudden enlightenment. This school competed with teachers from the Northern monastery where Shenxiu (the head monk in Hongren's poetry competition) had become abbot after Hongren's death. At a public council in 730 CE – 30 years after Shenxiu's death! – Shen-hui accused him of corrupting Hongren's dharma with an incorrect gradualist approach and usurping the rightful heir, Huineng (the winner of the poetry contest).

Until Shen-hui's diatribe, Huineng was at most an obscure figure in Zen; it's possible Huineng never even existed except in the story composed by Shen-hui. Furthermore, Shenxiu was not really a "gradualist" (McRae, 2003); although he advocated realizing Buddhahood in daily activities via constant, unremitting practice, Shenxiu also taught "it does not take long ... enlightenment is in the instant."

In the case of our conscience-burdened caregiver, it might look like spending a day going 'round and 'round a spiral escalator nudged Erica out of her oscillating ambivalence. However, Erica began her last session by saying: "I did drive to Nordstrom's and I did go around the escalator, but I didn't stay there very long, because while I was driving there, I realized – *I'd already made my decision*, before I even got in the car."

It appears that in this case the "cure" came before the "treatment task." Such a topsy-turvy sequence not only reminds us how difficult it is to predict when change will occur in therapy: it raises doubts about whether change occurs linearly, be it sudden *or* gradual.

When big changes occur in a small amount of time, we often resort to a "tipping point" model to explain it: many small alterations built up gradually, creating a configuration ripe for change. According to this thinking, mountain avalanches look sudden but occur only after years of incremental shifts: water falling on rocks, cracking them slightly during freezes, in alternating cycles of warm melts and cold ice until a single footfall triggers a massive rockslide (Figure 7.1).

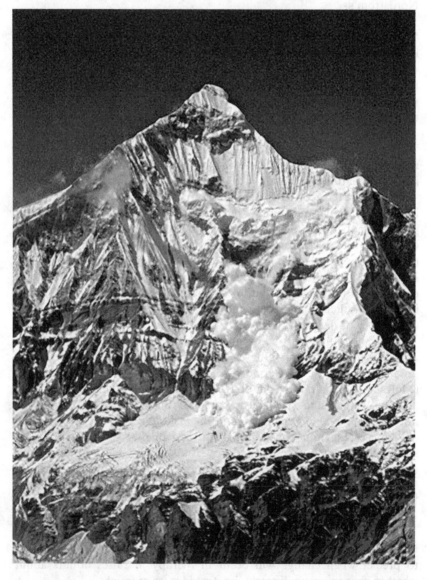

Figure 7.1 Gradual/Sudden (© R. Rosenbaum, 2014; used with permission.)

This "tipping point" process certainly occurs – but it doesn't take into account the moments when a perfectly stable slope is struck by lightning.

Sometimes psychotherapy can provide a tipping point for a client, but this doesn't explain all treatment changes. Most therapists have cases where clients experience unexpected, un-prepared for shifts in their lives, often surprising not only their therapist but also themselves.

The conundrum of how to reconcile discontinuous breakthroughs with processes of continuous change is not only found in psychotherapy. There are debates over gradual (Darwinian) versus punctuated (abrupt) evolution (Gould & Eldredge, 1977, p. 145); physics has difficulties reconciling measured phase transitions with stochastic quantum leaps. We still scratch our heads over Zeno's paradox of motion: to walk from point A to point B we must first traverse half the distance, but to do that we must move half of that half, and so on until we reach the conclusion that it's impossible. How can we traverse an infinite number of steps within a finite distance?

In psychotherapy, it may feel we need an infinite number of sessions to reach a distinct goal when we think clients change in neat step-by-step sequences. Even brief reflection reminds us how rarely our clinical caseload consists of a case where a problem appears suddenly; the client comes in; an intervention is applied; and the problem resolves. *People are ecologies, not things*: complex dynamical systems, fields of possible trajectories whose subjective pasts change depending on how they are viewed in the present, shaping futures anew.

Most therapists would agree that the process of change is rarely a straight line and often mysterious. Too often, though, we approach clinical phenomena with covert oversimplified assumptions: "gradual/sudden," "internal/external," "individual/relational." We unthinkingly assume our pasts are "outside" our present experience, and our current feelings are "inside" us.

That people "have" feelings "inside" them may seem incontrovertible; much of therapy depends on clients "owning" their feelings. However, this rests on an outdated classical view of emotion depicted in the popular recent Pixar film *Inside Out:* feelings are hard-wired inside us, and each emotion has its own neuro-physiological fingerprint; external events trigger these feelings, activating localized brain structures with distinct chemistries and channels of expression.

Recent neuropsychological research suggests none of these assumptions hold true (Barrett, 2017). Rather than being identifiable internal states, emotions are *emergent processes* that have no inherent existence outside of the interpretations we place on ever-fluctuating patterns of brain networks. The classical model of emotions, which posits seven independent core emotions hard-wired "in" an organism that light up selectively in response to specific stimuli, is unable to account for the wide variability in how brain states and environmental situations dance with each other. In contrast, a more systemic emerging paradigm treats emotions as continuously constructed, with no set number of basic emotions; the underlying neurological underpinnings are unique to each situation, so each emotion which arises in response is unique to its particular place and time. Emotions manifest along continuous dimensions of valences and intensities rather than discrete categories; emotions color our experience but they overlap and are often difficult to distinguish from each other, being more like the infinite shadings on a color wheel than a box containing six crayons. In short, emotions are not physiological facts but psychological interpretations arising within interpersonal cultural contexts.

When we approach emotions this way – as living systems rather than specified states – we see our feelings don't resolve into happy sunshine or disturbing thunderstorms. Our emotions are more like flowing weather fronts, and as changeable. Weather is continuously moving and morphing, wide in its possibilities: it encompasses sudden and gradual both. During a sudden squall, the temperature is gradually dropping. We may be in a chilly, foggy valley where warmth and visibility slowly improve as the sun rises; we may feel burning hot under a blue sky on a snowy high mountain slope, until the thin air turns suddenly cold when a single cloud obscures the fierce high-altitude sun.

If we want to come to grips with the issue of sudden versus gradual change over time, we need to re-visit not only how to weather emotions, but also to re-examine our ideas about time itself. Time, too, functions differently in the mountains than in the valley. This is true not only subjectively but literally (and has been verified in numerous experiments that measured clocks running faster at higher elevations where gravity was weaker). Most of us think of time as something separate from ourselves, a physical dimension we traverse from a start to a stop, a beginning to an end. We think of time as a quantity and complain about its restrictions: we feel we don't have enough time to do everything we want; we object to economic factors that pressure us to be more productive, to cram more and more work into shorter and shorter amounts of time. We view time as a tyrant that subjects all our loves to loss and decay:

> When I do count the clock that tells the time [...]
> then of thy beauty do I question make,
> that thou among the wastes of time must go.
> – Shakespeare (Sonnet 12)

In *The Hobbit* (Tolkien, 1937/1966), Gollum poses a dark riddle to the erstwhile Bilbo Baggins: "This thing all things devours: birds, beasts, trees, flowers; gnaws iron, bites steel; grinds hard stones to meal; slays king, ruins town, and beats high mountain down." The riddle freezes

Bilbo's brain: he is saved only because, as Gollum approaches to kill him, Bilbo gasps out "Give me more time!"

Feeling trapped in therapies that allot a certain number of minutes or sessions to resolve life problems, both therapists and clients might say, "Give us more time!" Better, perhaps, to make time our friend (Hoyt, 2017; Talmon, 2018; Young, 2018). After all, most people experience situations that clearly contradict our idea of time as an irrevocably fixed quantity: situations where we are so absorbed in what we are doing, or enjoying ourselves so much, that we lose track of time. We all also know the reverse, where time seems to crawl. Despite the vividness of such experiences, we treat our personal, subjective sense of time as if it's somehow less valid than clock time. The fact is, therapy takes place not in digital ticks and tocks but in the living heartbeats of *being* time.

The vividness of experiential time is certainly at least as pertinent to psychotherapy as the number of sessions or the number of minutes in a meeting. We get caught thinking change is sudden or gradual, therapy is short or long, when we mistake existential time for the time that is measured out in the teaspoons of clocks and calendars. We forget that moments are not brief intervals of time: *moments are meetings.*

Psychotherapy ceases to be short or long, gradual or sudden because when we engage in our human meetings, we enliven and, yes, enlighten each other: we sparkle, we realize ourselves in a way which is not separate from time, but manifests the incandescence of each moment. As Jorge Luis Borges wrote (1946/1964, p. 234): "Time is the substance from which I am made. Time is a river which carries me along, but I am the river; it is a tiger that devours me, but I am the tiger; it is a fire that consumes me, but I am the fire."

We exist not *in*, but *as* the time of our lives. This life-time is natural and immeasurable; it may look from one perspective like a step-by-step journey from birth to death, but this doesn't take into account how we are fully ourselves in the expression of each moment. Zen teacher Eihei Dogen (1233/2010) described this in his essay "The Time-Being":

> Firewood becomes ash, and it does not become firewood again. Yet, do not suppose that the ash is future and the firewood past. You should understand that firewood abides in the phenomenal expression of firewood, which fully includes past and future and is independent of past and future [...]

Birth is an expression complete this moment. Death is an expression complete this moment. They are like winter and spring. You do not call winter the beginning of spring, nor summer the end of spring.

Dogen's description accounts for our personal (and clinical) reality better than time-card accounting can. In the case of Erica's firewood and ash, she is complete as a dutiful daughter and as an autonomous adult; neither role turns into nor contradicts the other. In the case of the Zen student's *satori,* the moment of insight and its realization through lifetime practice coexist: they nurture each other continuously, so it doesn't make sense to say which comes first, the chicken or the egg.

Therapy is not confined by the minutes of a session: Because each of us is complete each moment, clients are changing every moment before, during, and after therapy. At the moments where clients and therapists meet, a vector emerges from all the life factors which are simultaneously at play.

Sometimes becoming aware of this play of life-time can be sufficient to resolve a client's presenting problem: we smile when we hear a 40-year-old mother of two who, surrounded by slim twenty-somethings in her ballet class, worries they will trigger a relapse of her teenage anorexia until she says in a moment of realization, "Oh! I'm a grown woman, in a grown woman's body" (Rosenbaum, 2014, p. 44). We rejoice when a client who has felt dragged down by childhood traumas feels liberated when she exclaims, "I'm *me* – I'm not what *happened* to me" (Rosenbaum, 1999, p. 207).

We are not just the memories of our desires and our hurts, residues of our pasts, or phantasms of our futures. We live our current lives as our self-of-the-moment, so realization is not sudden or gradual: it shimmers and glows.

Change does not take time. Change *is* time. Firewood is firewood, ash is ash. A little girl is not an incomplete version of an adult woman, and a wise crone is not a decayed version of a little girl (Rosenbaum, 2014). When we approach therapy sessions not as a limited number of minutes but as a living swirl, we open up a field far beyond short or long, near or far. We open the possibilities for each session and each moment to act as a pivot point for our entire life (Rosenbaum, Hoyt, & Talmon, 1990). As Eihei Dogen (1233/2010) describes:

> Each moment is all being, is the entire world. [...]
> [When] the moon [is] reflected on the water [...]although its light is wide and great, the moon is reflected even in a puddle an inch wide. The whole moon and the entire sky are reflected in dewdrops on the grass, or even in one drop of water.
> The depth of the drop is the height of the moon.
> Each reflection, however long or short its duration,
> manifests the vastness of the dewdrop,
> and realizes the limitlessness of the moonlight in the sky.

References

Barrett, L.F. (2017). *How Emotions Are Made: The Secret Life of the Brain.* New York: Houghton Mifflin Harcourt.

Borges, J.L. (1964). A new refutation of time. In *Labyrinths: Selected Stories & Other Writings* (pp. 217–234). New York: New Directions Press (work originally published 1946).

Dogen, E. (2010). Actualizing the fundamental point. In K. Tanahashi (Ed.), *Treasury of the True Dharma Eye: Zen Master Dogen's Shobogenzo* (pp. 29–33). Boston & London: Shambhala Publications. (original work 1233).

Gould, S.J., & Eldredge, N. (1977). Punctuated equilibria: The tempo and mode of evolution reconsidered. *Paleobiology, 3*(2), 115–151.

Hoyt, M.F. (2017). On time in brief therapy. In *Brief Therapy and Beyond: Stories, Language, Love, Hope and Time* (pp. 6–32). New York: Routledge (originally published 1990).

McRae, J. (2003). *Seeing Through Zen: Encounter, Transformation, and Genealogy in Chinese Chan Buddhism.* Berkeley and Los Angeles: University of California Press.

Rosenbaum, R. (1999). *Zen and the Heart of Psychotherapy.* Philadelphia: Brunner/Mazel.

Rosenbaum, R. (2014). The time of your life. In M.F. Hoyt & M. Talmon (Eds.), *Capturing the Moment: Single Session Therapy and Walk-In Services* (pp. 41–52). Bethel, CT: Crown House Publishing.

Rosenbaum, R., Hoyt, M.F., & Talmon, M. (1990). The challenge of single-session psychotherapies: Creating pivotal moments. In R.A. Wells & V.J. Giannetti (Eds.), *Handbook of the Brief Psychotherapies* (pp. 165–192). New York: Plenum.

Talmon, M. (2018). The eternal now: On becoming and being a single-session therapist. In M.F. Hoyt, M. Bobele, A. Slive, J. Young, & M. Talmon (Eds.), *Single-Session Therapy by Walk-In or Appointment: Administrative, Clinical, and Supervisory Aspects of One-at-a-Time Services* (pp. 148–154). New York: Routledge.

Tolkien, J.R.R. (1966). *The Hobbit.* New York: Ballantine Books (work originally published 1937).

Yampolsky, P.B. (1967). *The Platform Sutra of the Sixth Patriarch: The Text of the Tun-huang* (trans. by Philip B. Yampolsky). New York: Columbia University Press. ISBN 978-0-231-08361-4.

Young, J. (2018). Single session therapy: The misunderstood gift that keeps on giving. In M.F. Hoyt, M. Bobele, A. Slive, J. Young, & M. Talmon (Eds.), *Single-Session Therapy by Walk-In or Appointment: Administrative, Clinical, and Supervisory Aspects of One-at-a-Time Services* (pp. 40–58). New York: Routledge.

Section III

Implementation: Single Session Practice

8 Implementing Single Session Thinking in Public Mental Health Settings in Queensland: Part 1 – Introducing Single Session Family Consultations into Adult Inpatient and Community Care

Catherine Renkin, Karen Alexander, and Marianne Wyder

Family is personal for us. It is a source of inspiration, identity, and relationships. It is also a meaning-making experience we draw on heavily in all our work.

Mental health concerns impact individuals and their family across all domains of life. This is particularly so when the person's symptoms may be overwhelming or when they experience a crisis. While the focus of care is on the individuals, for many people living with a mental illness, the recovery journey is relational (Price-Robertson, Obradovic, & Morgan, 2017). It is the support of family and friends that enables the person to take responsibility for his or her own recovery (Wyder & Bland, 2014). There is now mounting evidence that families play an important part in their loved one's recovery and while this is generally acknowledged, they are not routinely included in provision of clinical care for consumers (Dixon, 2000; Parr, 2009). There is an increasing reference within policy to the rights of families and carers to have their own needs addressed alongside recognition of the role they play in consumers' lives and their recovery outcomes (Queensland Health, 2016; Department of Health, 2017).

In line with these research and policy developments, increasing the availability of family interventions has been part of the ongoing priorities of Metro South Addictions and Mental Health Service (MSAMHS), a large public mental health multi-site service in the state of Queensland. In recognition of the diversity and range of loved ones important to consumer recovery, "family" has been defined to include unpaid carers, relatives, and friends. Various programs comprised of psychoeducation and peer support have been made available to family members through leadership and support by social workers. While the evaluation of these various initiatives was positive, clinical records showed overall levels of engagement and inclusion of the family in care planning remained low and varied across the service. In addition, quality assurance review and feedback reports identified poor communication and lack of engagement with families as a common factor in analysis of complaints and adverse outcomes.

As a result, the social-work leadership at MSAMHS identified family engagement as a priority, highlighting the need to shift the focus from providing "add on" education and support for an identified relative or friend to supporting routine inclusion of families and a partnership approach to care as standard practice. Single Session Family Consultation (SSFC) or family-focused planning meetings were identified as one strategy to overcome some of the fragmentation in current approaches to engaging with families. SSFC is ideal as it aims to clarify the nature of family involvement with clients as well as helping the family to identify and respond to their own needs. In addition, it provides a brief or short-term treatment in the inpatient or community setting favored by an agency under pressure from increased service demands to reduce length of stay in inpatient units. The evidence for the benefits and feasibility of adopting SSFC in public mental health service settings (Fry, 2012; The Bouverie Centre, 2015; Poon, Harvey, Fuzzard, & O'Hanlon, 2019; also see Chapter 5 of this volume) made SSFC an identified intervention with potential to meet service goals for greater family engagement and improved consumer/family outcomes.

Piloting Phase of SSFC

In 2016, the SSFC was piloted at MSAMHS in the form of structured family meetings in an adult psychiatric inpatient unit and across a variety of community settings. Initial sites were chosen according to location of staff who possessed the knowledge and willingness to implement SSFC. The pilot was based on the formalized version of SSFC and a training package devised based on the Single Session Family Consultation Practice Manual (The Bouverie Centre, 2014; also see Chapter 5). SSFC has three stages:

1. Meeting with the client to decide on participants and topic, then the clinician calling the family to invite them and negotiate agenda
2. A facilitated session with client and family, focused on pre-identified issues
3. A follow-up phone call to family.

The training focused on this process, the principles of single session work, the family consultation approach, and skills for practice with families using an SSFC framework. Strategies and resources for introducing this new practice within each participant's current work setting were also included. Individual consultations upon request and structured group supervision were also set up and commenced within a month of the first training session. Supervision sessions were offered initially at monthly, then bi-monthly intervals and were co-facilitated by an external consultant from The Bouverie Centre.

The training package was delivered to a total of 46 self-nominated staff from various disciplines with 15% of the trained clinicians going on to offer the SSFC intervention to 31 families and deliver 25 family sessions in the inpatient and community settings. Feedback from consumers and their family indicated that this approach favorably addressed many of their concerns. Clinicians also reported beneficial outcomes for consumers and added that they have adopted many of the principles and process into their wider practice. We present three composite case vignettes to illustrate these experiences.

Three Illustrations

Vignette #1: Bridging Treating Team, Consumer, and Family Expectations

Dave had been working with Jane for over five years. Jane was in her 70s and her health and functioning had been deteriorating. The treatment team believed that the best option for Jane was to be moved into a nursing home. Dave was asked to relay this decision to the family. Dave arranged for a single session family consultation with the family. During this session, he spoke about the treatment team's concerns and gauged the family views. The family, while acknowledging that Jane's health was a concern, did not want her to go into care just yet and believed, with extra support, they could care for her at home. As a family, they were able to develop a plan that would provide Jane with the additional supports needed to safely stay home.

What did the SSFC approach bring? The SSFC allowed for Dave to share the treating team's concerns with the family in a way that invited collaboration and development of alternative solutions.

Vignette #2: SSFC to Enhance Family Communication

John, a 45-year-old man, had been an inpatient for four weeks and was about to be discharged. The family had concerns about John's past behaviors and future plans, and different views as to how best to support him. A family meeting was co-facilitated by Sally, the family peer support worker, and Mary, the social worker, with time allocated for John and family members to each voice their perspective. While the session was constructive, the facilitators felt that there was no tangible outcome and issues were left unresolved. At a phone follow-up, Mum thanked Sally for ensuring all family members had been heard at the meeting. She advised that the family had gone for coffee afterwards and discussed the issues raised during the session. While there were still differences in viewpoints, the family was able to come to a compromise and resolve some issues and now felt more confident they could work together to support John after discharge.

What did the SSFC approach bring? The single session approach allowed the family to strengthen their communication skills, share individual concerns and expectations, and find new ways to sort out differences.

Vignette #3: Finding Different Ways to Support Those Experiencing Chronic Suicidality

Sandra, who was in her late 30s, had been experiencing feelings of depression and suicidality for the past five years. She was often in distress and, while it was not the ideal solution, had presented to the Emergency Department on numerous occasions. Her distress had taken its toll on family members and they felt they were unable to continue supporting her. A Single Session Family Consultation at Sandra's home was suggested by Natalie, the Community Case Manager, and Sandra agreed, identifying multiple people she would like to be invited. While initially the focus of the session was on how to support Sandra, family members raised the many past encounters with the mental health care agency and talked about the trauma and difficulties associated with these. It became apparent that while the family was enduring secondary trauma, Sandra increasingly felt that her family did not care about her. Once the family had all been able to talk about their own reactions to distress, they were able to develop strategies and alternative ways to respond to Sandra. As a result, Sandra felt more supported and less in need to go to the Emergency Department.

What did the SSFC approach bring? The SSFC approach allowed the family to talk about the ongoing impacts of mental illness, including secondary trauma. It allowed a shift of focus from managing individual distress to understanding trauma and promoting recovery for the whole family.

Using Implementation Science to Introduce SSFC

The full introduction of SSFC into the service was informed by implementation science principles. Effective implementation of new interventions in healthcare needs to take into consideration the characteristics of the intervention and the service context as well as creating a thorough process to embed the intervention into practice (Damschroder et al., 2009). Implementation generally has two sets of outcomes (intervention outcomes and implementation outcomes). To aid planning and evaluation, the resources, activities, and outputs associated with implementation of SSFC were articulated in a program logic format. The resources required included trainers and trained clinicians as well as organizational support for greater family engagement. Table 8.1 provides the program logic developed for the project.

Table 8.1 SSFC Implementation Program Logic

What's the Problem?	Resources/Inputs	Activities	Outputs	Short & Long-Term Outcomes	Impact
Families not routinely engaged in planning for, or provision of, mental health service care to consumers.	• Clinicians • Trainers • Method/ intervention for engaging consumers and families • Organizational support for greater family engagement	• Lobbying for increased allocation of staff time and resources • Identify and promote appropriate intervention • Training for clinical staff in Family Intervention method • Implementation support for practice change	• Greater number of contacts with family across the service • Family meetings are inclusive of both consumer & family • Increased staff skills & confidence in providing SSFC • Consumers & families routinely rating meetings	• Greater family engagement across service • Reduced conflict & more positive family r/ships • Identification and mitigation planning of clinical risk inclusive of consumers and family • Better service-family-consumer communication	• Consumers and family are better supported to maintain own well-being • Earlier service response to family identified decline in mental health • Decreased burden for families
Evaluation		• Records of staff training and supervision • Clinician logs of SSFC activity • Number of service contacts with families • Session feedback evaluation from families		• Care Plans – identify input & role of carers • Reduced complaints and adverse events relating to family communication • Increased consumer and family service satisfaction	

To inform the implementation, an assessment of the factors across domains of the intervention characteristics, outer setting, inner setting, and characteristics of involved individuals was undertaken. The identification of barriers and enablers within these different domains formed a basis for choice of implementation strategies and actions to promote uptake of SSFC (Powell et al., 2015; Hateley-Browne, Hodge, Polimeni, & Mildon, 2019). The following implementation plan (Table 8.2) lists the identified barriers and enablers and implementation strategies adopted to address them.

In relation to the *Intervention Characteristics*, the main implementation strategy adopted was to promote the adaptability of SSFC. Educational materials were developed to raise awareness of the principles and benefits of SSFC as a flexible, adaptable, brief intervention. Processes for maintaining fidelity whilst allowing for adaptation were developed in conjunction with staff. Supervision sessions offered for all staff throughout the pilot phase provided feedback to inform adaptation of the intervention, training and development of additional implementation strategies. The formalized SSFC model of a pre-meeting discussion with consumer then family, meeting together with consumer and family, and a follow-up phone call was adapted as a result of feedback. Change in protocol so that the pre-meeting contact and the family meeting could be combined in one interaction meant that the intervention could be offered whenever the opportunity to meet with families arose.

Strategies to influence factors in the *Outer Context* included conducting a local needs assessment to demonstrate the need for improvement to practice with families and consolidate support at the system and organizational levels. Baseline data was collected from existing records of family engagement and staff capability in family work. Collation of this data increased awareness of the gaps between existing policy and standards and practice. As a result, a key performance measure of "Family Contact" was adopted by the agency that assisted in keeping family work on crowded staff, team, and wider agency agendas throughout implementation.

A multi-disciplinary implementation team was established, drawn from staff with leadership roles in family practice, single session work, workforce development, and research. In the absence of additional allocated funding, this team was able to identify and use existing structures and resources of the broader health service. For example, dedicated funding for individual professional development was used to pay for trainers, and external experts in Knowledge Translation projects were accessed via a pilot staff mentoring initiative offered by the Allied Health department of our district hospital.

To address barriers of the *Inner Context*, engagement with operational and professional leaders was prioritized to gauge support, identify champions, flag expected challenges, and provide feedback and updates on introduction of SSFC at pilot sites.

Implementation team members trained in SST and SSFC developed and delivered training suitable for a multi-disciplinary staff cohort

Table 8.2 SSFC Implementation Plan

Domain	Barriers	Enablers	Implementation Strategy
Intervention Characteristics: (SSFC Framework)	Skepticism regarding impact and effectiveness of brief family intervention.	SSFC evidence and resource materials available and accessible. SSFC is manualized intervention with built-in flexibility	Develop educational materials. Promote adaptability
Outer Context: (Public funded health service system)	Limited resources and competing priorities for health funding. High demand for MH services.	Policy, standards and legislation require service engagement with carers & families. Service reform drive at national and state level to improve efficiency and effectiveness of care.	Conduct local needs assessment. Access new funding
Inner Context: (Organizational structure and culture re family work and practice change)	Management reluctance to allocate staff time to train and provide family interventions. Staff carrying high caseloads and providing crisis response as well as treatment.	Executive support for intervention and practice change with families. Social work and carer peer workforce identify family work as integral part of role.	Conduct educational meetings & outreach visits. Assess for readiness & identify barriers and facilitators. Identify early adopters. Use train-the-trainer strategies
Characteristics of Individuals: Clients (Consumers & family) and Staff (Multidisciplinary workforce)	Reluctance of consumer and/or family to engage in family-focused intervention. Variation across disciplines, teams, settings of attitudes and skill in working with families	Large number of consumers with nominated carer. Families of consumers seeking engagement. Strong, active peer workforce (consumer & carer). Pool of existing staff with skills, knowledge, attitudes that aligned with SSFC framework.	Conduct ongoing training supervision. Make training dynamic. Provide clinical. Provide ongoing consultation

who could then become "champions" for family work in their teams. Social workers and carer peer support workers were targeted as the discipline groups most active/invested in family work. To ensure that clinicians were able to attend the training and minimize the time away from busy clinical schedules, the training was blended, including an online information module and a face-to-face component that was experiential and built on existing knowledge and skills in engaging with families.

Consistency of process and documentation of SSFC implementation was promoted through staff use of templates to record activity and outcomes. To address management reluctance for staff allocation of time to family work, these templates served dual purposes of tracking uptake of SSFC and meeting agency requirements for recording of all contacts with consumers and families. In addition, SSFC was promoted by trained clinicians who became champions within their teams and, where it was incorporated as a possible intervention into team clinical review processes, a greater number of referrals and sessions occurred.

Ongoing training, clinical supervision, and individual consultation were used to address the diversity of knowledge and skill of the workforce and practice contexts. Partnering with consumer and carer peer workers to implement SSFC has enabled lived experience workers to enrich the training and supervision. Professional leads/seniors (particularly social work and nursing) were invited to training to facilitate ongoing access to individual supervision for clinicians.

Positive staff evaluation of training led to provision of funding for further partnership with The Bouverie Centre to provide subsequent rounds of staff training and input into the supervision program. Staff have used the structured peer group supervision as a space for accessing support to get started, undertaking reflection and receiving feedback on practice with families as well as to access SSFC process and skills refresher sessions.

We used the process of training, mentoring, group expert-led, and peer supervision as opportunities to reiterate and develop shared understanding of the aims and elements of the framework that maximized effectiveness. We have also used evaluation to identify core elements of the method/intervention that are valued (from staff and family perspective) to inform our ongoing adaptation-fidelity dance!

Conclusions

SSFC provides a potentially unifying approach for family meetings that can be adopted by mental healthcare workers to engage with and empower families as partners in care. It is aligned with policy and organizational priorities, structured enough so that training and process guides can support fidelity, flexible enough to enable multiple disciplines to adapt and incorporate into their own practice, brief enough to be acceptable to families, and feasible for widespread use. All of these factors work to enhance the benefits of single session family consultation.

References

Damschroder, L.J., Aron, D.C., Keith, R.E., Kirsh, S.R., Alexander, J.A., & Lowery, J.C. (2009). Fostering implementation of health services research findings into practice: A consolidated framework for advancing implementation science. *Implementation Science, 4*(1), 50–64. Retrieved from https://doi.org/10.1186/1748-5908-4-50

Department of Health. (2017). *The Fifth National Mental Health and Suicide Prevention Plan.* Canberra, ACT: Australian Government Department of Health.

Department of Health. (2018). *NCEC Implementation Guide and Toolkit.* Dublin, Ireland: Department of Health. Retrieved from https://www.gov.ie/en/collection/cd41ac-clinical-effectiveness-resources-and-learning/

Dixon, L. (2000). Reflections on recovery. *Community Mental Health Journal, 36,* 443–447.

Fry, D. (2012). Implementing single session family consultation: A reflective team approach. *Australian and New Zealand Journal of Family Therapy, 33*(1), 54–69.

Hateley-Browne, J., Hodge, L., Polimeni, M., & Mildon, R. (2019). *Implementation in Action: A Guide to Implementing Evidence Informed Programs and Practices.* Melbourne, VIC: Australian Institute of Family Studies.

Parr, H. (2009). *Carers and Supporting Recovery.* Glasgow, Scotland, UK: Scottish Recovery Network.

Poon, W., Harvey, C., Fuzzard, S., & O'Hanlon, B. (2019). Implementing a family-inclusive practice model in youth mental health services in Australia. *Early Intervention in Psychiatry, 13*(3), 1–8.

Powell, B.J., Waltz, T.J., Chinman, M.J., Damschroder, L.J., Smith, J.L., Matthieu, M.M., ... Kirchner, J.E. (2015). A refined compilation of implementation strategies: Results from the Expert Recommendations for Implementing Change (ERIC) project. *Implementation Science, 21,* 10, doi:10.1186/s13012-015-0209-1.

Price-Robertson, R., Obradovic, A., & Morgan, B. (2017). Relational recovery: Beyond individualism in the recovery approach. *Advances in Mental Health, 15*(2), 108–120. doi:10.1080/18387357.2016.1243014

Queensland Health. (2016, October). Connecting Care to Recovery 2016–2021: A Plan for Queensland's State-Funded Mental Health, Alcohol and Other Drug Services. Brisbane, Australia: State of Queensland (Queensland Health).

The Bouverie Centre (2014). *Single Session Family Consultation Practice Manual* (Version 2). Melbourne, VIC, Australia: Latrobe University. (https://www.bouverie.org.au/images/uploads/Single_Session_Family_Consultation_Practice_Manual_2014.pdf)

The Bouverie Centre (2015). *Mental Health Beacon: Implementing Family Inclusive Practices in Victorian Mental Health Services: Project Report.* Melbourne, VIC, Australia: La Trobe University. https://www.bouverie.org.au/images/uploads/MH_Beacon_Project_Report_March_2015.pdf

Wyder, M., & Bland, R. (2014). The recovery framework as a way of understanding families' responses to mental illness: Balancing different needs and recovery journeys. *Australian Social Work, 67*(2), 179–196. https://doi.org/10.1080/0312407X.2013.8755

9 Implementing Single Session Thinking in a Public Mental Health Setting in Queensland: Part II – Adapting and Integrating Single Session Therapy into an Acute Care Setting

Jillian McDonald, Paul Hickey, and Marianne Wyder

In Australia, when people experiencing a mental health crisis come to the attention of a public mental health service, they are seen by an acute care team (ACT) in the community or at an emergency department. The primary role of these teams is to assess a person's immediate risk to themselves and the community. ACTs' core model of service prioritizes the assessment of a person's mental state and risk and places emphasis on medical interventions rather than interventions that are informed by psychotherapy models. Psychotherapies are generally offered only after this initial contact with the service. This overlooks the opportunity to respond psychotherapeutically from the start. Single Session Therapy (SST) was considered a practical approach to capture this opportunity. The single session model utilizes brief therapy skills to expedite solution finding and address psychological distress.

In 2015, Metro South Addictions and Mental Health Services (MSAMHS) trialed the Single Session Therapy model from The Bouverie Centre, Victoria, Australia. MSAMHS is a public metropolitan health service in Brisbane, Queensland, Australia, which provides treatment and support to people across all age groups. This trial affirmed that there was the potential for considerable benefit from a single session approach (Le Gros, Wyder, & Brunelli, 2018). During the trial, SST was offered to consumers as an additional appointment after a comprehensive mental health assessment. The evaluation of the trial indicated that while clinicians felt that the model enabled an opportunity to provide a brief intervention for those in crisis, there were challenges integrating the model within existing practice frameworks and service processes. This chapter describes these challenges and how they were overcome.

Consultation

Several consultations were undertaken to adapt the single session approach to be integrated within the acute care service model. These started in 2017. The Bouverie Centre's (Young & Rycroft, 1997) model of SST (described below) was presented to managers, team leaders, and ACT clinicians. The consultations focused on collecting their understanding and perceptions of SST. Discussion identified the strengths and benefits of the model, implementation barriers, challenges within this setting and sustainability. The model was presented as an opportunity for practice improvement; to bring a consistent, therapeutically informed approach to clinical work in this setting.

Single Session as a Framework Approach

Adopting the model focused on integrating the underlying principles of a single session approach into the assessment process. The practice principles of time, honesty, and prioritizing consumer identified needs remained critical elements to the approach. Above all other components, clinicians appreciated the component of openly conveying the time available, focusing conversation on the most urgent issues, which is important in this time-poor clinical setting. *Take-Aways* (Young, Rycroft, & Weir, 2006), a note written by consumers outlining the most important reminders and resources they'll take from the single session, was the only paperwork retained and was primarily used as a care planning resource.

Training was tailored to the needs of the ACT team. As workload is high and clinicians' professional development time is limited, a blended approach to training was developed. The training involved a prerequisite one-hour online module and a six-hour face-to-face workshop. To ensure consistency, the training was developed by staff who were trained by The Bouverie Centre. The online module focused on how to introduce brief interventions into the assessment process as well as the history, principles and components of an SST approach. The workshop focused on practicing the skills and discussion about how these principles could be translated into existing practice and team processes. While the training was aimed at the ACT staff members, practitioners from other parts of the service - of varied discipline and training backgrounds - attended, as well as staff in lived experience roles.[1]

Underlying Principles for Implementation

To ensure the effective implementation of this project, we adopted the Knowledge to Action Cycle (KTA) approach (Graham et al., 2006). KTA is easy to use and combines action theories and practice change processes to structure implementation. As part of this process, much of the knowledge creation was derived from stakeholder consultations and synthesized with existing experience of SST, including identifying implementation challenges. This knowledge was applied through the action cycle to tailor both the implementation of the intervention and the intervention itself.

Implementation Challenges and Solutions

Several challenges were experienced throughout the process of implementing this approach in an acute care setting.

Prioritization of Team and Clinical Functions

The ACT environment can be hectic. Furthermore, the ACT processes and paperwork required are extensive. Clinicians of the acute care team expressed concerns in incorporating psychotherapeutic interventions on top of their other obligations and responsibilities. These include mandated tasks, such as risk and mental health assessments. The clinicians' view of how SST fits with existing work practices varied widely. It ranged from seeing SST as aligning with existing work processes and practice, to being considered as outside of the assessment process. It was critical to consider the time pressure the ACT teams are under and that any new model or intervention had to be done within the existing assessment processes rather than an additional intervention conducted with the consumer after the assessment. To build their confidence in integrating the model, clinicians initiated practicing with peers. Some clinicians were able to bridge existing practice with SST and led others to provide it as an additional intervention.

Suitability with Consumers

Clinicians also expressed concern that a single session approach would not be suitable for all consumers, particularly those consumers with severe symptoms or those with immediate safety concerns (e.g., people with active symptoms of psychosis whose cognitive capacity is compromised or those whose physical safeguarding was paramount), overriding any other interventions.

Alignment with Assessment Work

The SST approach provided a session framework which allows clinicians to incorporate a psychotherapeutic intervention while conducting a mental health assessment. Generally, the assessment consists of a series of structured questions for the purpose of confirming or clarifying diagnosis, evaluating a person's self-harm risk and establishing a care plan. The way these assessments are conducted varies according to the professional discipline and training, as well as experience of the clinician. While many clinicians have identified that they already use similar skills to SST in their practice, the SST session framework was a way to formalize their approach and bring a consistency to the assessment process. This allowed the clinicians to shift their interactions away from conducting the assessment as a task-driven interaction and towards an approach that was directed by what the consumer wanted addressed, allowing for a brief psychotherapy intervention. The SST framework emphasizes what the consumer wants addressed and guides the interaction rather than being driven by an assessment document. Clinicians spoke about the meaningful participation that resulted from meeting the consumers' expectations.

Professional Identity

Clinicians welcomed the opportunity to deliver psychotherapeutic approaches. Some clinicians spoke about a loss of professional identity when their work is focused on risk assessment and diagnostics. Clinicians described SST as enabling them to reinvigorate their therapeutic skills in this practice setting as it provided a framework. The SST framework moved clinicians away from a somewhat rigid and structured inquiry approach and allowed clinicians more flexibility to engage their diverse professional and experiential skills in psychotherapeutic engagement.

Practice Change

A practical challenge for some clinicians has been to differentiate the SST approach from current practice and to move away from "We do that already." Clinicians identified existing skills that embodied the SST approach but did not have knowledge of the overall model. When clinicians began to understand the model through training and discussion, they appreciated the alignment and validation that it bought to their existing practice principles. Having the conversation on practice barriers and enablers in the training workshop also enabled clinicians to be reflective and plan for workable solutions to reset their practice. Clinicians continue to report being challenged with routinely using the SST framework as the process for assessment, although most are integrating SST skills into the way they currently conduct an assessment. Clinicians who are using an SST approach to conduct assessments explore records for historical information before the session to avoid unnecessary questions, follow the SST framework to explore, prioritize or park issues, and allow time for any unstated assessment information at the end of the session. Clinicians reported that rapport can be difficult with a questionnaire approach, whereas SST provided the consumer a sense of control, allowing the conversation to flow and information to be freely revealed.

Establishing Professional Development

SST is not a mandatory approach. It can be challenging for clinicians to prioritize it as part of their professional development. Management endorsement of the training led to greater uptake. The blended training also reduced the time clinicians are absent from clinical work.

To support staff in incorporating SST into practice, regular supervision sessions were offered. These supervision sessions provided staff with the opportunity to reflect on their practice. An hour session was provided monthly and accessible either in person, by phone or videoconference. As part of the process, brief practice reflection pieces were developed for electronic distribution to clinicians. These are skill reminders; each taking less than one minute to read. Each skill is presented with an explanation of its purpose and an example of its application. Skill examples:

> *Checking In.* Checking in avoids a loss of focus and direction during the interaction; to keep the interaction relevant and purposeful. Asking the consumer is the only way to know whether you're on track. How do you check in with the consumer? Simply ask, "*Is this what you wanted? Is this helpful?*"

> *Establishing the Consumers' Priorities (Not Ours).* Consumers have priorities to discuss. Clinicians also come with an agenda to complete set tasks. Establishing the consumers' priorities validates their distress, builds rapport and opens opportunity to explore influencing factors and solutions. Discreet questioning or inadvertent information can also be collected within this discussion to satisfy assessment tasks. How do you prioritize the consumer's needs? Do you ask, "*What is important for you to prioritize today?*"

Sustaining Practice

Investment in workforce development by the organization is required for staff to build and sustain practice. In addition to the supervision sessions, a Practice Development Matrix (PDM) was developed based on the therapy capability framework described by Lau, Meredith, Bennett, Crompton, and Dark (2017). The matrix is intended to help staff to reflect on their practice and identify available supports, which enhance and sustain their practice. The PDM is designed to support staff in achieving their desired practice level in SST. Levels of practice range from foundational knowledge through advanced practitioner level. The PDM describes what is required to meet, sustain, and support clinicians at each level of practice. The clinician, team leader, and service each have expected actions to support this process. Some of the strategies include observing the practice of colleagues, sharing practice experiences in team meetings, facilitating access to training and supervision, and promoting leaders. Table 9.1 provides an abridged version of the PDM.

Table 9.1 Single Session Therapy (SST) Practice Development Matrix (PDM)

Single Session Therapy (SST) Practice Development Matrix (PDM)		
To achieve SST Foundation Practitioner	To achieve SST Practice Informed Practitioner	To achieve SST Practitioner
Practice: Clinician will have SST knowledge.	**Practice:** Clinician will be developing their SST practice.	**Practice:** Clinician will be practicing and mentoring others in SST.
Attainment: Clinicians who have completed SST foundation knowledge training.	**Attainment:** Clinicians who have completed SST training.	**Attainment:** Clinicians report on SST practice.
Aim: To develop an induction schedule to identify and engage learning in SST.	**Aim:** To build confidence in individual practice and integrate SST within team processes.	**Aim:** To consolidate and expand individual and team practice in SST.
Actions:	**Actions:** In addition to SST Foundation Practitioner	**Actions:** In addition to SST Practice Informed Practitioner
Clinician Attain foundation knowledge within 3 months of commencement of service Familiarity through peer discussion & observed practice	**Clinician** Attend training within 3 months of attaining foundation knowledge Practice SST with SST Practitioner within 1 month of training Refresh knowledge within 12 months of training Practice individually or in pairs Share learning with peers, team & in supervision Supervision with SST Practitioner or clinical lead	**Clinician** Incorporate SST into daily practice. Expand brief therapy knowledge & practice. Lead peer practice, supervision & team discussions in SST
Team Leader Identify training needs Support access to SST training of all existing & new clinicians Facilitate SST team discussions	**Team Leader** Enable supervision Support learning needs in performance coaching goals	**Team Leader** Identify clinical site leads in SST Support advancing SST clinical practice through peer practice, supervision and case discussion.
Service Endorse SST as best practice Integrate SST into the induction to clinical services. Articulate training expectations Report for tracking and action Acknowledge learning achievements	**Service** Support a culture of peer learning Validate practice	**Service** Promote SST Practitioner roles as leaders. Invite SST Practitioners to contribute to formal evaluation and to confirm SST processes in service planning
Progression: Move clinician to Practice Informed Practitioners.	**Progression:** Move clinician to Practitioner.	**Progression:** Clinician may decide to advance practice, supervision and research in SST.

Developed using OTCEP Quick Reference Guide: Using Principles of Best Practice in Education with Health Learning Environments, March 2019 and MSAMHS Therapy Capability and Practice Framework. Lau, G., Meredith, P., Bennett, S., Crompton, D., & Dark, F. (2017), "A Capability Framework to Develop Leadership for Evidence-Informed Therapies in Publicly Funded Mental Health Services." *International Journal of Public Leadership*, 13(3), 151–165. ©Metro South HHS, MSAMHS. Used with permission.

Outcomes and Key Learnings

SST was first introduced within acute care settings with the purpose of providing mental health consumers with an immediate, supportive, and therapeutic approach to find solutions to their problems. We underestimated the complexity of implementing a new practice within this setting. While clinicians saw that SST could have a place within their clinical practice and was potentially useful within their clinical setting, they also identified the challenge of incorporating SST within their existing clinical practices and mandated team processes. This highlighted the vital task of meaningfully consulting with staff prior to introducing a new practice model.

Being responsive to the needs of clinicians and their work context were key components of successfully implementing SST into the acute care setting. The engagement with clinicians and their managers ensured that the SST framework was relevant to the acute care context and successfully adopted into practice. Validation was a critical element of engagement: this appealed to clinicians to adopt SST into their practice. Recognizing the clinicians' alignment to "We do that already" and validating their desire to bring more of their professional identity to their practice opened the opportunity to use the model to affirm their practice. Engaging peer practice also ensured that there was strong collegial respect and a shared understanding of the model. Furthermore, a flexible approach to professional development was also critical as clinicians need different opportunities for learning and reflective practice within this setting.

Respect for clinicians' practice and a willingness to engage their knowledge and perspectives has enabled the discussion of fit and sustainability within this practice setting. Clinicians embrace the opportunity to refresh and re-engage psychotherapeutic practice in this setting and view SST as offering this opportunity.

Note

1 Lived experience workers are people employed to use their personal experience of mental health distress to aid others.

References

Graham, I.D., Logan, J., Harrison, M.B., Straus, S.E., Tetroe, J., Caswell, W., & Robinson, N. (2006). Lost in knowledge translation: Time for a map? *Journal of Continuing Education in the Health Professions*, 26(1), 13–24.

Lau, G., Meredith, P., Bennett, S., Crompton, D., & Dark, F. (2017). A capability framework to develop leadership for evidence-informed therapies in publicly-funded mental health services. *International Journal of Public Leadership*, 13(3), 151–165.

Le Gros, J., Wyder, M., & Brunelli, V. (2018). Single session work: Implementing brief intervention as routine practice in an acute care mental health assessment service. *Australasian Psychiatry*, 27(1), 21–24.

Young, J. & Rycroft, P. (1997). Single session therapy: Capturing the moment. *Psychotherapy in Australia*, 4(1), 18–23.

Young, J., Rycroft, P., & Weir, S. (2006). *Continuing Education Workbook: Single Session Work*. Melbourne, VIC, Australia: The Bouverie Centre, La Trobe University.

10 One-Off Sessions to Address a Waitlist: A Pilot Study

*Henry von Doussa, Kelly Tsorlinis,
Kate Cordukes, Julie Beauchamp,
and Jennifer E. McIntosh*

The commitment to seek help and the motivation to change is highest when families first call a service (Schleider, Dobias, Sung, & Mullarkey, 2020). With ever-growing demand for mental health services, long wait-lists are common, and can be detrimental for a family seeking change. In search of an answer to enhanced accessibility and earliest engagement, The Bouverie Centre's Clinical Program embarked on a pilot project providing a "one-off session" to families on our waitlist. While the Centre has a long history of utilizing service delivery models responsive to families' help-seeking behavior, such as single session therapy (SST; see Young, Weir, & Rycroft, 2012; Young, Rycroft, & Weir, 2014; Young et al., 2018), the provision of a one-off session as a waitlist management strategy was untested in the service.

Background

Client waitlists are a perennial problem in mental health services, both internationally and in the local Australian context. Long waitlists have been shown to have negative impacts for clients and service providers alike. They are associated with reduced service accessibility (Iskra, Deane, Wahlin, & Davis, 2018; Boyhan, 1996); dropouts and negative attitudes toward the service for prospective clients (Ewen, Mushquash, Mushquash, Bailey, Haggarty, & Stones, 2018); and stress for therapists trying to manage over-demand for services (Lan, Lin, Yan, & Tang, 2018; Lloyd, Mckenna, & King, 2005). Recent research in both adult and youth contexts, however, has shown that timely interventions with brief therapy approaches have positive impacts on service accessibility and, in turn, accelerate opportunities for families to address and often resolve presenting issues (Schleider et al., 2020; Ewen et al., 2018).

In the context of ever-increasing service demand, these findings were a driver for The Bouverie Centre to seek ways to respond immediately to referrals so as to "capture the moment" (Rycroft & Young, 1997; Hoyt & Talmon, 2014) and take advantage of the window of opportunity for client change while offering a more consumer-friendly service. Keeping families engaged and providing a responsive holding service for clients on the waitlist became a key concern for the organization. In 2016, the Centre began a waitlist process for the first time. The waitlist was capped at 30 families to keep it manageable, in the hope that families would not wait more than three months. Nevertheless, we still had many families waiting beyond three months, given that returning families also sought access.

In an attempt to address waitlist problems, one-off sessions based on single session thinking were piloted. SST, of course, was not new to The Bouverie Centre. A single session family therapy approach, based initially on the work of Talmon (1990, 1993) and the Dalmar Centre (Price, 1994), had been offered to families since 1994 (Boyhan, 1996; O'Neill, 2017; Young et al., 2018). However, over time, the demand for our service grew (approximately 1,000 intake calls for 200 new places per year) and hence the pilot to offer one-off sessions to client families on the waitlist was initiated. The evaluation undertaken as part of the pilot research focused primarily on whether one-off sessions were an effective way to address the waitlist. Secondly, we focused on the feasibility and acceptability of this approach with families, including how they responded to the invitation of a one-off session without the guarantee of immediate follow-up sessions.

Method

During the month of October 2018, one-off sessions were offered to all 37 families on our Clinical Program waitlist. Generally, this session was conducted by a single therapist and sometimes with two co-therapists, and ran for about 90 minutes. Three family therapists took part in the pilot, all trained and experienced in Single Session Therapy (SST).

The one-off sessions were guided by the following SST principles (Rycroft & Young, 1997; also see Chapter 3 of this volume):

- Making the most of the time available
- Focusing on clients' hopes and goals for change
- Establishing the clients' priorities
- Staying on track
- Checking in with the clients about the focus of the session
- Investigating attempted solutions and listening for clients' resources
- Offering towards the end of the session any thoughts or reflections, clear feedback, and direct tentative advice
- Listening clearly for client responses to therapist feedback and allowing for any last-minute issues that the family might raise.

At the end of the one session, a follow-up phone call with a nominated family member (usually the person who made the initial contact) was planned. The call was usually 14 days after the session, with the purpose of determining if the family wished to remain on the waitlist for further therapy, if the one-off session in itself had been enough to address their presenting issues, or if referral to another service was needed. No opportunity for further waitlist sessions was offered as part of the pilot, unless risk issues were identified in the one-off session – in which case they were responded to immediately, as they would be in ongoing work. If families declined a one-off session, they simply remained on the waitlist in their current position, and if they accepted the offer of a one-off session and chose to return to the waitlist after the one-off session, they also retained their position on the waitlist.

For all participating families, the follow-up phone call also included post-session evaluation questions. These questions corresponded with the pre-session questionnaire that all families complete before the first session of our regular family therapy service. In the main, questions ask family members to describe their most significant problems, what is working well in their family and what they would like addressed, including any specific questions they would like answered during the session.

Summarized group data of the participating families are given in Table 10.1.

Table 10.1 Participant Families (figures rounded, may not total 100%)

Total families on waitlist offered a one-off session	Families who accepted	Families who declined	Families attending the allocated session	Families who did not show for allocated session
37	33 (89.1%)	4 (10.8%)	25 (75.7%)	8 (24.2%)

Results

We will first report what participants indicated were their reasons for choosing to attend the offered one-off session, then will report what attendees said were their experiences of the sessions.

Reasons for Accepting the One-Off Session

The 33 families who accepted a one-off session were asked to identify the reasons they agreed to participate in the one-off session rather than wait for the regular family therapy service. Predominately, the family member who had initiated the session responded to the question on behalf of the family group (70% mothers; 30% fathers). The following themes emerged:

- Wanting to be seen as soon as possible
- Hoping to address issues in just the one session

- Having had therapy before at The Bouverie Centre and wanting to return as soon as possible
- Wanting to see what the service is like
- Being in crisis
- Simply a good opportunity.

The 25 families who ultimately attended a session presented with an array of family conflict and communication problems between family members, or problems related to a parent with a mental illness, and/or associated with a child's behavior or mental health concerns. Twenty-four of the 25 presentations were categorized by intake staff as "complex"; that is, a range of co-occurring presenting issues including bipolar disorder, schizophrenia, PTSD, family violence, and/or drug and alcohol issues. For 16 of the 25 families, "trauma" was the key presenting issue.

Feedback from Families After the One-Off Session

In the two-week post-session follow-up phone call, families were asked about their experience of the one-off session, including what they liked and disliked about the session, and whether the session helped them to resolve the problems they brought to the session. The majority (88%) of respondents (22 of 25 families) who attended the one-off session reported that the session was a helpful and positive experience.

The major themes were:

- Improved sense of being valued and not judged
- Increased safety
- Immediate improvement in communication
- Being able to see the bigger picture
- Reduced conflict.

Three families (12%) reported negative responses. The key themes were lack of change and the need for more assistance than a one-off single session could provide. All of these families presented with severe, acute difficulties, including recent hospitalization of a family member due to mental illness.

Families were also asked to identify some of the practical ways the one-off session had helped in resolving the problems they brought to the session. Families highlighted:

- The practical nature of the session
- Resources and communication tools learned
- Safe experimentation through role play with different strategies for communicating
- Reframing of and novel approach to problems.

Return to Waitlist: Pilot and Comparison Clients

Of the 25 families who attended a one-off session, 24 (96%) elected to return to the waitlist. Only one family reported that the one-off session was enough while on the waitlist. All families were allocated to the regular service for ongoing sessions within 12 weeks. When the time came for their next appointment, four further families (16%) declined an appointment, citing adequate improvement of the initial problem. Thus, for 20% of the initial sample, a single session had met their needs to the extent of their not seeking a further session.

Thirteen of the intervention group families engaged in one further session (52%) and seven families (28%) attended ongoing family therapy.

The total number of client families who decided to have either one or two sessions was eighteen (72%).

To understand more fully the pilot results, we constructed a comparison group of all 25 families who were on the waitlist immediately prior to the pilot, to contrast the sessions utilized in the regular family therapy service where families are offered a single session or ongoing therapy. Both groups presented in the same calendar quarter and had a similar range of presenting issues.

Results for the two groups are presented in Figure 10.1. In the comparison group, four families (16%) attended one session, another four families (16%) attended two sessions, and 17 families (68%) had three or more sessions.

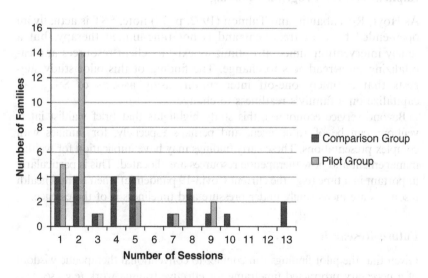

Figure 10.1 Post-waitlist attendance for comparison and pilot families.

Discussion

This pilot study was undertaken to explore the utility of offering a single session to client families on the waitlist, with the major outcome of interest being the perceived adequacy of a timely early intervention in the single session modality, and associated economies of service. We found that the waitlist session did not reduce the waitlist, but for most families, it did attenuate the subsequent length of treatment, and reduced numbers of families seeking more than two sessions.

Only one family in the intervention group left the waitlist after the single session. This finding differs from other non-waitlist studies in the SST literature (Hoyt, Bobele, Slive, Young, & Talmon, 2018; Hoyt, Rosenbaum, & Talmon, 1992) and prior Bouverie Centre SST research (Boyhan, 1996; O'Neill, 2017; O'Neill & Rottem, 2012) that found 50% of families did not require further therapy after one session, even when offered additional sessions. Our finding that only one family left the waitlist may be related to the difference between the non-waitlist literature cited above where families were offered a single session *alongside* the offer of further sessions (at the families' choice), and the time-limited "one-off" session offered to the pilot group. Findings may also reflect reluctance to lose a valued place on a long waitlist, given families in the intervention group had been waiting for several months prior to being offered the one-off session.

The data show that when early, timely sessions are offered, the total treatment period is reduced.

Implications for Program Planning

As Hoyt, Rosenbaum, and Talmon (1992, p. 75) note, SST is actually an open-ended form of treatment and is not time-limited therapy, but a timely intervention aimed at optimizing existing client resources and capitalizing on a readiness to change. The finding of this pilot study suggests that a timely one-off intervention, using aspects of SST, can capitalize on a family's readiness to change.

Beyond service economies, this study highlights that brief waitlist interventions can be of value even, and perhaps especially, for families with complex presentations. These early findings may have implication for waitlist management and how therapeutic resources are allocated. This is particularly important in a time (e.g., the current Covid-19 pandemic) when mental health resources are increasingly under pressure and timeliness is of the essence.

Future Research

Given that the pilot findings run counter to conventional therapeutic wisdom of a necessary protracted timeframe for effective trauma work (e.g., see van der Kolk, 2003; Courtois, 2004; Perry, 2008), there is a need to test the assumption that families who did not return after one or two sessions had their needs met; and to identify those families for whom this was not true. Follow-up research may also investigate "dosage" effects on waitlist management, for example, for whom two sessions may be more helpful than one, and whether two sessions may give families confidence to work on deeper issues and set more significant goals than one session permits. Additionally, mechanisms driving the attenuated treatment period following a timely one-off session could be articulated through depth case studies.

Conclusion

This pilot study supports the value of a one-off session for families on the waitlist. Using elements from SST can help to meet the aims of making therapy more responsive, accessible, and timely; provide early containment of family distress; and shorten the subsequent total length of treatment.

References

Boyhan, P.A. (1996). Clients' perceptions of single session consultations as an option to waiting for family therapy. *Australian and New Zealand Journal of Family Therapy, 17*(2), 85–96.

Briere, J.N., & Scott, C. (2014). *Principles of Trauma Therapy: A Guide to Symptoms, Evaluation, and Treatment (DSM-5 Update)*. Los Angeles, CA: SAGE.

Courtois, C.A. (2004). Understanding complex trauma, complex reaction, and treatment approaches. *Psychotherapy: Theory, Research, Practice, and Training, 41*(4), 412–425.

Ewen, V., Mushquash, A.R., Mushquash, C.J., Bailey, S.K., Haggarty, J.M., & Stones, M.J. (2018). Single-session therapy in outpatient mental health services: Examining the effect on mental health symptoms and functioning. *Social Work in Mental Health, 16*(5), 573–589.

Hoyt, M.F., Bobele, M., Slive, A., Young, J., & Talmon, M. (Eds.). (2018). *Single-Session Therapy by Walk-In or Appointment: Administrative, Clinical, and Supervisory Aspects of One-at-a-Time Services*. New York: Routledge.

Hoyt, M.F., Rosenbaum, R., & Talmon, M. (1992). Planned single-session psychotherapy. In S.H. Budman, M.F. Hoyt, & S. Friedman (Eds.), *The First Session in Brief Therapy* (pp. 59–86). New York: Guilford Press.

Hoyt, M.F., & Talmon, M. (Eds.). (2014). *Capturing the Moment: Single Session Therapy and Walk-In Services*. Bethel, CT: Crown House Publishing.

Iskra, W., Deane, F.P., Wahlin, T., & Davis, E.L. (2018). Parental perceptions of barriers to mental health services for young people. *Early Intervention in Psychiatry, 12*(2), 125–134.

Lan, Y.L., Lin, Y.C., Yan, Y.H., & Tang, Y.P. (2018). Relationship between work stress, workload, and quality of life among rehabilitation professionals. *International Journal of Healthcare and Medical Sciences, 4*(6), 105–110.

Lloyd, C., McKenna, K., & King, R. (2005). Sources of stress experienced by occupational therapists and social workers in mental health settings. *Occupational Therapy International, 12*(2), 81–94.

O'Neill, I. (2017). What's in a name? Clients' experiences of single session therapy. *Journal of Family Therapy, 39*(1), 63–79.

O'Neill, I., & Rottem, N. (2012). Reflections and learning from an agency-wide implementation of single session work in family therapy. *Australian and New Zealand Journal of Family Therapy, 33*(1), 70–83.

Perry, B.D. (2008). Child maltreatment: A neurodevelopmental perspective on the role of trauma and neglect in psychopathology. In T.P. Beauchaine & S.P. Hinshaw (Eds.), *Child and Adolescent Psychopathology* (pp. 93–128). New York: Wiley.

Price, C. (1994). Open days: Making family therapy accessible in working class suburbs. *Australian and New Zealand Journal of Family Therapy, 15*(4), 191–196.

Rosenbaum, R., Hoyt, M.F., & Talmon, M. (1992). Planned single-session psychotherapy. In S.H. Budman, M.F. Hoyt, & S. Friedman (Eds.), *The First Session in Brief Therapy* (pp. 59–86). New York: Guilford Press.

Rycroft, P., & Young, J. (1997). Single session therapy: Capturing the moment. *Psychotherapy in Australia, 4*(1), 18–23.

Schleider, J.L., Dobias, M.L., Sung, J.Y., & Mullarkey, M.C. (2020). Future directions in single-session youth mental health interventions. *Journal of Clinical Child & Adolescent Psychology, 49*(2), 264–278.

Stalker, C.A., Riemer, M., Cait, C.A., Horton, S., Booton, J., Josling, L., ... Zaczek, M. (2016). A comparison of walk-in counseling and the wait list model for delivering counseling services. *Journal of Mental Health, 25*(5), 403–409.

Talmon, M. (1990). *Single-Session Therapy: Maximizing the Effect of the First (and Often Only) Therapeutic Encounter.* San Francisco: Jossey-Bass.

Talmon, M. (1993). *Single-Session Solutions: A Guide to Practical: Effective and Affordable Therapy.* Reading, MA: Addison-Wesley.

van der Kolk, B.A. (2003). The neurobiology of childhood trauma and abuse. *Child and Adolescent Psychiatric Clinics, 12*(2), 293–317.

Young, J. (2018). Single-session therapy: The misunderstood gift that keeps on giving. In M.F. Hoyt, M. Bobele, A. Slive, J. Young, & M. Talmon (Eds.) *Single-Session Therapy by Walk-In or Appointment* (pp. 40–58). New York: Routledge.

Young, J., Rycroft, P., & Weir, S. (2014). Implementing single session therapy: Wisdoms from Down Under. In M.F. Hoyt & M. Talmon (Eds.), *Capturing the Moment: Single Session Therapy and Walk-In Services* (pp. 121–140). Bethel, CT: Crown House Publishing.

Young, J., Weir, S., & Rycroft, P. (2012). Implementing single session therapy. *Australian and New Zealand Journal of Family Therapy, 33*(1), 84–97.

11 The Story of the Eastside Family Centre: 30 Years of Walk-in Single Session Therapy

Nancy McElheran

There is compelling evidence that walk-in single session therapy is efficient and effective in meeting the immediate need(s) of a broad spectrum of people in today's society (Hoyt & Talmon, 2014; Hoyt, Bobele, Slive, Young, & Talmon, 2018). The Eastside Family Centre (EFC), operated by Wood's Homes, in Calgary, Canada, led the way in developing this type of service that is now employed nationally and internationally. Wood's Homes is a nationally accredited and recognized mental health treatment center for children and their families and has been serving the Calgary area since 1914. This chapter will highlight key points in developing a walk-in service for individuals, couples and families of all ages who are seeking more immediate access to mental health services.

Developing the Service

The Eastside Family Centre, launched in 1990, pioneered the development of a community-based walk-in single session approach to the delivery of mental health services in Canada. The idea of an immediately accessible and economically feasible walk-in service, where people could meet with a therapist and receive a single session of therapy (SST) at moments of need, emerged from discussions Wood's Homes' senior management and governing board had with local community, provincial, and political leaders. These discussions focused on developing a service that would address growing concerns about a lack of social-service infrastructure for a rapidly growing, ethnically diverse, and high-needs community on the east side of the city.

A volunteer advisory committee, comprised of local business, police and community leaders assisted in the formation of the walk-in service. This advisory body addressed the Centre's community mandate, its location, and hours of operation. The advisory committee also assisted in consolidating community connections by developing partnerships with key agencies and groups and by highlighting the principles of immediate, affordable and accessible mental health walk-in services as central themes.

Centre staff worked alongside the advisory committee, meeting with local physicians, key school personnel, and community resource center staff. Like-minded community services were invited to utilize space at the Centre, increasing collaboration which in turn created a seamless service delivery system (Slive, MacLaurin, Oakander, & Amundson, 1995). Services such as Wood's Homes' Community Resource Team (CRT), a mobile crisis response team, as well as a local agency offering longer-term therapy to children and families are co-located at the Centre. Recently, the EFC launched an e-therapy service for those who are not able to attend the walk-in but could benefit from a single session of therapy.

In the spring of 2019, the research department of Wood's Homes undertook a cross-Canada web search of walk-in single session mental health services in Canada. The web search uncovered over 200 such services. Remarkably, every province and territory had, or was in the process of developing, walk-in and/or single session services in their communities. This web search was followed by phone calls from EFC staff to some of these services. Interestingly, the principles of immediacy, accessibility, and affordability, the foundations of the EFC, are also the principles guiding the development of this type of service elsewhere in Canada. The comments by managers of these services were that their wait lists were impeding care for critical issues and that the development of walk-in and/or single session therapy services at strategic locations both reduced wait lists and significantly addressed the immediate mental health needs/crises of their clientele. Additionally, they expressed that their staff really enjoy the work in that they find that the focus on the most pressing client need requires a new way of thinking about and conducting a therapy session!

These principles are aligned with the original needs identified by the Calgary community: that waitlists for traditional services are lengthy; that emergency rooms are often overcrowded with people who are in a mental health crisis; that clients choose to walk in at a time of significant need; that walking in should not require an appointment; that prior knowledge of the client or their situation is not required; that clients can return as often as they feel is necessary, and that a walk-in single session therapy service is a safety valve for the community (Slive, McElheran, & Lawson, 2008). Recent Canadian research supports this knowledge (Reimer et al., 2018).

The Therapeutic Approach

The foundation of the therapeutic approach at the EFC has been consistent with the therapy research literature over time. For example, Talmon (1990) found that the majority of clients tend to come for only one session. Duncan, Miller, and Sparks (2004) and Bloom (2001) proposed that rapid change is both possible and common in the human experience, and that individuals and families have strengths they have yet to access. They also describe how the greatest opportunity for change comes early in the therapy process and that a therapist's beliefs regarding the possibility of change are communicated to the client in both overt and covert ways.

Central to this approach is the concept that the therapist is a consultant to the client in the spirit of collaboration and mutual respect. The therapist endeavours to create with clients a context that facilitates the client uncovering their own resources as well as ways to utilize them. The therapist offers ideas for the client to consider and the client responds to the therapist regarding the feasibility of the suggestions. Most importantly, clients set the goal(s) based on their need(s) and beliefs regarding how change happens while the therapist creates the context for developing a therapeutic alliance that focuses on the here and now.

Consistent with these ideas are the theoretical perspectives that inform the EFC walk-in SST. As noted by Slive et al. (2008), the model that has evolved over time was developed through practice experience, teaching, and the clinical supervision of others. Integration of theoretical approaches such as systems theory/thinking, postmodernism, social constructivism, solution-focused, narrative, brief approaches, and the clients' theory of change are joined with common factors research to create a flexible, client-centered approach to each session (Boscolo, Cecchin, Hoffman, & Penn, 1987; Hoyt 1998; White & Epstein 1990; Hubble, Duncan, & Miller, 1999; Lipchik, 2002). Since no one model fits every client, the job of the therapist is to uncover what the client will find most useful in the current session and to find ways to co-create workable solutions to the immediate presenting concern. Consistent with the literature and the EFC strengths-based team approach, commendations are offered during and at the end of each session that highlight the client's strengths, resources, and capacity for change (Houger-Limacher, 2003; McElheran & Harper-Jaques, 1994).

Creating a consistent format for each session is valuable for both the client and the therapy team, providing structure for each session that all find useful. Not all walk-in SST services in Canada and elsewhere have adopted a team approach. Nor do they offer learning for students or professional volunteers. Rather, they offer services based on their staffing capacity and offer consultation to one another on an as-needed basis. The EFC has, however, employed therapy teams from the outset.

Guided by the work of the Milan group (Boscolo et al., 1987), each session has five parts:

- The *pre-session* where the therapy team receives information from the person who has walked in, enabling it to focus on what the client perceives as their most pressing issue

- The *session* itself where the therapist guides the process, using therapeutic questions, to uncover what would be most useful
- The *inter-session* where a team of three or four professional colleagues hear the client's story and offers suggestions to the therapist regarding interventions that might be helpful
- The *intervention* where the client gets to hear and consider what the team has offered regarding possible ideas/solutions including an action they can incorporate into their day-to-day life if they wish. As noted above, consistent with the literature and the EFC strengths-based team approach, commendations are offered during and at the end of each session (Houger-Limacher, 2003; McElheran & Harper-Jaques, 1994)
- The *post-session de-briefing* where the team reflects upon the fit of its ideas with the client's needs and makes suggestions for future sessions should the person return.

EFC Infrastructure

The supportive infrastructure of the EFC, proven to be effective over time (Stewart et al., 2018), includes both administrative and therapy staff. Hours of operation – six days/week, including evening hours – are structured to optimize accessibility for clients.

Clients walk in, are greeted by a receptionist, and are asked to complete a user-friendly form that asks for some demographic information, followed by questions concerning what the client wants from this particular session, what strengths and resources they see themselves bringing, what would be most useful for them to leave their session thinking about, and what would define success for them. Completion of this form varies from 5 to 15 minutes depending on how detailed clients are with their information. Some clients ask for specific advice, while most indicate they would like to see positive change to their current situation.

In addition to questions asking clients to specify what they want from their session, clients are asked to rate their distress. In recent years, forms have been added that ask clients to rate their anxiety, depression, and potential for risk of self-harm. Clients are also asked if they would like information regarding domestic violence. It has been found that having clients address these specific mental health and safety issues early, over and above what they request, assists the therapy team with its pre-session briefing. When identified, risk and safety issues are addressed directly by the therapist and team with a solution to the risk issue(s) emerging from the session. The solution could include the involvement of family members and/or Emergency Medical Services (EMS) assisting a client with getting to a hospital if that is required. When there is a child at risk, local Children's Services authorities are involved and assist with making a decision as to the most appropriate intervention. In situations where domestic violence is an immediate concern, clients are assisted with attending a shelter. In less urgent situations, safety plans are created that fit with the clients' need.

Therapy Teams

Therapy teams are comprised of three to four graduate-level professionals from varied backgrounds, including Wood's Homes' clinical staff and graduate-level students receiving clinical supervision. Typically a team is comprised of two paid staff/consultants and two students/volunteers. Staff and students come from the disciplines of social work, psychology, nursing, family therapy, and medicine. In addition are graduate-level community professionals who donate their time to the service in exchange for opportunities of working with a diverse team to advance their single session skills.

Each team works a four-hour shift and has a clinical lead (shift coordinator) who has advanced knowledge of walk-in SST. This clinician holds responsibility for the quality of the service delivered, including the management of risk/safety issues as noted above. Psychiatric consultants, available several days per week, supervise the work of the medical residents and provide consultation to the therapy teams. The psychiatrist's role is limited to consultation, as distinct from providing formal psychiatric diagnoses and/or prescribing medications. Clients are referred to community doctors for this purpose. The clinical energy that is created by this team diversity adds to the conversation and potentiates favorable outcomes for the client (McElheran, Stewart, Soenen, Newman, & MacLaurin, 2014).

Sessions are frequently conducted using a one-way mirror where team members observing from behind the mirror designate one member who phones in questions to the therapist as needed. Clients are asked at the outset if they would like the opportunity of a mirror team. Clients who prefer a no-mirror session still receive a team consultation as the therapist conducting the session meets with the team to present the issues raised by the client and generate an intervention. Outcome data indicate that both mirror and no-mirror consultations are highly rated by clients, with particular satisfaction for the former (Wood's Homes Research Department, 2019).

Supervision and Training

The EFC is a leading graduate and post-graduate training center. Local university faculties, including Social Work, Psychology, and Medicine, report that students receive a rich experience and solid preparation for becoming therapists following their supervised experiences. Stewart et al. (2018) note that students at the EFC learn therapy skills that meet their goals, have the opportunity of participating in multi-disciplinary teams, and receive supervision specific to their respective disciplines.

EFC senior management and staff have emphasized the importance of reciprocity in relationships with the community. This has included health professionals who have graduate degrees and a desire to learn this therapy model. Professionals who donate their time to the walk-in service are called volunteer community therapists; they do this in exchange for teaching and/or supervision. While they may not have an assigned supervisor, volunteer community therapists are guided and/or supervised by an EFC staff member, depending on their need and request.

The training process includes students and volunteers being offered selected readings specific to the EFC walk-in SST model and research, followed by conversations that focus on the application of theory to the walk-in SST practice. They observe a minimum of four sessions from behind the one-way mirror, observing clients who are presenting with a range of concerns across the severity, risk, and acuity spectrum. The student/volunteer has the opportunity to hear senior staff asking questions of the therapist leading the session that highlight key aspects of the client situation. The student/volunteer also observes the development of the collaborative relationship with the client that is central to the model. This experience is often followed by conversations, either in the inter-session break or post session, that provide additional learning.

The five-part session has many benefits, including the opportunity for the student/volunteer to participate in team conversation either at pre-session, during the intersession break or at the post-session de-briefing. Depending on the skill level of the individual trainee, this is another opportunity for learning, based on their knowledge and experience. Once the student/volunteers (and staff overseeing their work) are comfortable and confident with the process, they are supported to conduct initial sessions with therapy staff who supervise from behind the mirror. A tool called the Supervisor Evaluation Form (Matheson & McElheran, 2016), assists with highlighting the development of the skills needed by a particular student and can be used as required with a volunteer. As the student/volunteer becomes more proficient and comfortable with conducting sessions and consulting with the therapy team, the supervisor/team becomes less specific in helping with case conceptualization. The goal of this training/supervision model is for the student/volunteer to become a fully contributing member of the therapy team.

Training programs for professionals interested in establishing walk-in SST and/or SST approaches in their agencies have been offered at the EFC and across the country since 1994, when a year-long certificate training program was provided to a multi-disciplinary group of agency leaders and physicians. Since then, workshops that vary in length and intensity from a half-day overview to a full-week intensive with both theory and supervised practice components are offered to local agencies and across Canada, both online and in person. A recent example is a week-long workshop for a community agency that is launching an SST by-appointment service and wanted to benefit from the knowledge and experience of the EFC walk-in approach. Another example is an online teaching workshop that was offered to a group in northern Canada.

Research Highlights

Wood's Homes developed a research department in the early 2000s that gathers and analyzes data for all of the agency's programs. An outcome study conducted in 2015 indicated the EFC serves the acute needs of an ethnically diverse population and that the therapy received significantly reduces distress, addresses the most pressing client concern(s), and offers useful ideas for clients to take away. The data indicate that about 40% of clients return. They report they find the structure and approach to the delivery of the service meets their particular need(s). Clients like the idea of "walking in" for a session at moments of need, and many indicate they would attempt to access hospital emergency departments if the EFC walk-in were not available. Levels of service satisfaction have remained consistently high over time (Stewart et al., 2018). These findings, as well as earlier studies (e.g. Hoffart & Hoffart, 1994), indicate that the community has found the EFC walk-in SST to be efficient, effective, and a much needed service.

Acknowledgment

Many thanks to my good colleagues and friends, Ann Lawson, Dr. Arnie Slive, and Sandy Harper-Jaques for their astute comments. Thanks also to Harry Park, Dan Neuls, Chris Scissons, Janet Stewart, and Drs. Maureen Pennington and Margie Oakander for their valuable contributions over time.

References

Bloom, B.L. (2001). Focused single session psychotherapy: A review of the clinical and research literature. *Brief Treatment and Crisis Intervention, 1*(1),75–86.

Boscolo, L., Cecchin, G., Hoffman, L., & Penn, P. (1987). *Milan Systemic Family Therapy: Conversations in Theory and Practice.* New York: Basic Books.

Duncan, B.L., Miller, S.D., & Sparks, J. (2004). *The Heroic Client: A Revolutionary Way to Improve Effectiveness Through Client-Directed, Outcome Informed Therapy.* San Francisco: Jossey-Bass.

Hoffart B., & Hoffart, I. (1994). *Program Evaluation of Eastside Family Centre.* Calgary, AB, Canada: Synergy Research Group.

Houger-Limacher, L. (2003). *Commendations: The Healing Potential of One Family Systems Nursing Intervention.* (Unpublished doctoral thesis). Calgary, AB, Canada: University of Calgary.

Hoyt, M.F. (Ed.) (1998). *The Handbook of Constructive Therapies*. San Francisco: Jossey-Bass.

Hoyt, M.F., Bobele, M., Slive, A., Young, J., & Talmon, M. (Eds). (2018). *Single-Session Therapy by Walk-In or Appointment: Administrative, Clinical and Supervisory aspects of One-at-a-Time Services*. New York: Routledge.

Hoyt, M.F., & Talmon, M. (Eds.). (2014). *Capturing the Moment: Single Session Therapy and Walk-In Services*. Wales: Crown House Publishing.

Hubble, M.A., Duncan, B.L., & Miller, S.D. (Eds). (1999). *The Heart and Soul of Change: What Works in Therapy*. Washington, DC: APA Books.

Lipchik, E. (2002). *Beyond Technique in Solution-Focused Therapy*. New York: Guilford Press.

Matheson, J., & McElheran, N. (2016). *Supervision Evaluation Form*. Calgary, AB, Canada: Wood's Homes.

McElheran, N., & Harper-Jaques, S. (1994). Commendations: A resource intervention for clinical practice. *Clinical Nurse Specialist, 8*(1), 7–10.

McElheran, N., Stewart, J., Soenen, D., Newman, J., & MacLaurin, B. (2014). Walk-in single session therapy at the Eastside Family Centre. In M.F. Hoyt & M. Talmon (Eds.), *Capturing the Moment: Single Session Therapy and Walk-In Services* (pp. 177–194). Bethel, CT: Crown House Publishing.

Reimer, M., Stalker, C., Dittmer, L., Cait, C.A., Horton, S., Kermani, N., & Booton, J. (2018). The walk-in counseling model of service delivery: Who benefits most. *Canadian Journal of Community Mental Health, 37*(2), 29–47.

Slive, A., & Bobele, M. (Eds.). (2011). *When One Hour is All You Have: Effective Therapy for Walk-In Clients*. Phoenix, AZ: Zeig, Tucker & Theisen.

Slive, A., & Bobele, M. (2018). The three top reasons why walk-in/single sessions make perfect sense. In M.F. Hoyt, M. Bobele, A. Slive, J. Young, & M. Talmon (Eds.), *Single-Session Therapy by Walk-In or Appointment: Administrative, Clinical, and Supervisory Aspects of One-at-a-Time Services* (pp. 27–39). New York: Routledge.

Slive, A., McElheran, N., & Lawson, A. (2008). How brief does it get? Walk-in single session therapy. *Journal of Systemic Therapies, 27*, 5–22.

Slive, A., MacLaurin, B., Oakander, M., & Amundson, J. (1995). Walk-in single sessions: A new paradigm in clinical service delivery. *Journal of Systemic Therapies, 14*, 3–11.

Stewart, J., McElheran, N., Park, H., Oakander, M., MacLaurin, B., Jing Fang, C., & Robinson, A. (2018). Twenty-five years of walk-in single sessions at the Eastside Family Centre: Clinical and research dimensions. In M.F. Hoyt, M. Bobele, A. Slive, J. Young, & M. Talmon (Eds.), *Single-Session Therapy by Walk-In or Appointment: Administrative, Clinical, and Supervisory Aspects of One-at-a-Time Services* (pp. 72–90). New York: Routledge.

Talmon, M. (1990). *Single-Session Therapy: Maximizing the Effect of the First (and Often Only) Therapeutic Encounter*. San Francisco: Jossey-Bass.

White, M., & Epstein, D. (1990). *Narrative Means to Therapeutic Ends*. New York: Norton.

Wood's Homes Research Department. (2019). *Eastside Family Centre Wood's Homes Outcome Measurements (WHOM). Report: January–December 2019*. Calgary, AB, Canada: Wood's Homes.

12 Embedding Single Session Family Consultation in a National Youth Mental Health Service: headspace[1]

Suzanne Fuzzard

headspace[2] is a National Youth Mental Health Service that commenced in 2006 with funding from the Australian federal government of the day and continues to receive bipartisan support. The vision for headspace was to provide a one-stop shop for young people (ages 12–25 years) with mild to moderate mental health concerns in order to provide early intervention and community engagement and awareness around mental health issues (Rickwood et al., 2019). headspace has grown to having 150 sites established across Australia, with many sites receiving additional primary health money to provide services to young people presenting with complex care needs and at risk of developing serious mental health issues.

In 2013, I commenced my journey into headspace when I took on the position of Clinical Lead for headspace Murray Bridge in rural South Australia. As a clinical family therapist coming into a youth mental health service, I was surprised to notice families sitting in the waiting room or doing drop-offs in the car park and rarely being invited into the room. I questioned my colleagues across the headspace network as to why many did not include the families in the young persons' care. Most commented that their job was to work with the young person and be youth centered. They seemed to suggest that in order to be youth centered you had to be family excluding. Many noted they did not have any training in working with families and in fact their youth training had oriented them toward seeing the family as often the problem in a young person's life. They feared how including the family might jeopardize their relationship and alliance with the young person. Many just did not feel confident to work with families and in particular how they would deal with the conflict that might arise in the session. Those that did see families described a process of inviting a family in for some assessment information, then having them leave the room, and later at the end of a session informing them what had occurred in the session (within limits of confidentiality with the young person) and how they could be helpful to the young person. It did not appear to be consultative and rarely invited family members to discuss what they themselves might need in order to be the best support for their young person.

When headspace National created an opportunity for internal staff to put forward an idea for a new initiative grant, I decided to apply around the idea of increasing family inclusive practices within the headspace service. Relationships and interactions between people have been the central theme across all my 30-plus years of working, whether it was in mental health, community health, or the domestic violence sector. Professional working relationships have also been equally important. It was from my longstanding connection to The Bouverie Centre and the staff who worked there that it became clear that their Single Session Family Consultation (SSFC) framework would be ideal to pilot in a headspace context. My first contact with Single Session Therapy (SST) had occurred in 2002 when I was working in a busy inner-Melbourne health service and the manager of our team decided to trial single session therapy days, offering clients on the waitlist the opportunity to have a single session. All staff were trained in SST and we worked in pairs offering SST for a full day each week. What has stayed with me most about this experience is my first client in SST. A woman in her 50s, with a life history of contact with the tertiary mental health services – inpatient and outpatient. What remains with me was not what we did in the session but in fact her comment to us that day: that she of all people had been invited into a single session and as such we must have held a belief that she, a long-term mental health patient, could be helped in merely one session. I often reflect that if this woman took nothing more from the session than the message that we believed she had the resources and skills to live her life with just a small amount of intervention, this was an extremely helpful session! Thus, began my passion for single session work and the power of brief interventions. This, combined with my belief in working with people's social network, has made Single Session Family Consultation an ideal fit for me and I believed an ideal fit for headspace.

Why Did I Think SSFC Was So Ideal?

There were several reasons:

1. SSFC offered a framework in which clinicians could still use their trained models and skills when working with young people and families. This framework gave nervous clinicians a structure in which to conduct the session and draws on single session therapy skills to manage the session. (Please see Chapter 5 for more regarding the SSFC model)
2. It was not promoted as "family therapy" but rather as a meaningful family meeting that was consultative and sought to provide focused assistance around the goals of the young person and the family members in a timely manner

3. It is a framework that is do-able and very teachable to workers from a variety of professional backgrounds. It could be modified for online delivery in part, allowing for sustainability given the headspace workforce changed regularly

4. Outcomes are measurable – client satisfaction is the key, meeting clients' nominated goals for the session being the overall aim

5. Since getting the whole family together can be logistically challenging, focusing energy on trying to have a *single* session seemed more achievable for many families and practitioners. Often a young person and/or the family were reticent to have a family session – offering this as a *one-off* gave many the opportunity to try it out without any further "strings attached"

6. It enables headspace sites to position themselves as services that worked meaningfully with families in the care of young people without identifying themselves as a specialist family therapy service and risking the clinicians' sense of working outside of their scope of practice. (See Chapter 5 for further description of the Pyramid of Care.)

The key component in getting such a project off the ground for a large national organization was to pilot it first. It was important to not only trial the framework for acceptability for clients but also for the workforce. We needed to establish evidence to support its usefulness for young people and families, to show that young people did not feel alienated from the service or their worker in the process of attending an SSFC. We needed to establish evidence that workers of all levels of experience and training would be able to take on this training and deliver an SSFC. We also needed to explore how one might embed such a framework into the day-to-day practice of head-space services and ensure it was sustainable despite the staffing changes.

It was essential to have a team of people and organizations to address these needs: we required the expertise of a training team to deliver the framework – The Bouverie Centre, a research team, local headspace centers, and headspace National office input. We all shared an implementation focus as well as specific skills in delivering unique outputs.

So How Did We Go?

Outcomes from 129 youth clients and their family members (N = 191) completing the feedback forms following a SSFC demonstrated mean ratings 5.0 or higher (out of a maximum of 6.0), as shown in Table 12.1.

For practitioners, six months post-training had statistically significant improvements in:

• Practitioners' confidence in providing family interventions and familiarity with approaches to working with families

Table 12.1 Feedback from Clients and Their Families. (All Ratings on a 0–6 Scale.)

	Clients (N = 129)		Family Members (N = 191)	
	Mean	SD	Mean	SD
1. *Subject:* Relationship *Question:* "I felt heard, understood, and respected."	5.0	1.4	5.6	0.8
2. *Subject:* Goals and Topics *Question:* "We worked on and talked about what I wanted to work on and talk about."	5.1	1.3	5.4	0.9
3. *Subject:* Approach or method *Question:* "The therapist's approach is a good fit for me."	5.2	1.1	5.5	1.0
4. *Subject:* Helpfulness *Question:* "Session was helpful in addressing some of my needs."	5.2	1.2	5.4	0.9
5. *Subject:* Overall *Question:* "Overall, today's session was right for me."	5.2	1.1	5.2	1.3

Source: From Poon, Harvey, Fuzzard, and O'Hanlon, 2017; used with permission.

Note: SD = standard deviation.

- Practitioners' perception of significant improvement in organizational support for working with families.

Some themes from the six-month follow-up interviews with practitioners and managers highlighted the following:

- Training and ongoing supervision were important, with an experienced family therapist identified as most advantageous as was managerial (top-down) support in encouraging this work to be part of best practice
- A team approach to practicing was also noted to be helpful in uptake of SSFC by practitioners, with a specific internal worker identified as the champion being the most potent means by which to ensure sustainability
- Support by management and funders to ensure that rooms were big enough to see families and that caseloads were limited, in order to enable a new practice to be adopted.

However, despite these findings, in Australia, due to a significant component of the headspace workforce being private practitioners funded via Medicare, there is limited financial incentive for these practitioners to provide longer sessions that include the family. Much of this workforce is predominantly trained in providing individualized therapies. They receive mental health care plans identifying a diagnosis for the young person that is generally individual pathology such as anxiety and depression.

Nevertheless, as a result of a successful and well-researched pilot study by headspace, ongoing funding was obtained by headspace National from the federal government for a national roll-out across 50 headspace centers in Australia.

What Has Worked and How Has This Occurred?

What has worked and been helpful in embedding SSFC in these headspace centers has been the multiple organizations and layers within the centers, all working together with a strong implementation focus, not merely offering training. The national organization has delivered consistent and strong messages to all the headspace centers regarding the importance of family inclusive practice in the headspace model. SSFC has gained brand recognition across the network as the means by which to achieve this. In order to operate as a headspace service, strict licensing conditions need to be satisfied and one of the criteria is evidence of family-inclusive practice.

Through provision of an online training program, developed by The Bouverie Centre, headspace sites can deliver in-house training on an ongoing basis, thus supporting sustainability. Also, data collection that better recognizes family work has been developed on the national platform.

Moreover, centers are supporting each other in the growth of SSFC. This was made evident in a recent audit exploring how much SSFC was being done in centers. This was found to be higher than the number of centers trained by national office funding.

Where Do the Challenges Lay?

The ongoing challenges observed are around how to sustain staff training internally and build capacity of a workforce predominantly trained in individualistic therapies and long-term work. Online options have been helpful, but for many novice practitioners, family work remains mysterious and frightening and opportunities for face-to-face support and supervision is still crucial. I would suggest family therapists need to consider ways in which their training and skills can be integrated into undergraduate training, seen as common practice rather than a speciality that is considered postgraduate. We might then begin to see practice in services reflect this ideal.

Other challenges include the ways in which services are measured and funding is obtained, both of which currently privilege individual treatment services and a pathologizing of the young person. This creates pressure on clinicians to deliver an individualized service with high targets per day. It also orientates young people, the family, and the services toward seeing the young person as the owner of the problem.

Young people attending a headspace setting come in with as varying a range of issues and concerns as there are young people. All of them, however, exist within a social network, often a *family*. This family, whether considered to be helpful or unhelpful to the young person, is often the group of people that are around that young person most of the time. They often struggle to know how to be helpful in the care of their young person and, unless clinicians are going to take home all of the young people they meet, surely the way we assist young people is to support their social system to be as helpful as possible. SSFC provides clinicians of all training and experience a clear and structured way in which to work meaningfully and collaboratively with young people and their families to meet their goals. It conveys a strong sense of belief in the young person and their social network that they can do this with just a small amount of assistance.

Above all, the Single Session Family Consultation framework builds a sense of success and usefulness around help seeking that is likely to see a young person return when needed.

Notes

1 The opinions expressed herein are those of the author and don't necessarily reflect those of headspace.
2 headspace is branded in lowercase to appeal to youth.

References

Poon, A.W.C., Harvey, C., Fuzzard, S., & O'Hanlon, B. (2017). Implementing a family-inclusive practice model in youth mental health services in Australia. *Early Intervention in Psychiatry*, *13*(3), 1–8.

Rickwood, D., Paraskakis, M., Quin, D., Hobbs, N., Ryall, V., Trethowan, J., & McGorry, P. (2019). Australia's innovation in youth mental health care: The headspace centre model. *Early Intervention in Psychiatry*, *13*(1), 159–166.

Section IV

Single Session Thinking and Practice in Different Clinical Contexts

13 Introducing Single Session Therapy at a University Counseling Center

*Alexandra M. Robinson, Grace Harvey,
Molly McDonald, and Turi Honegger*

Over the past three decades, student mental health centers have noted an increasing demand on services, due to the severity and complexity of presenting concerns and the increase in the number of students accessing services (Center for Collegiate Mental Health, 2020). The requirement for services often surpasses the availability of clinical resources. Recently, the University of California Santa Barbara (UCSB) incorporated Single Session Therapy (SST) as an option to address clinical, student, and organizational needs. We describe the process of implementing SST at our center and offer an explanation of the clinical and organizational adaptations that contributed to its successful implementation at our campus.

Identifying the Need

The year prior to the introduction of SST at UCSB Counseling and Psychological Services, the center implemented a triage system in response to the increasing demand and severity of problems faced by students requesting services. In this system, students were offered a walk-in Brief Assessment (BA). The goal of the BA was to evaluate presenting concerns and help students connect to the most appropriate treatment option(s) based upon their clinical presentation, needs, and resources (see Bratby & Hull-Styles, 2017). Despite increased efficiency, demand continued to surpass clinical availability. Given the need for innovative responses to the "new normal" of college mental health, the SST model was raised during a triage team meeting as a potential solution. One of the postdoctoral fellows, the first author (AMR), had previous SST experience at the Eastside Family Center (EFC) in Calgary, Canada (see Chapter 11 of this volume), which uses the Five-Part (pre-session, session, inter-session consult, intervention delivery, post-session) Milan Model for sessions. She, along with the Clinical Director, Turi Honegger, and the Clinical Coordinator, Grace Harvey, began to identify ways to adapt and implement the EFC SST model for the UCSB counseling center.

Integrating SST with Existing Structures and Organizational Culture

As we considered how to integrate SST with services already offered at our center, it became clear that the BA appointment would serve as the primary referral source. Unlike a typical walk-in model, single sessions are scheduled following a referral from the walk-in BA. To ensure appropriate referrals, we provided training on SST to the whole agency. To our surprise, the training and explanation of SST services was met with significant resistance. Worries were expressed that this model, which was being implemented by primarily white, female therapists, may not be culturally sensitive for traditionally underrepresented and underserved populations (Van Loon, van Schaik, Dekker, & Beekman, 2013). Staff raised concerns that the fairly directive recommendations and inter-session consult, which involves pausing the session for the clinician to meet with a consultation team, could increase the sense of vulnerability, especially amongst Latinx and African American students who had experienced generations of systemic discrimination and betrayal by people in authority. In response to the thoughtful concerns raised, the authors adapted the explanation of SST to be culturally responsive: extra time was devoted at the introduction of each session to explaining confidentiality, the benefit of the consultation was explained, and the therapist spent additional time to answer any other questions or concerns. We also incorporated a multicultural lens in which the therapist makes a conscious effort to understand and respect both cultural and experiential differences (Brown, 2018).

Difficulty in adopting the model due to other unspecified reservations was demonstrated by a few staff members who seemed confused about the model. This resulted in referrals that were not appropriate and/or where the referred client did not receive an accurate description of the service prior to the session. One of the issues that continues to surface is the misconception that the model is an abbreviated substitute for regular therapy rather than a deliberate therapy intervention developed intentionally and based on worldwide data on the benefits of SST (Slive & Bobele, 2011; Green, Correia, Bobele, & Slive, 2011; Hoyt & Talmon, 2014a; Hoyt, Bobele, Slive, Young, & Talmon, 2018; Stewart et al., 2018; Alfred Health, 2020). Following suit from single session pioneers Hoyt and Talmon (2014b; p. 4, italics added), the implementation team realized the agency needed more information to *"view each encounter as a whole, complete in itself."* To increase support and understanding of SST, we continued to engage with staff and leadership about existing research conducted in other agencies and disseminated preliminary data of pre- and post-session outcomes and case examples gathered at our clinic. While some residual skepticism remains, SST has been embraced by the staff as evidenced by a growing SST team and a steady flow of referrals.

Gradual Implementation

Single session services were gradually introduced over a six-month period with only two of the coauthors (AMR and GH) initially offering direct services. This allowed the team to refine the referral process, train other staff through direct observation and debriefing of sessions, and collect outcome data to demonstrate that the SST services were meeting clinical needs. Gradual introduction was also effective in addressing a number of issues: lack of staff trained in SST; uncertainty about how the students would respond; concern over human resource support to administer the service; determining how best to refer students and how best to fit this model into the current system; responding to student diversity; identifying the best way to collect pre- and post-session surveys; scheduling; and gathering of initial data. Once these details were resolved, the agency was ready to launch SST on a larger scale. Leadership further incentivized therapists concerned about their caseload by offering a novel "trade-off" of a routine intake for a single session, so that therapists who joined the SST team would have one fewer intake on their schedule for every single session they offered.

Due to our decision to offer the single session option using the Five-Part Milan Model used at EFC and elsewhere (see Slive & Bobele, 2011), which includes team consultation, one of the most challenging aspects of implementing SST was *scheduling*. With great effort, we were able to identify times in therapists' schedules that would best adapt to a 90-minute block, allowing for a buffer time in our packed schedules. We sought to group at least two sessions at a time, offset by approximately 15 minutes, to optimize the consult team availability for both sessions. (The SST process is described in the next section.)

Refining the Referral Process

To place the student in a position of authority regarding their service options, SST is offered as an option that students can self-select during their BA appointment. Similar to the Stepped Care 2.0 model (Cornish et al., 2017), this empowers students to be engaged in planning their treatment. In presenting SST as a treatment option during the referral portion of the BA, the therapist might say:

> *A lot of people find that just one session is enough for them. You could choose to work on your concern with a Single Session appointment, which is a stand-alone meeting with a therapist focused solely on your goal, and it would be scheduled within the week. If you're interested in this option, I can tell you more.*

For interested students, we further describe the format of the session and support them with identifying their goal for the session:

The first 30 minutes of the session is the time when you and the therapist discuss what has been going on and what you are hoping to get help with. Then, there is a break in the session for 10–15 minutes during which time the therapist will consult with a team of therapists and brainstorm recommendations for you based on your goals. The remainder of the time is used to review the team's ideas with you and hopefully you will find some of the team's ideas helpful!

A small SST information sheet (see Table 13.1), which briefly explains Single Session Therapy, what to expect, and how to make the most of their session, is also provided at the time of referral. Students looking for concrete, immediate steps to address their mental health needs tend to be most interested in SST.

Table 13.1 SST Information Sheet

What is Single Session Therapy?
A goal-oriented therapy session intended to provide you with strategies
  and solutions to help improve your overall mental health and wellness.

What is this service most helpful for?
Students find it useful to help manage a range of concerns such as stress, anxiety,
  depression, situational crisis, grief, difficulty adjusting to college, lifestyle
  concerns, etc.

What should I do to prepare for my appointment?
Come to your appointment with a goal in mind! Arrive at CAPS 15 minutes early
  to allow time for paperwork. Please allow for 90 minutes, including paperwork.

What can I expect during the session?
You will spend the first ~30 minutes discussing the nature of why you are
  here and what you are hoping to get help with. Then, the clinician takes
  10–15 minutes to meet with a consultation team to brainstorm ideas based on
  your goals for the session (believing two heads are better than one!). After
  this, the clinician will return to share the team's thoughts and ideas with you,
  which concludes the session.

Students unfamiliar with the single session approach often ask questions, such as: *"What if I need more than one session?"* to which we reply:

Often, one session is enough. If at the end of the session, you and the therapist determine that ongoing therapy would be beneficial, that will be one of the interventions discussed.

To a similar question: *"Can I see that therapist more than once?"* our reply is:

Each session is one-at-a-time, and after each session it is best to try implementing the strategies for a period of time before returning for more help. If you do return, often you will be working with a different therapist due to the stand-alone nature of the service.

To increase consistency in the referral process and to ensure student-client understanding, we engage in ongoing conversations with the referring therapists. As we have a limited number of sessions to offer, we decided that it was important to identify "appropriate" and "inappropriate" referrals. The most important exclusionary criterion was a preference for ongoing or long-term therapy. Other "inappropriate" referrals at our agency are ambivalence, and no specific goal. This pre-screening referral process seems to be unique to our center as others offering SST have found it difficult to identify appropriate referrals (Young, 2018; Young, Rycroft, & Weir, 2014). Additionally, we instituted a one-week cutoff for scheduling, as we identified a higher rate of no-shows if the appointment is booked more than a week in advance. Unfortunately, what this means is that our SST spots fill quickly, and if we are unable to offer SST as an option we refer student-clients to other available services.

How We Adapted the Five-Part Model

As noted previously, we utilize the EFC model as the basis of our single session structure: each session is treated as a whole therapy, we focus on client-centered theory of change, and we use the Five-Part Milan Model (Boscolo, Cecchin, Hoffman, & Penn, 1987; see Stewart et al., 2018). One of the key shifts in focus using this modality is to emphasize the clients' capacities rather than deficits while focusing on the clients' strengths and resources to assist them in solving their problems (Clements, McElheran, Hackney, & Park, 2011). To illustrate, we include a case study of the third coauthor's (MMcD) first independently conducted SST with a student-client, whom we will name Amber. The therapist is a staff psychologist who adopted the model and joined the team after positive experiences participating on the single session consulting team.

Pre-Session: Paperwork

Upon arrival for her session, Amber was asked to complete pre-session paperwork that was adapted from the intake paperwork used at EFC, along with the Counseling Center Assessment of Psychological Symptoms-34 (Locke et al., 2012), which is a self-report measure of psychological symptoms and distress that is required at all clinical appointments at the agency. The therapist was also able to review the Brief Assessment note ahead of time and, if indicated, organize a colleague with specific expertise (e.g., eating disorders, ADHD, trauma) to be available for the consultation, as we do not have the capability to always refer directly to a single session therapist who has a particular specialty.

Using the intake information collected prior to the start of Amber's session, the therapist knew that Amber was a 20-year-old Chinese American lesbian-identified woman, who was a first-generation college student at the university. Amber's identified goals for the single session included: wanting strategies to cope with family distress; learning how to respond better to her romantic partner; and help with knowing how/ whether to continue contact with a "difficult" parent. Upon reviewing the intake information, the therapist thought to herself, "How is a single session possibly going to be sufficient?" She sought out consultation with AMR and GH prior to beginning the session, during which she received reminders to focus on the student's goals for the session and explore the client's strengths and resiliency factors.

The Session

After a brief consultation with team members, the therapist greeted Amber in the waiting area and escorted her to the office. She introduced the session by orienting Amber to the structure of the single session, both to ensure that the expectation of a one-time session was established and to frame the structure and focus for the hour. She reviewed the intake questionnaire with Amber and asked clarifying questions to better understand Amber's goals and identify where she felt "stuck."

Amber explained that she had a complicated family-of-origin. She reported that her father had been diagnosed with borderline personality disorder and that due to consistent conflict within the home while she was living there, she was repeatedly placed in foster care. Although Amber reported being aware that continued contact with her father was harmful, she felt she needed to maintain contact so that she could have access to her aunt, who was living with her father. She also expressed concern about behaviors she has enacted in her own romantic relationship that she felt were similar to her father's behaviors (e.g., reactivity, irritability, demanding of attention, etc.). During this portion of the session, it was important for the therapist to maintain a focus on solutions, goals, strengths, and the most recent symptoms in order to obtain only the necessary information while avoiding the temptation to gather too much extraneous data.

Inter-Session

After approximately 30 minutes of discussion, Amber was invited to wait in the lobby while the therapist met with "the consultation team."

Sometimes the team is simply the one available therapist, while at other times as many as five therapists may be available. In this case, the consultation team included three other clinicians. The therapist began the consultation introducing the student's demographics and goal for the session and other relevant information related to presenting concern and case conceptualization. The team discussed where the client was stuck and considered what resources might be helpful and realistic based on the therapist's impressions of the client's readiness for change (Prochaska, Redding, & Evers, 2015). Utilizing a strengths-based focus and client-centered orientation, the team first identified commendations, such as what Amber was already doing well and what the therapist and team appreciated about their experience with her. This format is used to help decrease defensiveness and increase client receptiveness to the team recommendations (Slive & Bobele, 2011). Interventions often include a variety of techniques and resources, handouts, thought restructuring exercises, mindfulness strategies, and psychoeducation. The consultation team identified specific interventions based on Amber's goals:

1. *Commendations for insight, use of resources, and valuing of relationships*
2. *Reading material regarding having parents with personality disorders*
3. *Use of a scale to monitor her distress level in order to manage distress response*
4. *Grounding strategies and soothing rituals*
5. *Normalization and instilling hope that she could re-wire her attachment patterns*
6. *Identification of methods of contact with father associated with the least distress*
7. *Psychoeducation and handouts on effective communication and "fighting fairly."*

To improve the efficiency of the consultation process, our team developed a "handout folder" in a shared drive from which we can readily print a hard copy to give to the student. The folder includes psychoeducational materials as well as information regarding other campus, community, and online resources. It is important to recognize that some therapists are able to adapt to this type of consultation quite effectively, while others need more guidance in order to remain focused on the goal for the session. To standardize the consultation process, we created a reference page (see Table 13.2) for the consultation team with simple intervention guidelines to maximize the effectiveness of the consultation process.

Table 13.2 Inter-Session Consultation Guidelines

Single Session Consultation Structure
1. Clinician highlights student-client's identified goal for the session, which will guide the focus of the interventions. (one to two minutes)
2. Clinician presents summary of case, including what strengths they have and things they've tried. (three to five minutes)
3. Team and clinician first identify commendations: what can we commend this student-client for? What can we validate or normalize? (one to two minutes)
4. Team and clinician identify 2–4 interventions that are in line with student-client's identified goal and strengths. (five to six minutes).
(Team to print/gather handouts as needed while discussion occurs.)

Intervention

After about a 15-minute consultation, the therapist gathered the handouts and printed a "takeaway" page, adapted from The Bouverie Centre (Young, Weir, Rycroft, & Whittle, 2006), to reference recommendations and referrals. She then invited Amber back to the office to share the team's ideas with Amber. While receiving the list of interventions, Amber eagerly wrote down the ideas and strategies on the takeaway page and appeared excited at the handouts/articles printed for her. Prior to leaving, she said, *"I've done a lot of therapy before, and this was the most helpful thing I've ever done!"*

Post-Session Feedback: How Do We Know It Is Working?

At the conclusion of each single session, the student-client is invited to fill out a Post-Session Feedback form (adapted from the Session Rating Scale [SRS]; Duncan et al., 2003). The survey is on a computer in the waiting area and student-clients are asked to "take a minute" to fill it out before they leave. The pre- and post-surveys have been particularly helpful with implementing, justifying, and expanding SST services at our counseling center. Student-client average pre-session distress level indicated on a rating scale is 7.1 (out of a possible 10) with post-session distress reduced to 3.2 (out of possible 10, n = 195). Consistent with our findings, Amber experienced a significant reduction in distress after just one session. Amber's self-reported pre-session distress was 9 (out of 10) and post-session she indicated her distress was 0. She also reported "very high" overall satisfaction with the service. To date, 100% of students (n = 195) who have accessed SST at UCSB reported high or very high satisfaction with the service. As previously mentioned, one of the main concerns with this model amongst our colleagues and leadership was how this model may or may not be appropriate for our diverse campus community. Using the demographic data collected for each student, the feedback received has been overwhelmingly positive, regardless of race, gender, or migration status.

The Team Experience

For many of us, psychotherapy can be an isolating profession. A main benefit of using a team approach is that it affords the opportunity to work closely with our colleagues and learn from each other's expertise in both implementation and consultation. Therapists have expressed appreciation for the direct feedback provided post-session about what worked well and how impactful a single session can be for students. Using the traditional service model, Amber would typically have had a two- to three-week wait for an intake, followed by several appointments. Just as this team had hoped, SST has provided an opportunity for student-clients to access services quickly and capitalize on their existing strengths. Further, it has proved to be a sustainable, positive experience for the clinicians.

References

Alfred Health. (2020). *Child and Youth Mental Health Services (CYMHS)*. Retrieved from https://www.alfredhealth.org.au/services/single-session-family-consultation/.

Bratby, K., & Hull-Styles, M. (2017). The role of triage in a regional university counselling services. *Australia and New Zealand Student Services Association Newsletter*, December, 30–32.

Boscolo, L., Cecchin, G., Hoffman, L., & Penn, P. (1987). *Milan Systemic Family Therapy: Conversations in Theory and Practice*. New York: Basic Books.

Brown, L.S. (2018). *Feminist Therapy* (2nd ed.). Washington DC: APA Books.

Center for Collegiate Mental Health. (2020, January). *2019 Annual Report* (Publication No. STA 20-244).

Clements, R., McElheran, N., Hackney, L., & Park, H. (2011). The Eastside Family Centre: 20 years of single-session walk-in therapy, where we have been and where we are going. In A. Slive & M. Bobele (Eds.), *When One Hour is All You Have* (pp. 109–127). Phoenix, AZ: Zeig, Tucker, & Theisen.

Cornish, P.A., Berry, G., Benton, S., Barros-Gomes, P., Johnson, D., Ginsburg, R., … Romano, V. (2017). Meeting the mental health needs of today's college student: Reinventing services through Stepped Care 2.0. *Psychological Services*, *14*(4), 428–442.

Duncan, B.L., Miller, S.D., Sparks, J.A., Claud, D.A., Reynolds, L.R., & Johnson, L.D. (2003). The Session Rating Scale: Preliminary psychometric properties of a working alliance measure. *Journal of Brief Therapy*, *3*, 3–12.

Green, K., Correia, T., Bobele, M., & Slive, A. (2011). The research case for walk-in single sessions. In A. Slive & M. Bobele (Eds.), *When One Hour is All You Have: Effective Therapy for Walk-In Clients* (pp. 23–36). Phoenix, AZ: Zeig, Tucker, & Theisen.

Hoyt, M.F., Bobele, M., Slive, A., Young, J., & Talmon, M. (Eds.). (2018). *Single-Session Therapy by Walk-In or Appointment: Administrative, Clinical, and Supervisory Aspects of One-at-a-Time Services*. New York: Routledge.

Hoyt, M.F., & Talmon M. (2014a). What the literature says: An annotated bibliography. In M.F. Hoyt & M. Talmon (Eds.), *Capturing the Moment:*

Single-Session Therapy and Walk-In Services (pp. 487–516). Bethel, CT: Crown House Publishing.

Hoyt, M.F., & Talmon, M. (2014b). Editors' introduction: Single session therapy and walk-in services. In M.F. Hoyt & M. Talmon (Eds.), *Capturing the Moment: Single Session Therapy and Walk-In Services* (pp. 1–26). Bethel, CT: Crown House Publishing.

Locke, B.D., McAleavey, A.A., Zhao, Y., Lei, P.-W., Hayes, J.A., Castonguay, L.G., … Lin, Y.-C. (2012). Development and initial validation of the Counseling Center Assessment of Psychological Symptoms–34. *Measurement and Evaluation in Counseling and Development, 45*(3), 151–169.

Prochaska, J.O., Redding, C.A., & Evers, K.E. (2015). The transtheoretical model and stages of change. In K. Glanz, B.K. Rimer, & K.V. Viswanath (Eds.), *Health Behavior: Theory, Research, and Practice* (pp. 125–148). San Francisco: Jossey-Bass.

Stewart, J., McElheran, N., Park, H., Maclaurin, B., Fang, C., Oakander, M., & Robinson, A. (2018). Twenty-five years of walk-in single sessions at the Eastside Family Centre: Clinical and research dimensions. In M.F. Hoyt, M. Bobele, A. Slive, J. Young, & M. Talmon (Eds.), *Single-Session Therapy by Walk-In or Appointment: Administrative, Clinical, and Supervisory Aspects of One-at-a-Time Services* (pp. 72–90). New York: Routledge.

Slive, A., & Bobele, M. (2011). Making a difference in 50 minutes: A framework for walk-in counselling. In A. Slive & M. Bobele (Eds.), *When One Hour is All You Have: Effective Therapy for Walk-In Clients* (pp. 37–63). Phoenix, AZ: Zeig, Tucker, & Theisen.

Slive, A., & Bobele, M. (2014). Walk-in single session therapy: Accessible mental health services. In M.F. Hoyt & M. Talmon (Eds.), *Capturing the Moment: Single Session Therapy and Walk-In Services* (pp. 73–94). Bethel, CT: Crown House Publishing.

Van Loon, A., van Schaik, A., Dekker, J., & Beekman, A. (2013). Bridging the gap for ethnic minority adult outpatients with depression and anxiety disorders by culturally adapted treatments. *Journal of Affective Disorders, 147*, 9–16.

Young, J. (2018). Single-session therapy: The misunderstood gift that keeps on giving. In M.F. Hoyt, M. Bobele, A. Slive, J. Young, & M. Talmon (Eds.), *Single-Session Therapy by Walk-In or Appointment: Administrative, Clinical, and Supervisory Aspects of One-at-a-Time Services* (pp. 40–58). New York: Routledge.

Young, J., Rycroft, P., & Weir, S. (2014). Implementing single session therapy: Practical wisdoms from Down Under. In M.F. Hoyt & M. Talmon (Eds.), *Capturing the Moment: Single Session Therapy and Walk-In Services* (pp. 121–140). Bethel, CT: Crown House Publishing.

Young, J., Weir, S., Rycroft, P., & Whittle, T. (2006). *Single Session Work Implementation Resource Parcel.* Melbourne, Victoria, Australia: The Bouverie Centre.

14 Sign Up, Meet Up, Speak Out: Single Sessions in the Context of Meet-Up Groups

Windy Dryden

For the past six years, I have been running a meet-up group in London from a CBT perspective. A typical group lasts two hours and includes me giving a lecture on a psychological theme and two single sessions where I work with people from the audience (predominantly professional, but with some non-professionals in attendance) who seek help for problems related to the theme of the lecture. In this chapter, I will present data on the themes raised by volunteers and outline how I tend to work in these sessions.

The Context

The single session work that I discuss in this chapter takes place in the context of a meet-up group known as the "UK CBT" Meet-up Group. Meet-up is a service used to organize online groups that host in-person events for people with similar interests. The UK CBT Meet-up Group is for people interested in Cognitive Behavior Therapy and Coaching (CBT) and Rational Emotive Behavior Therapy and Coaching (REBT). Everyone is welcome. Currently, people pay £20 entry fee. This covers the hire of the room and related expenses.

At each meeting, attended by about 50 people, I give a presentation on a psychological theme, followed by two single sessions with volunteers from the audience. Each evening runs for two hours – usually 7 p.m.–9 p.m. with a 15-minute intermission (see Table 14.1).

I see the work that I do in the lectures and sessions as having three functions. First, it has an educational function. It is a form of psychological education where people can learn about a problematic psychological issue (Tables 14.2 and 14.3) and how it can be tackled from a CBT perspective. Second, it has a therapeutic function. Two people per evening are entrusting me with their problems, and I want to be as helpful as I can to them while being mindful that they are discussing these problems in a public setting. Third, it has an entertainment function. My goal is to hold the attention of everyone in the room and to this effect, I introduce humor as much as I can into my lecture and sessions while preserving the seriousness of the work. In what follows, I will focus on the single session work that I do rather than on the lectures that I give.

The Single Sessions

The single sessions that I do follow in the tradition of the public demonstrations carried out by Alfred Adler and Albert Ellis. From 1965–2015, Ellis carried out live demos of REBT in New York in what was called the "Friday Night Workshop" (Ellis & Joffe, 2002) which continues to this day under the name "Friday Night Live" (FNL) with sessions run by leading therapists at the Albert Ellis Institute. The format remains the same, however, with two volunteers from the audience being helped with their "problems in living." Lectures are not given at FNL.

Getting a Volunteer

When people sign up for a UK CBT meeting, they are asked if they have an interest in volunteering as a client. At the meeting, I stress that a volunteer should have a problem relevant to the topic of the lecture that they are keen to address and are willing to do so in front of the audience. Preference is given to someone who has not volunteered before.

Dealing with the Volunteer and the Audience

Before I start, I ask the audience to abide by the ethical rule, "What is seen and heard here, stays here." I ask them to observe silence during the sessions and stress that they will be able to ask the volunteer and me any questions that they wish after the session.

I ask permission from the volunteer to record the session, and they are sent the recording and transcript afterward on request. If the volunteer needs aftercare, I will make some recommendations to them. So far, this has never been necessary, and I have done over 100 demonstrations since June 2012. A few people have volunteered more than once for help with different problems. Table 14.1 presents information about the first 100 sessions that I have conducted and session timings.

Table 14.1 The First 100 Single Sessions in the UK CBT Meet-Up Group: Session Times

• From June, 28, 2012 till October 25, 2018
• 74 females and 26 males

The average time of the session was 16 minutes 31 seconds
Session times ranged from 5 minutes 16 seconds to 29 minutes 46 seconds

• From 5 minutes to 9 minutes 59 seconds...........................5 sessions
• From 10 minutes to 14 minutes 59 seconds..................... 35 sessions
• From 15 minutes to 19 minutes 59 seconds.....................40 sessions
• From 20 minutes to 24 minutes 59 seconds.....................15 sessions
• From 25 minutes to 29 minutes 59 seconds.......................5 sessions

Problems Discussed by Volunteers

At the outset, it is important to realize that the problems discussed by the volunteers will reflect the themes of the lectures that I have given. Tables 14.2 and 14.3 list the problems raised by volunteers by gender.

Table 14.2 Problems Discussed by Volunteers by Gender

Problem	Female	Male
Anger	8	4
Anxiety & Phobia	10	2
Uncertainty	4	2
Lack of Control	4	1
Procrastination	17	4
Relationship Problems	5	3
Self-Esteem Problems	12	2
Other Emotional Problems	14	8
Total	74	26

Table 14.3 Other Emotional Problems by Gender

Problem	Female	Male
Guilt	3	2
Shame	3	3
Hurt	4	2
Jealousy	2	0
Envy	1	1
Obsessive-Compulsive Disorder	1	0
Total	14	8

How I Work in These Demonstration Sessions

In this part of the chapter, I want to provide a sense of how I work during the demonstration sessions. While I will outline a template of the way I work, not all points that I cover will be present in all the demonstration sessions. What I do depends on the time available, the nature of the problem brought by the volunteer, and what they want to achieve from the session.

My main orientation is Rational Emotive Behavior Therapy to which I bring the single session mindset (Dryden, 2019a). Both the volunteer and I go forward knowing that the session that we will have will be our only therapeutic encounter. A possible referral is not discussed at the outset. About 5% of the volunteers ask me later if I can recommend a therapist who can take things further with them, which I do. I never recommend myself. However, the volunteer knows that I will send them, on request, an audio copy of the session, and later, a transcript of the session for later review. Approximately 70% of volunteers email me to request a copy of the recording and transcript.

Selecting the Issue

At the very beginning of the session, I ask the volunteer what issue they want to address with me. If they mention more than one issue, I ask them to select *one* which I refer to as the target issue. I then help the person to formulate the target issue.

Establishing a Goal-Orientation

I will then seek to adopt a goal-orientation with the volunteer. Here, it is important to distinguish between a *problem-related goal* – what the volunteer wants to achieve with respect to the target issue and a session goal – what the person wants to achieve by the end of the session.

I encourage the volunteer to see that the achievement of a session goal is a stepping stone to achievement of a problem-related goal. This fits well with my stated objectives of SST, which are to (i) help the person address a specific issue; (ii) to help the client get "unstuck"; and (iii) to help the client take a few steps forward, which may help them to travel the rest of the journey without professional assistance (Dryden, 2019b).

Understanding Past Attempts at Dealing with the Issue

As is common practice in SST, I ascertain how the volunteer has tried to deal with the issue in the past and understand the outcome of these attempts. I encourage the volunteer to distance themself from unhelpful components of these attempts and capitalize on helpful components.

Dealing with a Specific Example of the Target Issue, if Relevant

If the client's target issue lends itself to the examination of a specific example, then I help them to select such an example. In doing so, I want to discover specific information concerning who was present, what happened, and where did it happen. While the chosen example can be recent, typical, or vivid, I encourage the volunteer to select one that is imminent, if relevant. The value of a future example is that the work done on it lends itself to the implementation of any solution chosen by the volunteer.

Assessing the Specific Example: The Situational ABC Model

When I am working with a specific example of the volunteer's target issue, I will assess it using the "Situational ABC Model" that stems from Rational Emotive Behavior Therapy (REBT). Briefly, this model states that when a problem occurs, it does so in a situational context. Here, the person responds unconstructively (at "C") to a feature of the situation which is for them an adversity (at "A"). The core of the REBT model is that these unconstructive responses are best explained by the rigid and extreme basic attitudes (at "B") that the person holds toward the adversity. REBT argues that the person's best solution to their target issue is to develop an alternative set of flexible and non-extreme attitudes (at "B") toward the adversity (at "A"). This will result in them dealing with the adversity in a more constructive manner (at "C"). This is summarized in Table 14.4. Please note that I do not use this framework explicitly or formally with the volunteer. Rather, I keep it in mind while doing the assessment and when planning interventions.

Table 14.4 REBT's Situational ABC Framework

Situation = Description of context
A = Adversity (The aspect of situation to which the person responds emotionally, cognitively, and behaviorally)
B = Basic attitude (Rigid/Extreme or Flexible/Non-Extreme)
C [e] = Emotional consequence (Healthy or Unhealthy)
　[t] = Thinking consequence (Negative and Highly Distorted or Balanced and Realistic)
　[b] = Behavioral consequence (Dysfunctional or Functional)

The following steps, which are notional rather than fixed, should help to clarify what happens during such an assessment.

Step 1: Situation. Here, I get a brief description of the situation in which the episode occurred.

Step 2: Emotional "C." Here, I identify the person's most troublesome negative emotion and the behavior and thinking that accompany it, if necessary.

Step 3: Adversity. I am now ready to identify the aspect of the situation that the volunteer was most troubled about. This represents the adversity at "A." At this point, I encourage the person to assume temporarily that the adversity happened. Even if the adversity can be shown to be inaccurate, the point is that the person responded to it as if it were true and thus we go forward on that basis, but only if doing so makes sense to the person. If not, I will take a different tack. In Table 14.5, I outline the most efficient way that I have found of identifying "A" if this is not clear at the outset.

Table 14.5 Windy's Magic Question (WMQ)

The purpose of this technique is to help the volunteer to identify the "A" in the ABC framework as quickly as possible (i.e., what the person is most disturbed about) once "C" has been assessed and the situation in which "C "has occurred has been identified and briefly described:

- **Step 1:** I have the person focus on their disturbed "C" (e.g., "anxiety").
- **Step 2:** I then ask the person to focus on the situation in which "C" occurred (e.g., "about to give a public presentation to a group of consultants").
- **Step 3:** I then ask the person, "Which ingredient could we give you that would eliminate or significantly reduce 'C' [here, anxiety]?" (In this case, the person said, "my mind not going blank.") I take care that the person does not change the situation (i.e., that they do not say: "not giving the presentation").
- **Step 4:** The opposite to this ingredient is probably "A" (e.g., "my mind going blank"), but I check this. Thus, I ask, "So when you were about to give the presentation, were you most anxious about your mind going blank"? If not, I use the question again until the person confirms what they were most anxious about in the described situation.

Step 4: Adversity-Based Goal. Before proceeding to helping the volunteer understand the role that their attitudes play in both their problem and the potential solution to their problem, I help them to set a realistic adversity-based goal. This involves helping them to see that they can still have an emotion that feels bad but is healthy and is at the heart of a constructive response to the adversity (e.g., concern rather than anxiety about facing a threat). Identifying such a goal will help me when I take an attitudinal focus.

Step 5: Identifying Basic Attitudes. I now shift focus and help the volunteer understand the role that rigid/extreme basic attitudes at "B" play in their problem and the potential role of flexible/non-extreme basic attitudes in the solution to their problem, which should be the same as their adversity-based goal identified above. In Table 14.6, I outline the most efficient way that I have found in doing this work.

Identifying the Solution

By now it should be clear that REBT offers the volunteer an attitude-based solution to their target issue. In short, this is that if the person develops and acts on a set of flexible and non-extreme attitudes toward the adversity, they will achieve their problem-related goal. If the volunteer accepts this, then we can proceed to the next step. If not, I will help them to develop a non-attitude-based solution.

Implementing the Solution

The first step to implementing an attitude-based solution is to help the person strengthen the flexible/non-extreme attitudes that they have

Table 14.6 Windy's Review Assessment Procedure (WRAP)

Once "C" (e.g., "anxiety") and "A" (e.g., "my mind going blank") have been assessed, I often use this technique to identify both the client's rigid/extreme and flexible/non-extreme basic attitudes and help the person to understand the two relevant "B"–"C" connections.

- **Step 1:** I begin by saying, "Let's review what we know and what we don't know so far."
- **Step 2:** I then say, "We know three things. First, we know that you were anxious ('C'). Second, we know that you were anxious about your mind going blank ('A'). Third, and this is an educated guess on my part, we know that it is important to you that your mind does not go blank. Am I correct?" Assuming that the person confirms my hunch, what I have done is to identify the part of the attitude that is common to both the person's rigid attitude and alternative flexible attitude.
- **Step 3:** I continue by saying, "Let's review what we don't know. This is where I need your help. We don't know which of two attitudes your anxiety was based on. So, when you were anxious about your mind going blank was your anxiety based on Attitude Number 1: 'It is important to me that my mind does not go blank and therefore it must not do so' ('Rigid attitude') or Attitude Number 2: 'It is important to me that my mind does not go blank, but that does not mean that it must not do so ('Flexible attitude')'?"
- **Step 4:** If necessary, I help the person to understand that their anxiety was based on their rigid attitude if they are unsure.
- **Step 5:** Once the person is clear that their anxiety was based on their rigid attitude, I make and emphasize the rigid/extreme attitude-disturbed "C" connection. Then, I ask, "Now let's suppose instead that you had a strong conviction in attitude number 2, how would you feel about your mind going blank if you strongly believed that while it was important to you that your mind did not go blank, it did not follow that it must not do so?"
- **Step 6:** If necessary, I help the person nominate a healthy negative emotion such as concern, if not immediately volunteered, and make and emphasize the flexible/non-extreme attitude-healthy "C" connection.

chosen (see above). There are a variety of ways that this can be done in the session. These include:

- Asking them to imagine teaching their selected attitude to their loved ones
- Helping them to identify and respond to any doubts, reservations or objections they have about their selected attitude
- Encouraging them to engage in attitude-based in-session practice of the solution (e.g., through role-play, imagery and chair-work).

Helping the Volunteer Understand the Change Process

It can be useful to outline a realistic view of the change process with the volunteer. This includes the importance of rehearsing healthy attitudes, and regularly acting in ways that are consistent with this developing attitude.

Helping the Volunteer to Develop a Cognitive-Behavioral Plan

With the above points in mind, the next step is to help the person develop a cognitive-behavioral plan so they can implement their selected solution in their life. This involves being clear with themself how they can best integrate the solution in their life and when, where, and how frequently they are prepared to implement this plan.

Ending

As with other forms of Single Session Therapy, it is important to have a good ending (Hoyt & Rosenbaum, 2018). I do this by encouraging the person to summarize what they are going to take away from the session and to voice any last-minute issues or ask any questions they might have wished they had asked me once they have gotten home.

Audience Input

Once the session has finished, I invite members of the audience to ask myself and the volunteer suitable questions or make any relevant observations as they see fit. My role here is to encourage discussion and to preserve what the volunteer will take away from the session. Questions encompass both the content of the session and the process of the intervention. This format could conceivably be used widely in the training of single session therapists.

Clinical Example

"Eloise" (not her real name) is a woman in her mid-40s who volunteered for help at a meet-up group where the theme was "Dealing with Anxiety." The following is an edited transcript of the highlights of the interview. The ellipses indicate missing conversation.

Selecting the Issue

Windy: What problem can I help you with this evening?
Eloise: I get worried and anxious if my 18-year-old son comes home late from college or from a night out.
Windy: What do you do when you're worried?
Eloise: I keep calling in on the phone …

Establishing a Goal Orientation

Windy: What would you like to take away from the session that would give you a sense that you were glad you volunteered this evening?

Eloise: A way of not worrying ...

(I return to the issue of goals later.)

Understanding Past Attempts at Dealing with the Issue

Windy: What have you done in the past to address the problem?
Eloise: I have tried to distract myself or do what I do now, which is to phone him when he is five minutes late.
Windy: What effect have these two methods had on you?
Eloise: They help me in what you called in the lecture "the short term" but not in the longer term ...

Dealing with a Specific Example of the Target Issue, if Relevant

Windy: When is your son next going to college or going out?
Eloise: He has a week off from college, but he is going out with his mates tomorrow night.
Windy: Do you anticipate having the problem tomorrow?
Eloise: For sure, if he is late.

Assessing the Specific Example: The Situational ABC Model

Windy: Let's assume that he will be late, shall we? ("Situation")
Eloise: OK.
Windy: What would you be worried about? ("Emotional C" = worry – see above)
Eloise: That he will be harmed in some way...
Windy: What one ingredient would take your worry away?
Eloise: Knowing he is safe ...
Windy: So, are you most worried about not knowing that he is safe?
Eloise: Yes. ("A" = not knowing that my son is safe.)
Windy: So, we know that you are worried and that you would prefer to know that he is safe. But we don't know what your attitude towards this uncertainty is when you are worried. Shall we find out?
Eloise: Yes, please.
Windy: Is it, attitude 1, "I want to know that my son is safe and therefore I absolutely must know this"; or attitude 2, "I want to know that my son is safe, but I don't absolutely have to have this certainty." Which attitude is your worry based on?
Eloise: Put like that, definitely number 1. ("Rigid basic attitude at B" = "I want to know that my son is safe and therefore I absolutely must know this.")

Clarifying the Adversity-Based Goal and Identifying a Solution

Windy: And how would you feel if you really believed attitude number 2? (Potential solution = "Flexible basic attitude at B" = "I want to know that my son is safe but I don't have to have this certainty.")

Eloise: I'm not sure of the word for it but my worry would be manageable.

Windy: Remember in the lecture, I distinguished between worry and worry-free concern?

Eloise: Yes, but for me as a Jewish mother I need to see myself worry.

Windy: So, how about manageable worry rather than unmanageable worry? (Adversity-based goal)

Eloise: Perfect!

I then helped Eloise to anchor the following constructive behaviors with her new flexible basic attitude: (a) asking her son to call her if he was going to be late; (b) calling him 45 minutes after he was expected home if he forgets to call; (c) not checking her phone in the interim period even if she feels the urge to do so; and (d) getting on with whatever she would be doing if she knew he was safe. I then took her through an imagery rehearsal of these components and she agreed to implement this cognitive-behavioral plan in imagery twice a day and in actuality whenever her son was late. I ended by asking her to review the session from her perspective and seeing if she had any questions to ask or points to make. I then asked the audience for their comments and questions.

References

Dryden, W. (2019a). *Single-Session 'One-at-a-Time' (OAAT) Therapy: A Rational Emotive Behaviour Therapy Approach*. Abingdon, Oxon, U.K.: Routledge.

Dryden, W. (2019b). *Single-Session Therapy: 100 Key Points and Techniques*. Abingdon, Oxon, U.K.: Routledge.

Ellis, A., & Joffe, D. (2002). A study of volunteer clients who experienced live sessions of rational emotive behavior therapy in front of a public audience. *Journal of Rational-Emotive & Cognitive-Behavior Therapy, 20*, 151–158.

Hoyt, M.F., & Rosenbaum, R. (2018). Some ways to end an SST. In M.F. Hoyt, M. Bobele, A. Slive, J. Young, & M. Talmon (Eds.), *Single-Session Therapy by Walk-In or Appointment: Administrative, Clinical, and Supervisory Aspects of One-at-a-Time Services* (pp. 318–323). New York: Routledge.

15 Making the Leap with Couples in Sweden: One-at-a-Time Mindset in Action

Martin Söderquist, Malena Cronholm-Nouicer, Lars Dannerup, and Karin Wulff

How do we know when it is time to make a change in our lives or in our work? What leads to us realizing the need or necessity to start a new habit? Once we have the realization, how do we get there? What are the first steps? Are there any risks involved in making these changes? What will other people say? Couples deciding to schedule a counseling session are often asking themselves these sorts of questions.

It's the same for counselors developing new methods. Introducing a One-at-a-Time (OAAT) approach to couple counseling – in which a therapist and client meet with the understanding that it will be for a single session – has given couples easy access to counseling without waiting lists or the need for intake procedures and after that session, another session if they want.

Couple Counseling in Malmö, Sweden

In Sweden, couple counseling is mandated by law and with absolute confidentiality, no registration, and no filing of records. Many Swedes know about couple counseling and we do not need to advertise. Couples find us on the internet and many couples are recommended by friends and relatives.

Our group in Malmö, Couple Counseling Team,[1] is a small team of eight counselors. When we introduced single session therapy (SST) several years ago, we were most of all inspired by the mindset described in Talmon's (1990) book. We implemented, followed up, and evaluated our sessions with good results (Söderquist, 2018). After a few years, we found that we wanted to further develop our service. We wanted to offer couples access to a session within a week, with the possibility to have additional sessions combined with a range of other options.

Today we offer couples several choices when they make appointments over the phone:

- Traditional couple counseling – the possibility to have several sessions with the same counselor. This option involves a waiting list of several weeks with periods of two to three months between appointments. It is the choice of 70–75% of couples
- OAAT – a session within a week. This is the choice of 25–30% of couples. There is the possibility to return for one or more sessions if the couple wants. Sessions are held on Tuesdays. Couples can schedule OAAT and also be put on the waiting list for traditional counseling; it is possible to cancel the traditional counseling if not needed after the OAAT session
- One-day multi-couple training day focused on conflict and communication
- One-day multi-couple training day focused on sex and desire.

We consider it important for couples to have a choice. They know best what they need and want.

Couples and OAAT

There are many reasons for couples to choose OAAT, such as:

- Relational crisis/emergency
- Session within a week
- "We think one session is enough"
- "We want to try counseling"
- "We want to start something together"
- One partner persuades the reluctant partner to attend one session.

Scheduling an OAAT session within a week is optimal whatever reason since the couple are in the "window of change" when they phone us.

It is also important that the couples are given options after the OAAT session, such as continuing on their own, returning later to OAAT, scheduling regular traditional counseling or coming to the conclusion that counseling doesn't suit them. If one or both partners need individual therapy, we recommend individual therapists and if their problems are related to dangerous levels of intimate partner violence we guide them to a specialist service for the best help they can get. Currently we don't do any follow-up – we leave the decision to the couple to decide how they want to proceed.

Counselors and OAAT

Couples coming to counseling very often see problems and blame each other, and see few or no possibilities. They typically assume counseling will require many sessions but hope for immediate (and often brief) outcomes. Opening up possibilities for small changes in their relationship, making plans for the immediate future, and creating hope in one session are important. It is a challenge best faced collaboratively with the couple.

To work well as a couple counselor you need to be trained in family and couple therapy and be experienced in brief therapy work. In Sweden, 75–80% of couples attend one to four sessions (Socialstyrelsen, 2020; https://www.mfof.se/familjeradgivning/statistik.html). The important shift from an *individual to relational mindset* was introduced by family therapy pioneers like Erickson, Satir, Minuchin, and Haley in the 1960–70s (see Satir, 1967; Haley, 1973, 1976; Minuchin, 1974). This had an enormous impact on the field – clients were seen in their social contexts and family members were accepted as important and helpful to the clients. The next mindset shift, in the 1980–90s, was to *brief* relational work. de Shazer (1985, 1988), Berg and Dolan (2001), Hoyt (1994, 1996, 1998), White and Epston (1990), and many others were leading proponents.

Although brief relational work is now accepted, going from *brief* to *OAAT* relational work, beginning in the 1990–2000s, was another giant leap. Going from serial thinking about processes to *one-off sessions in OAAT* is a great challenge. The idea of scheduling one session, collaboratively doing the best in that session and leaving the decision to the client – to make a new appointment, to find another counselor, or to take care of their situation on their own – is for many couple therapists very much "outside the box."

When you have made the OAAT leap, there are forces working against you. The diagnostic culture currently dominates in Sweden. Organizations and managers/colleagues demand that counselors and therapists use assessments, diagnoses, and more traditional models of counseling and therapy.

The mindset of OAAT is to believe in clients' resources and really trust them. It also means that you believe in the possibility of sudden or unexpected changes and that important moments can occur in one session. As counselors, we are not always so important as we might think – the couple can do much or all of the work with a small amount of support (Slive & Bobele, 2011; Hoyt & Talmon, 2014; Hoyt, Bobele, Slive, Young, & Talmon, 2018).

How Did We Make the Leap to Embracing an OAAT Approach as Couple Counselors?

There are many different roads to Rome, as the saying goes, and there are many ways for couple counselors to make the leap to an OAAT mindset. It is impossible to describe them all but inspired by the collection *Therapist Stories of Inspiration, Passion, and Renewal: What's Love Got to*

Do with It? (Hoyt, 2013), we want to share some stories of our own. We all had a head start – we were already trained in family and brief therapy.

Martin Söderquist: When I first read Talmon's book in the beginning of the 1990s I was thrilled and excited. In a way, it was a perfect fit – I and my colleagues already worked in a family-oriented and solution-focused way. I wanted to implement Single Session Therapy immediately. This wasn't possible for many reasons and it wasn't until I began working as a couple counselor in the beginning of the 2000's that I really could start planning SST/OAAT.

What finally got me going was a telephone follow-up that we did with 68 unplanned single session couples. Many couples told us "one session was enough." Some of the couples reported that "we had decided to attend one session" – but they didn't tell the counselor. I realized that some couples asked – not always in a direct manner – for one session and not more. This reminded me of how important it is to offer clients what they want and when they ask for it instead of making clients fit into your preferred therapy model or the administration of the organization.

This was my leap more than ten years ago and for me, there is no way back.

Karin Wulff: Paradoxically, it's been a long and slow process for me to embrace brief OAAT. Trained in solution-focused theory and after a decade of daily Solution Focused Brief Therapy (SFBT) sessions with individuals one might think it would be easy. It was trickier than I expected.

I started implementing the mindset of OAAT in 2015, in the context of couple counseling. Hard work and a lot of practice made me overcome the challenging parts and enjoy the energy and possibilities in each session.

To me it's a question about timing. Timing in several aspects: if a client can get help when they need it, you offer the right question, affirmation and intervention in the right moment of the session. I find it slightly more challenging to work with couples compared to individuals. Practicing OAAT I've become more disciplined with focus and timing, which I also find helpful in other forms of clinical work.

It's a privilege to work in a context that offers counseling when people ask for it. My readiness to be there when a couple is looking for change is something to aim for in every session.

A lot of things can change if your timing is good.

Lars Dannerup: How do we know if things we talked about were useful? How do we know anything about the future? How do we know if change happens quickly or slowly? The simple answer to that is, we don't know it until after it has happened. That means that we can only do our best in the single moment.

In the beginning of my career as a therapist I had the good fortune to be a member of a team which on several occasions was trained and supervised by Steve de Shazer and Insoo Kim Berg. Especially two things made a huge impact on me. One thing to remember is that "every session could be the last session" and another thing is to always "ask the client where they want to go: don't get started until you know their destination."

Many years ago a woman in her late twenties stepped into my office. The only thing I knew about her was that she had been a heroin addict since the age of 13 and been in and out of treatment since then. It would have been easy to think that one session couldn't possibly make a difference. And, of course, I did. With de Shazer and Insoo Berg in mind, I just started out with where she wanted to go and some minutes into the session I asked the Miracle Question. She started by saying: "I'll get up in the morning, have a cup of coffee and then I'll be off to work." The session continued with us exploring her thoughts and feelings regarding the work she had pictured herself doing.

I meet her on and off in the community. She's now a teacher in a high school. Once she told me it was that one session that made the miracle.

Thirty years down the road it still can be hard work, but through her help and many others I now understand how helpful one single session can be.

Malena Cronholm-Nouicer: Therapists still don't know very much about how change happens. What we know is that life is constantly in motion whether we wish or not. For me, OAAT makes it a possibility to collaboratively create with the couple a space for hopes of relational movement. Sometimes this can be an intensive deep dive into something important for the couple, or a careful dipping of a toe in the water.

I work with OAAT, convinced that one single session can make a difference. My experience is that OAAT requires curiosity and careful attention to capture the first glimpse of what a move in the right direction could be or how a small change could ripple for the couple.

I will never forget the man who spontaneously said after the session: "Good God, what a relief! I thought you [his partner] were going to end our relationship in this session." Together we noted and realized that, on the contrary, the session was focused on the couple's desire for closeness. The session had given them more hope of such a possibility.

Creating Conditions for New Possibilities

Couples scheduling OAAT sessions do so for a variety of reasons, such as these:

- "We want to tell you how we handled a family crisis and want feedback from you"
- "We have decided to separate. We agree but we are very uncertain and worried for our children – how do we talk with them?"

- "Our teenage girl discovered two days ago that my husband has seen another woman for a long time and I am devastated now and don't know how to hold myself together"
- "The police told us to schedule an appointment with you after our last fight"
- "I have lost my feelings for my partner and he/she must change"
- "Our individual therapists both told us to see a couple counselor and that it was urgent."

An OAAT session needs to give the couple something new, giving hope and a sense of a plan for the immediate future. Pivotal moments and important turning points in therapy and consultations are very hard - sometimes impossible - to deliberately produce; they are more spontaneous and only possible to discover afterward. Pivotal moments for the couple and for the counselor can also be very different.

If couple counselors can't "produce" pivotal moments – then what can they do to help couples make a desired turn? You can lead the horse to water but you can't force the horse to drink. Virginia Satir expressed it like this many years ago: "No one can convince anyone else to change. Every one of us guards a door of change that only can be opened from inside" (Satir, personal communication with Martin Söderquist, 1977). We can *create conditions for change*; we can have the dialogue with each couple in an accepting, respectful and closely listening way to help the couple see their situation differently and maybe do something constructively together. It is all about following the couple's lead closely and at the same time asking questions and affirming them. In that way the couples are gently given the chance to reflect, to have new ideas, and maybe to start planning something new together.

Some couples coming to an OAAT session see each other as "the problem" (individual thinking) and have ideas about counseling as a process over time – the session not as potentially a single session or as OAAT but as the first in a planned series. This is a challenge for an OAAT counselor. We address this by saying: "Many people find one or a few sessions enough – let's come back to this after the session." We consider it possible to create conditions for change and at the same time help the couple plan and start the relational work. What has been said so far highlights the impossibility to manualize or make a program for OAAT sessions with couples. The couples, their situations, their contexts, their presenting problems, and their hopes are very diverse and varied. Every couple must be seen, talked with, and affirmed in unique ways precisely tailored to them.

We share the SST/OAAT mindset with others in this book. We want to point out three aspects especially important in our work with couples.

- *Beginnings and endings.* How we start and end sessions is very important (see Budman, Hoyt, & Friedman, 1992; Hoyt &

Talmon, 2014b; Hoyt & Rosenbaum, 2018). It frames the session as a whole. "Welcome" and introducing the context – "one hour" and "Let us do our best to make it helpful and useful to you" – is of utmost importance at the start. Couples most often want feedback, reflections, and constructive ideas (often expressed as "tools") from the counselor and they are entitled to have them. The counselor can give these reflections during the session and/or summarize at the end of the session, after a brief team break or "individual reflection time" (see Sharry, Madden, Darmody, & Miller, 2001; Hoyt, 2015, p. 310) – the counselor leaving the session room for some minutes. These reflections mark the end of the session and the start of the couple's own continued work toward their goals.

- *Invitations.* Inviting the couple to briefly talk about their problems and in more detail about their hopes and goals most often generates positive and creative possibilities.
- *Focusing on doing/behavior.* When asking more about what people *do* it is easier to get to what they are good at, their competencies and their strength to resist oppression, violence, and problems (Wade, 1997).

Helpful in describing what is collaboratively constructed in an OAAT is the "Interventive Interviewing – Full Expanded Framework" model, revised and expanded from Karl Tomm's model from the 1980s (Tomm 1987a,b; 1988) and presented (in Danish) by Tomm and Danish colleagues (Hornstrup, Tomm, & Johansen, 2009). Some examples of questions derived from their model:

- "What are your most urgent problems right now?" *(Situational question)*
- "The person who knows you the best as a couple – what would he or she say about your situation?" *(Perspective question)*
- "What is the best imaginable result of this session?" *(Possibility question)*
- "What can you do to go in the direction of your goals?" *(Initiative question)*

In OAAT sessions, the main focus is on Possibility and Initiative questions. A question often used by us is: "How will your partner/your children/the persons that know you very well – tomorrow/this weekend/next week – notice the changes you talk about/things going in the right direction for you/ your collaboration is the way you want?" This question is categorized as a "Context Initiative Question" (Tomm, personal communication, 2019).

There are some couples who start the session with "We want to tell our story and our problems!" This is a special challenge since the session is about 1–1.5 hour and you can't answer "No" or spend the whole session listening to problem talk. There are many ways for counselors to focus our listening in these cases, by asking for example:

- "How would you like me to listen to your story?"
- "What in your story would you prefer me to listen specifically to and what questions and reflections from me will you appreciate?"
- "When you have told your story – what are your best hopes this will mean to you?"

Some clients and couples already have a plan for the session. It is important to follow their lead – their plan might be very constructive.

Closing Reflections

During the years we have offered couples SST/OAAT, we have received a lot of comments and feedback from the couples in telephone interviews, evaluations (protocols before and after the OAAT sessions), and comments made by the couple when leaving the session room. They have told us they feel validated, have a plan, and are more confident of being able to handle their situation, and are grateful for the chance to have the session when they needed it. This has been important and inspiring for us and told us we are on the right track. A few quotes exemplify this:

- *"The session was overwhelming and really worked for us"*
- *"You focused on what was most important to us and that was helpful"*
- *"We do not need any more sessions – your confirmation of what and how we had done everything right to handle our family crisis was what we needed to hear"*
- *"This must be the best service in Malmö! We just called you and in less than a week we had this session. Fantastic! Just what we needed – in time at the right time."*

An OAAT mindset is not something you get easily – it is something you have to work hard to achieve. It is a giant leap and it can be challenging for yourself, your colleagues, and your organization. OAAT is about closely following the couple's lead; simultaneously inviting them to express their hopes, goals, and what they do that works for them. OAAT also requires the discipline of staying away from inviting the couple to explore what they haven't asked for and from focusing on ideas and plans for next sessions.

Most of all, OAAT is beneficial to many couples and counselors.

Note

1 Visit https://malmo.se/Service/Stod-och-omsorg/Familjefragor/Samtalsstod-och-radgivning/Familjeradgivningen.html

References

Berg, I.K. & Dolan, Y.D. (2001). *Tales of Solutions: A Collection of Hope-Inspiring Stories*. New York: Norton.

Budman, S.H., Hoyt, M.F., & Friedman, S. (Eds.). (1992). *The First Session in Brief Therapy*. New York: Guilford Press.

de Shazer, S. (1985). *Keys to Solution in Brief Therapy*. New York: Norton.

de Shazer, S. (1988). *Clues: Investigating Solutions in Brief Therapy*. New York: Norton.

Haley, J. (1973). *Uncommon Therapy: The Psychiatric Techniques of Milton. H. Erickson, M.D.* New York: Norton.

Haley, J. (1976). *Problem-Solving Therapy: New Strategies for Effective Family Therapy*. San Francisco: Jossey-Bass.

Hornstrup, C., Tomm, K., & Johansen, T. (2009). "Sporgsmal – der gor en forskel" ("Questions that make a difference"). *Erhvervspsykologi (Business Psychology)*, 7(3), 2–16. (In Danish)

Hoyt, M.F. (Ed.). (1994). *Constructive Therapies*. New York: Guilford Press.

Hoyt, M.F. (Ed.). (1996). *Constructive Therapies* (Vol. 2). New York: Guilford Press.

Hoyt, M.F. (Ed.). (1998). *The Handbook of Constructive Therapies*. San Francisco: Jossey-Bass.

Hoyt, M.F. (Ed.). (2013). *Therapist Stories of Inspiration, Passion and Renewal: What's Love Got to Do with It?* New York: Routledge.

Hoyt, M.F. (2015). Solution-focused couple therapy. In A.S. Gurman, J.L. Lebow, & D.K. Snyder (Eds.), *Clinical Handbook of Couple Therapy* (5th ed., pp. 300–332). New York: Guilford Press.

Hoyt, M.F., Bobele, M., Slive, A., Young, J., & Talmon, M. (Eds.). (2018). *Single Session Therapy by Walk-In or Appointment: Administrative, Clinical and Supervisory Aspects of One-at-a-Time Services*. New York: Routledge.

Hoyt, M.F., & Rosenbaum, R. (2018). Some ways to end an SST. In M.F. Hoyt et al. (Eds.), *Single Session Therapy by Walk-In or Appointment: Administrative, Clinical and Supervisory Aspects of One-at-a-Time Services* (pp. 318–323). New York: Routledge.

Hoyt, M.F., & Talmon, M. (Eds.). (2014). *Capturing the Moment: Single-Session Therapy and Walk-In Services*. Bethel, CT: Crown House Publishing.

Hoyt, M.F., & Talmon, M. (2014b). The temporal structure of brief therapy: Some questions often associated with different phases of sessions and treatment. In M.F. Hoyt & M. Talmon (Eds.), *Capturing the Moment: Single Session Therapy and Walk-In Services* (pp. 517–522). Bethel, CT: Crown House Publishing.

Hubble, M.A., Duncan, B.L., & Miller, S.D. (Eds.). (1999). *The Heart and Soul of Change. What Works in Therapy*. Washington, DC: APA Books.

Minuchin, S. (1974). *Families and Family Therapy*. Cambridge, MA: Harvard University Press.

Satir, V. (1967). *Conjoint Family Therapy*. Palo Alto, CA: Science & Behavior Books.

Sharry, J., Madden, B., Darmody, M., & Miller, S.D. (2001). Giving our clients the break: Applications of client-directed, outcome-informed clinical work. *Journal of Systemic Therapies*, 20(3), 68–76.

Slive, A., & Bobele, M. (Eds.). (2011). *When One Hour is All You Have: Effective Therapy for Walk-In Clients*. Phoenix, AZ: Zeig, Tucker, & Theisen.

Socialstyrelsen (Swedish Board of Health). (2020). Statistik. https://www.mfof.se/familjeradgivning/statistik.html.

Söderquist, M. (2018). Coincidence favors the prepared mind. Single sessions with couples in Sweden. In M.F. Hoyt, M. Bobele, A. Slive, J. Young, & M. Talmon (Eds.), *Single Session Therapy by Walk-In or Appointment: Administrative, Clinical, and Supervisory Aspects of One-at-a-Time Services* (pp. 270–290). New York: Routledge.

Talmon, M. (1990). *Single-Session Therapy: Maximizing the Effect of the First (and Often Only) Therapeutic Encounter*. San Francisco: Jossey-Bass.

Tomm, K. (1987a). Interventive interviewing: Part I. Strategizing as a fourth guideline for the therapist. *Family Process, 26*, 3–13.

Tomm, K. (1987b). Interventive interviewing: Part II. Reflexive questioning as a means to enable self-healing. *Family Process, 26*, 167–183.

Tomm, K. (1988). Interventive interviewing: Part III. Intending to ask lineal, circular, strategic, or reflexive questions? *Family Process, 27*, 1–15.

Wade, A. (1997). Small acts of living. *Contemporary Family Therapy, 19*(1), 23–39.

White, M., & Epston, D. (1990). *Narrative Means to Therapeutic Ends*. New York: Norton.

16 Complex and Challenging Issues in SST: Reflections on the Past and Learnings for the Future

Patricia A. Boyhan

Single session therapy (SST) is an integral part of my practice. However, back in 1994 I was a master's student on placement at The Bouverie Family Therapy Centre (now known as The Bouverie Centre) and I had no knowledge of the concept. One of my supervisors attended a family therapy conference in 1993, where SST was presented by Dalmar Child and Family Therapy Services as an option for clients on their waiting list (see Price, 1994). After reading Talmon (1990) and researching the culture of over-demand for service that challenged mental health services in Australia at the time (Boyhan, 1996, p. 85), I went to Penrith, New South Wales to train with Dalmar. After returning to Bouverie I became part of a pilot to trial SST with a new clinical specialist team, which became the focus of my master's thesis.

This paper reflects on two case examples involving eight-year-old children – an early Bouverie case and a more contemporary one. Pseudonyms are used throughout. They demonstrate the evolution of SST across the years, including the implementation of SST in one-off consultations to support work in multi-disciplinary teams (Boyhan & Gerner, 2007). They also reinforce the need for reflective practice and supervision which encourages mindful consideration, safety, shared vulnerability, curiosity, awareness, support, and consolidation of new learning into practice (Hewson & Carroll, 2016). They encourage us to be mindful of culture at micro (within families) and macro (broader community) levels, which are influenced by ethnicity, education, socio-economics, gender, religion, demographics, customs, social behavior, and laws.

Example #1

Bouverie was contacted by Jodie who had recently remarried and moved to Melbourne with her new husband, Sean, and Joshua, her eight-year-old son from her former marriage. Jodie told the intake worker that since relocating, her previously happy son had become uncooperative, rude, oppositional and defiant towards Sean, had not made friends at his new school and had recently developed encopresis, which had resulted in bullying by his fellow students. Their family doctor was unable to identify physical causes and suggested family therapy. Jodie chose to attend the SST Program rather than be put on a four-month waiting list, and an SST questionnaire (Boyhan, 1996, p. 94) was sent to her.

Summary of the Session

David and I were the therapists assigned to the case, and after reading the responses to the SST questionnaire, we invited the family to join us in the therapy room. Jodie presented as anxious, Sean as angry and fed up, and Joshua had a cap pulled down over his eyes – clearly a reluctant participant. (For another example of working with a reluctant youth in SST, see Boyhan, 2014.) Jodie repeated what she had told the intake worker, and added she had been separated from Joshua's biological father (Brad, who was an interstate truck driver living in Melbourne) for many years. Occasionally Brad would stop on his way to Adelaide, but his visits were unpredictable. Since relocating, there had been no contact between Joshua and Brad.

Joshua was being identified as "The Problem" and nothing positive was said by Jodie or Sean. David and I were worried about the lack of parental emotional attunement so, rather than expose Joshua to further criticism, we moved to a more systemic focus by exploring what life was like in their previous town. There was a large extended family of Italian origin (maternal grandparents, aunts, uncles, and cousins) with whom they enjoyed sharing Italian family traditions; Joshua had friends, was involved in sporting activities and a church group, had been doing well at school, and had significantly more freedom as he could ride his bike to see his family and friends.

Although I tried to engage Joshua, he refused to respond. Eventually I said gently, "It seems you are VERY angry." He immediately looked up and yelled, "I AM." I then said, "I wonder if you might also be VERY sad." He stood up, went to the window, looked out with his back to everyone, then started to sob and shake. I waited for Jodie to respond, but she remained in her chair, so I said, "Perhaps you would like to comfort Joshua." She then brought him back to sit next to her and offered reassurance.

At this point, we summarized Joshua's recent experiences:

- He had not seen his Dad since coming to Melbourne, and although previous contact was unpredictable, there was always the hope Dad would visit on his way to Adelaide
- He had left behind his extended family, friends, sporting interests, school, and the freedom to ride his bike around town

- He had not settled at school, and the development of encopresis had resulted in bullying and teasing.

Jodie and Sean acknowledged these issues but explained they had needed to relocate because of Sean's work. David and I expressed understanding and empathy regarding their decision, and then posed the following questions to facilitate discussion on how life might be improved for Joshua:

- Perhaps Jodie could contact Brad and arrange to set up a visiting schedule?
- Would it be possible for Joshua to stay with extended family for weekends or school holidays?
- Had they explored options for sporting activities in Melbourne?
- Did Joshua have a friend they could invite home after school or on weekends?

Joshua became animated and was able to identify a friend at school, Jake, with whom he played basketball. Jodie and Sean committed to follow up on the strategies which had been jointly developed. They would contact Brad and discuss contact visits, arrange for Joshua to visit extended family during next school holidays, check out basketball teams locally, and invite Jake home one weekend.

David and I finished the session by asking if it had been helpful. Jodie and Sean responded positively and Joshua said rather guardedly, "It was OK." We checked if they wanted to return to the waiting list with the option to call Bouverie if there were any concerns. Jodie and Sean said they would try the strategies and then make a decision for the future. David and I arranged a follow-up phone call to check how things were going and to evaluate the session. After the family left we debriefed and felt we had done a pretty good job with this family.

Our response to the family was informed by:

- White (1984/1989, p. 115), who published a paper in which pseudo-encopresis was considered from the perspective of second cybernetics: "In families where these symptoms feature, all members are considered to be inadvertently participating in an uncontrolled avalanche of events. All members appear powerless to affect the course of these events, and experience the symptoms of encopresis as oppressive"
- Webber (1989), whose book and parenting program provided a positive approach for step-families
- Moloney (1993), who researched and published papers focusing on post-separation issues, and the rights and needs of children to maintain ongoing contact with parents and other significant people
- Biddulph (1994), who focused on the importance of fathers and male role models in children's development.

Follow-Up Phone Call. This was in the early development stage of SST at Bouverie, and another therapist conducted the follow-up phone call. Jodie reported she and Sean did not find the session as helpful as they hoped. While they now had a greater understanding of *why* Joshua was behaving badly, they still didn't know *what to do* about his behavior. When this was reported to David and me, we realized we had missed the most important aspect *for the parents* who wanted behavioral strategies to manage Joshua's acting-out behavior. We had helped them understand the possible *causes* of his distress and suggested some *longer-term strategies*, but we had not responded specifically to what they had come for, namely *what to do now* when Joshua was angry, uncooperative, and misbehaving at school.

I contacted Jodie, thanked her for her honest feedback, and acknowledged we had been distracted by Joshua's anguish triggered by my intervention, and in doing so had failed to respond to their goals which they had identified in their telephone intake and on the questionnaire. I invited Jodie and Sean for a second SST – which they understood would be another one-off meeting. During this session, we developed some immediate strategies to manage Joshua's negative behavior such as: setting boundaries around what would and would not be tolerated; introducing logical consequences for misbehavior; and time out to allow him to calm himself down when his anger was heightened. We also tried to instill hope and confidence that his behavior would improve once he felt more settled in his new environment.

Second Follow-Up Phone Call. I contacted Jodie four weeks later and she reported she and Sean had tried the behavior management strategies we suggested in the second session and they felt less frustrated with Joshua and more in control. She had also acted on the plans developed in our first session to reconnect Joshua to family and friends. Brad had agreed to visit Joshua; Joshua planned to visit extended family during the next school holidays; he had joined a local basketball team with Jake and had made other friends; his behavior was less confrontational, his relationship with Sean had improved, and Sean was taking him to his basketball games; the symptoms of encopresis were under control and he rarely had "accidents" at school.

Learnings for Practice

Reflection on this case provides a constant reminder to read carefully the pre-session questionnaire, which invites family members to nominate both what are their greatest problems and what outcome they would want from the therapy session. It also highlights how important it is to check back during the session to ensure I am on track and to make adjustments as needed, and near the end to ensure clients have got what they came for. If clients identify something has been missed I offer another session quickly to take advantage of the clients' readiness for change, which Hoyt, Rosenbaum, and Talmon (1992, p. 64) identified "as a state of *potential imminence* (not inevitability) in which various conditions are near a threshold that can, with recognition and skillful facilitation, be assisted and potentiated into actuality."

Additionally, as therapists we know that understanding *causes* for misbehavior has the potential to assist in its *management*. However we should not presume stressed parents will take that step without clear instructions and some psycho-education. Sometimes this will entail focusing on their cultural context, which in this case included the Italian background of the mother's family of origin and changes in their close-knit family structure. Furthermore, when I reflect on the high divorce rate which impacts many of my clients, I am reminded to keep up to date with changes to the Family Law Act which focus clearly on the "rights of the child" to have ongoing contact with both parents and other significant people, and to ensure children are protected from chronic post-separation conflict between parents. Helpful publications and presentations in the intervening years include Boyhan and Gerner (2007), Smyth and Moloney (2010), Sroufe and McIntosh (2011), Siegel and McIntosh (2011), Moloney (2014), and Smyth and Moloney (2019).

Example #2

More recently I worked for a large non-government agency that is funded to provide counseling and mediation/conciliation to individuals and families. The suite of services offered to separated parents included Conjoint Mediation and Therapy, known as the CoMeT Model (Boyhan, Foster, Grimes, & Jaffe, 2004) and Child Inclusive Practice, known as CIP (McIntosh, 2000):

- CoMeT was developed to support mediators working with high-conflict separated parents who are "stuck" and unable to resolve post-separation parenting issues. A mediator may request a counselor to join him/her to assist parents to identify and process the emotional wounding and pain that is preventing them from focusing on their children (Boyhan et al., 2004, p. 116)
- CIP involves children being interviewed separately, usually in a one-off session, by a trained child interviewer who then presents the children's views to the parents in the presence of the mediator and/or the counselor (McIntosh, 2000; Boyhan and Gerner, 2007).

As the following will illustrate, I found my SST training prepared me to work in the CoMeT model as well as helping me to keep focused on the limitations of my role in CIP.

Summary of the Session

Jenny and Sam presented for mediation, bringing very different cultural backgrounds. Jenny was Australian-born and Sam was a refugee from Iran. They had an eight-year-old daughter, Melanie. At intake they disclosed to the mediator, Jonathon, that they had been separated for two years and despite attempts to develop post-separation parenting arrangements they continued to experience high levels of conflict, and that contact between Melanie and Sam was constantly breaking down. Jenny blamed Sam for the "failure" of their marriage and expressed concern about the way he parented and punished Melanie. Sam said he felt a responsibility to ensure Melanie was brought up to be respectful and admitted he occasionally smacked her hand, although he denied he would ever seriously hurt Melanie. Jonathon discussed CoMeT with Jenny and Sam, and with their permission, invited a counselor, Juliette, to join the next session. Jonathon and Juliette had previously developed a good working relationship, and by using both counseling and mediation skills, they were able to explore the intense emotional issues which kept Jenny and Sam negatively attached, and also the cultural differences which underpinned their ongoing disputes. Juliette explained Australian laws relating to the protection of children and suggested that Sam might benefit from attending a parenting program to develop alternative ways to discipline Melanie. To assist them to understand the impact their disputes might have been having on Melanie, CIP was offered and they agreed to bring Melanie in for a session.

Child Inclusive Practice. I was appointed as the child interviewer and, after engaging with Melanie, I asked her to draw a picture of her family. She handed me the drawing shown in Figure 16.1. She explained one house (pointing to the one on the left) was Mum's and the other was Dad's. She then took back the picture and added "Help! I'm stuck!"

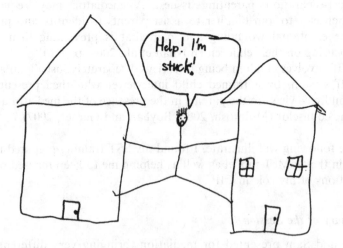

Figure 16.1 Melanie's Drawing of Her Family.

When I asked Melanie why she felt "stuck," she said her parents always fought and they frequently asked her to deliver messages from one to the other, but after she told them the message they would usually call on the telephone and have another fight. She then cried and said, *"Sometimes I think I don't tell it properly."* I reassured Melanie it was not her fault her parents fought. I asked her permission to take her drawing into a session with her Mum and Dad and to tell them she was worrying she may not be delivering messages properly. I then explored the different styles of discipline she experienced at Mum's house/Dad's house and I felt reassured she was not being physically abused by Sam.

Feedback to Parents. Two weeks later I met with Jonathon, Juliette, Jenny, and Sam. I complimented the parents on Melanie, and said she had been open and responsive in the session. However, I told them I believed Melanie was experiencing a high level of anxiety and shared her drawing. Both parents were visibly shocked. I then gently gave further feedback by telling them Melanie did not want to be a messenger any more as she worried she was not telling the messages properly and felt responsible when they rang each other and continued the fights. Jenny immediately started crying and Sam was also distressed. Neither understood how much pressure their fighting was putting on Melanie. I encouraged them to continue working with Jonathon and Juliette to build a parental alliance which would free Melanie from taking responsibility for their disputes. I also reinforced the "open door" policy that would allow them to contact me if they believed I could be helpful for Melanie in the future.

Therapeutic Outcome. Jenny and Sam continued with CoMeT and identified several cultural and family-of-origin differences, which were triggering their current conflict, and had probably been at the root of their marital discord. Eventually they were able to develop a post-separation parenting plan and a six-month follow-up revealed it had remained stable.

Learnings for Practice

Reflection on this case encourages me to continue to explore innovative uses for SST, especially to support work in multi-disciplinary teams. Both CoMeT and CIP require "consultant" clinicians to be available quickly to support the work of the mediator and counselor, to be able to focus on clients' needs accurately, and to be aware of the limitations of their role. They need to be able to *tolerate* withdrawing and leaving the outcome to be managed by the primary therapists, despite sometimes feeling *emotionally involved* with the family.

Additionally, both cases identify powerful systemic influences and the challenges for therapists to meet the needs of all family members. In Example #1 it was essential to address the goals of the parents, as well as developing strategies to relieve the distress of the child. In Example #2 the mediator and the counselor brought a range of skills from their individual professions to help release the impasse and unpack the emotional wounding of the separated parents. However, they also identified the potential for distress experienced by a child caught up in parental conflict and used a third practitioner to interview the child and report back to the parents.

Additional Reflections and Summary

These cases provide excellent examples of the importance of cultural influences at micro (family culture, altered structures in families and demographics) and macro levels (family law and protection of children). Additionally they illustrate how essential it is for therapists to really elicit and listen to what clients want *right now*. Moreover, 26 years of SST practice has taught me to expand my thinking about SST as a waiting list management strategy, and helped me to recognize what a valuable tool SST is for responding and providing help quickly (Boyhan, 1996); has demonstrated how SST can be expanded to support multi-disciplinary teams (Boyhan et al., 2004); and can be used to encourage reluctant participants to *engage* and to *respond* in counseling (Boyhan, 2014).

Furthermore, I frequently reflect on notes I wrote after a discussion with Moshe Talmon when he visited Australia in 1997. He said that allowing people to open up is intrinsically healing, and that when a professional acknowledges a client's pain, permission is given to review it and then let it go. He also encouraged the use of "constructive minimalism," remembering that people "do not get cured" but rather, life cycles continue to bring challenges and problems, and therapy across the life span assists clients with problem solving. He said SST practitioners need to be versatile and flexible in their skills; optimistic, respectful and warm in their attitude to clients; intrigued by partnership (over hierarchy), psychohealth (over psychopathology); and solution and change focused (over problems and more of the same). He emphasized the basic principle of SST is to be *present*.

SST allows us to be *present* when our clients are at the height of readiness for change, and reflective practice encourages us to be *present* and focused on what *the client* is aiming to achieve, and to innovatively consolidate new learnings into practice.

References

Biddulph, S. (1994). *Manhood*. Sydney, Australia: Finch Publishing.
Boyhan, P. (1996). Clients' perceptions of single session therapy consultations as an option to waiting for family therapy. *Australian and New Zealand Journal of Family Therapy, 17*(2), 85–96.

Boyhan, P. (2014). Innovative uses for single session therapy: Two case studies. In M.F. Hoyt & M. Talmon (Eds.), *Capturing the Moment: Single Session Therapy and Walk-In Services* (pp. 164–175). Bethel, CT: Crown House Publishing.

Boyhan, P., Foster, L., Grimes, A., & Jaffe, R. (2004). Conjoint mediation and therapy: Emergence of the CoMeT Model. *Australasian Dispute Resolution Journal, 15*(2), 108–118.

Boyhan, P., & Gerner, F. (2007). Doing what it takes: A family dispute resolution case study using a multidisciplinary approach. *Journal of Family Studies, 13*, 236–244.

Hewson, D., & Carroll, M. (2016). *Reflective Practice in Supervision.* Hazelbrook, NSW, Australia: MoshPit Publishing.

Hoyt, M.F., Rosenbaum, R., & Talmon, M. (1992). Planned single-session psychotherapy. In S.H. Budman, M.F. Hoyt, & S. Friedman (Eds.), *The First Session in Brief Therapy* (pp. 59–86). New York: Guilford Press.

McIntosh, J. (2000). Child-inclusive divorce mediation: Report on a qualitative research study. *Mediation Quarterly, 18*(1), 55–69.

Moloney, L. (1993). A children's rights approach to post-separation parenting. *Australian Journal of Family Law, 7*(3), 249–259.

Moloney, L. (2014, September 14). Parenting and parental absence after separation. *Australian Institute of Family Studies.* www.aifs.gov.au/cfca/2014/09/04/caring-children-after-separation-or-divorce

Price, C. (1994). Open days: Making family therapy accessible in working class suburbs. *Australian and New Zealand Journal of Family Therapy, 15*(4), 191–196.

Siegel, D., & McIntosh, J. (2011). Family law and the neuroscience of attachment, Part II. *Family Court Review, 49*(3), 521–528.

Smyth, B., & Moloney, L. (2010, May 14). *Practice Issues in Post-Separation Disputes over Children.* Family Law Pathways Conference. Coffs Harbour, NSW, Australia.

Smyth, B., & Moloney, L. (2019, June 4). *Post-Separation Decisions About Children. Engaging with Hidden Parental Motivations.* Keynote address at the Family Relationship Services Australia, Child Inclusive Practice Conference. Darwin, NT, Australia.

Sroufe, A., & McIntosh, J. (2011). Divorce and attachment relationships: The longitudinal journey. *Family Court Review, 49*(3), 464–473.

Talmon, M. (1990). *Single-Session Therapy: Maximizing the Effect of the First (and Often Only) Therapeutic Encounter.* San Francisco: Jossey-Bass.

Webber, R. (1989). *Living in a Stepfamily.* Melbourne, VIC, Australia: Australian Council for Educational Research (ACER).

White, M. (1989). Pseudo-encopresis: From avalanche to victory, from vicious to virtuous cycles. In M. White, *Selected Papers* (pp. 115–124). Adelaide, SA, Australia: Dulwich Centre Publications (work originally published 1984).

17 Strengthening Family Resilience Using a Single Session Mindset Following a Child's Diagnosis of Autism

Aspasia Stacey Rabba[1]

Coping with a young child's diagnosis of autism and navigating the pathway to early intervention presents many challenges for families. From the emotional experience of coming to terms with the diagnosis (e.g., loss, denial, acceptance) to the practical decisions that follow (e.g., identifying what supports are required), the post-diagnostic journey can lead to distress and uncertainty for families (Crane, Chester, Goddard, Henry, & Hill, 2016; Feinberg et al., 2014; McGrew & Keyes, 2014; Stuart & McGrew, 2009). Given the difficulties experienced by parents post-diagnosis, family-based interventions utilizing practical and effective therapeutic techniques are fundamental to addressing parental and family needs, enabling them to make the next steps confidently. Conventional parent interventions typically include multiple sessions or group therapy, with little regard for the time commitment required by parents to participate. With previous research identifying excessive time commitments as a specific challenge that impacts caregivers' psychosocial strain (Phelps, Hodgson, McCammon, & Lamson, 2009), it is important that we do not add to these constraints, but instead work to alleviate them. To address a family's needs and provide immediate support, it is important to identify a model of care that would be suitable, effective, and practical for parents following their child's diagnosis, and at the same time one that promotes a strengths-based approach to supporting families, thereby building resilience.

This chapter considers the use of Single Session Therapy (SST) with parents following their child's diagnosis of autism. This proactive approach to supporting families will also likely be beneficial to a diverse range of families, including those of children with other diagnosed conditions.

Family Resilience

Family resilience is defined here as a family's ability to adapt to risk and adversity by drawing on protective factors and internal and community resources (Mackay, 2003; Walsh, 2002). Strengthening family functioning and capacities in the face of adversity is the process by which to build family resilience. A family's response and adaptation to adversity (i.e., coping mechanisms) is an important element to consider as it may provide the initial indication of a family's ability to "bounce back." Family resilience provides a framework to guide prevention and intervention and to support and strengthen vulnerable families. It can serve as an important foundation for SST. By using focused brief intervention, we can help families identify their risks and protective factors to better understand their vulnerabilities and their strengths that could help them through the difficult times. Family resilience is more than managing crises and stressful life events – it is about recognizing potential for personal and relational transformation and growth, and a heightening of attention to what really matters. By fostering the underlying processes for resilience, families can become stronger and more resourceful.

Processes for resilience operating at the family level – including strong emotional attachments, effective communication, use of coping strategies, and family belief systems, especially those grounded in spiritual and religious values – are all important means by which families manage to cope with adversity (Mackay, 2003). Resilient families are described as those that show active persistence, perseverance, maintenance of hope and optimism, and confidence that they can overcome difficult situations.

Existing evidence has shown that the best approaches to instill family resilience involved early intervention that is sensitive to families' cultures and values, and that assist in relieving families' ecological stresses (Mackay, 2003). The period immediately post-diagnosis could be referred to as the "early intervention period." In the resilience literature, *intervening early* has been identified as a hallmark of successful intervention programs (Mackay, 2003). Given this recognition, a brief family clinic intervention built on single session therapy may be the most appropriate and realistic pathway to promote family resilience post-diagnosis. In addition to focusing on parents' reactions to diagnosis, the proposed single session model seeks to enhance family resilience by helping families tap into their existing resources and increase individual and family protective factors (e.g., social support, effective coping strategies, parenting self-efficacy).

Why Consider Single Session Therapy?

Single session therapy has evolved on the premise that the first session of psychotherapy is potentially the most therapeutic and has the greatest influence on outcome, with a single session being the most common length of psychotherapy (Hoyt, Bobele, Slive, Young, & Talmon, 2018; Hoyt & Talmon, 2014; Talmon, 2012; Young & Rycroft, 1997). Prior to researching families, I supported them in my role as a family counselor at one of the leading autism organizations in Melbourne, Australia. Over my years of practice, one thing became more and more evident: families were certainly time-poor and overwhelmed after receiving a child's diagnosis. Despite this, they were receptive to compassionate care that offered clear and direct information at this critical time in their lives. I provided families with face-to-face and telephone counseling. Although there was the option to access more than one counseling session for free due to government funding, I noticed that most parents attended one session and did not return for any subsequent appointments. One might think that this was a product of poor therapeutic alliance. However, when followed up, the most common response was "that was enough" to get them started on their journey. This did not mean that they never con-tacted the service again, although for some this was the case. However, more importantly, families consistently reported that in that first and often only session they received useful and sufficient information to make the next steps.

After systematically examining the various interventions available to families, including parent-training and group programs, numerous bar-riers that reduce parent participation in long-term psychotherapy were identified, including (a) inability or unwillingness to take the time and energy to complete longer-term programs, (b) concerns that individual problems will not be adequately addressed in group settings, and (c) privacy issues (Campbell, 1993; Johnson, Harrison, Burnett, & Emerson, 2003; Phelps et al., 2009).

Acute and immediate family support can be provided using SST, with the opportunity to shift parents' orientation toward greater family resi-lience and coping and improve family well-being post-diagnosis. An SST model is not only a more acceptable option for some parents, but it can provide a positive, short-term, cost-effective, and economically viable option to supporting families at this vulnerable time (Perkins, 2006; Talmon, 2012).

Single Session Therapy and Its Potential to Improve Families' Lives

Despite findings showing that a single session of therapy reduces symp-toms of depression, anxiety, and stress and improves confidence in par-enting skills (Hymmen, Stalker, & Cait, 2013), there are only a few published studies using SST with parents. Sommers-Flanagan (2007) examined general child-rearing strategies and measured parents' out-comes following a single consultation. After the session, parents rated themselves as less stressed and more capable of managing their child's behaviors. Parents also reported very positive reactions to their brief consultation experience. Several other studies have explored SST within a solution-focused family therapy approach in mental health settings, and consistently showed significant improvement in clinical psychopathology, satisfaction with service, and sustained positive outcomes over a 6- and 18-month period (Perkins, 2006; Perkins & Scarlett, 2008; McGarry et al., 2008). However, to my knowledge only one study exists which evaluated the efficacy of brief or single session counseling for parents of children diagnosed with autism. Ryan and O'Connor (2017) examined the feasibility of a single session psychology clinic for parents of children on the spectrum. It revealed a good attendance rate (88%) by parents and high satisfaction (76%), but no measures of parental anxiety, stress, or child outcomes were reported.

How to determine (and who decides) whether one session or multiple sessions of therapy are required is a universal challenge in psychotherapy, as is deciding when *"enough is enough."* For parents at the time of diagnosis, providing choice and empowerment regarding therapy is essential to making therapy a success. It is important to understand that the end of a single therapeutic session does not necessarily indicate that all problems have been completely and permanently resolved (Hoyt & Rosenbaum, 2018).

Instead, a single session of effective therapy provides an opportunity for a significant piece of psychological work to be accomplished that permits clients to then manage on their own. Being able to *re-enter society* (to their new normal) after receiving a child's diagnosis of a lifelong disability, such as autism, is an important consideration for parents. Specifically, a single focused session may assist parents of newly diagnosed children to begin their journey through early intervention.

Understanding the impact of diagnosis also adds to this argument. Previous research has identified that parents who receive a child's autism diagnosis for the first time experience significantly more distress than parents receiving subsequent diagnoses (Rabba, Dissanayake, & Barbaro, 2020). Supporting families when they are first exposed to autism is important as this first encounter may set the threshold for their coping and family resilience moving forward.

A Family Clinic

A specialized Family Clinic was developed to support parents after receiving their child's diagnosis of autism. Table 17.1 highlights the relevance of the SST model to these families. Its development was guided by previous qualitative research highlighting parents' experiences following a child's early autism diagnosis (Rabba, Dissanayake, & Barbaro, 2019).

A key factor identified by parents was the need for professional tailored support. The Family Clinic aimed to address these service gaps by providing parents with the opportunity to tailor the session to address their current needs, using the following five goals as a framework.

Table 17.1 Key Elements of SST and Relevance to Parents Following a Child's Autism Diagnosis

Key Elements of SST	Relevance to Parents
Actively find a focus for the session	Helps parents to actively focus on what matters to them most at the time
Check in to ensure the conversation is on track	Tailored session, addressing parents' priority needs in a timely manner
Be responsive to what clients want and share thoughts or ideas with them	Compassionate care that communicates an understanding of families' thoughts, ideas, and circumstances
Allow for the possibility that one session may be enough	A single session may not be enough for all families; it is therefore essential to provide relevant referral pathways for further support
Decide on the next steps together with the client/s	Develop an action plan with families that is realistic for them to achieve and empowers them to make the next steps
Addresses waiting lists and makes services more accessible; less costly than multiple sessions	Financially and economically viable

Note: Adapted from *Single Session Therapy* (The Bouverie Centre, La Trobe University, 2020).

Main Goals of the Family Clinic

1. Promote family well-being
2. Improve emotional well-being
3. Enhance family interaction
4. Improve satisfaction and efficacy in the parenting role, and promote self-care
5. Improve skills at seeking information, support, and resources regarding the child's diagnosis and services for the parents and child.

A Single Session in Action: Post-Diagnostic Support for Parents

A single session model of intervention helps the therapist focus on key factors associated with family well-being and resilience - primarily promoting protective factors (e.g., social support, coping strategies) and subsequently alleviating risk factors (e.g., depression, stress) associated with significant life events, such as receiving a child's diagnosis. By utilizing a strengths-based approach, the therapist can enhance parents' confidence to maintain and improve their family well-being. Clinicians also need to be sensitive and attentive to a family's ethnic-cultural values, whilst considering the implications of these on their experience post-diagnosis. The purpose of the Family Clinic is to improve the well-being and functioning of the entire family; therefore, it is recommended that when there are two caregivers/parents within the family unit, both attend this session together.

A case vignette (below) showcases the key elements of the post-diagnostic Family Clinic and how it is put into action.

Case Vignette

Marcella and Peter are parents of 2.5 year-old Lucas, recently diagnosed with autism. Although Marcella identified delays in Lucas' development early on (~9 months old), she thought he was "just a shy and quieter boy." Both Marcella and Peter are in their late-30s and of Italian heritage. Lucas is their first child. Following their son's assessment, Marcella and Peter were offered to attend a Family Clinic, which was described as a two-hour single session of therapy to focus on their needs moving forward. Two weeks after the diagnosis, Marcella and Peter attended the Family Clinic. An after-hours appointment was offered to accommodate the parents' busy schedule.

When Marcella and Peter arrived, they were greeted by the therapist and invited into a quiet and confidential space. Uncertainty was evident in their facial expressions; they did not know what to expect and "how to make the most of this session" as they soon shared with the therapist. The therapist explained the general layout of the session as she had done previously over the phone when booking the appointment and emphasized that the session would be tailored to their needs. Marcella and Peter were given three initial questionnaires to fill out. A form was provided where parents identify their two main concerns or challenges at present to help steer the way for the single session. Marcella and Peter recorded "Understanding autism" and "Where to now?" A list of various topics frequently associated with the period post-diagnosis was also presented to the family. From this list, parents rank in order of priority what they identify as most relevant/important to them. The top four topics are discussed together with the therapist and create the foundation for the single session, guiding parents to prioritize their difficulties and identify their focus. Marcella and Peter highlighted: (1) Knowledge of autism, (2) Coping and moving on, (3) Adapting to the diagnosis, and (4) Problem solving. Although these priorities guided therapy, they were not discussed in isolation.

Throughout the two-hour period of intervention, it became more and more evident that Marcella and Peter were coping with their own grief and so we detoured and steered towards acceptance of the diagnosis. Psychoeducation about autism was provided and how it presented in Lucas, drawing on both his strengths and difficulties. The parents identified their current coping strategies, including use of peer support (other parents), accessing early intervention services, and practicing self-care (e.g., yoga/exercise). The therapist used these opportunities to highlight the family's inner strengths and resources, reinforcing the value in what they were already doing. Mindfulness was employed by the therapist and practiced in-session with both parents to assist them in focusing on the here and now.

An Action Plan was devised collaboratively between the parents and therapist. This Action Plan enables parents to consolidate what was discussed in SST and apply some of this newfound knowledge to their everyday lives to make a genuine difference to their coping, adaptability, and ultimately resilience during significant life events such as a child's diagnosis.

Marcella and Peter were followed up via phone call two weeks after the Family Clinic. At this point, feedback was sought and post-evaluation completed. Both parents indicated how the session provided them with the opportunity to sit together and think about what this diagnosis meant to them, something they had not done prior to the appointment. It also gave them the space to discuss the unspoken grief that existed for both and how they had individually been managing this grief. Marcella and Peter noted that their Italian background played a key role in how they were coping with the diagnosis, stating that the stigma still attached to disability in their ethnic community made it challenging to discuss autism with family. However, during the session they identified close friends with whom they felt comfortable to share the diagnosis and from whom to seek social support. Although the session did not answer all the questions regarding Lucas' diagnosis, Marcella and Peter were able to leave with a better understanding of autism, clarity on their individual strengths and coping, and a practical and realistic action plan.

What Is Key to SST Practice with Families of Children on the Autism Spectrum?

Creating a safe space for parents to be heard and validated is essential for families at this critical post-diagnosis time. The single session provides parents with an opportunity to develop a greater understanding of what it means to them to be a parent of a child on the autism spectrum. The initial questionnaires are fundamental to the process of SST as they identify the short-term and long-term goals of this individual session and more broadly for the family moving forward.

An important element that contributes to building a strong therapeutic alliance in parents of children on the spectrum, and dare I say for any individual, is compassion. Most importantly, research shows that parents seek therapists who instill a sense of hope in families (Abbott, Bernard, & Forge, 2012; Woodgate, Ateah, & Secco, 2008). Parents also demonstrate a preference for a therapist who has knowledge in autism to help explain the diagnosis relative to their child and to guide them through the service system (Rabba et al., 2020).

Conclusion

Everyone's experience post-diagnosis is unique, and therefore their journey will be different. As therapists, it is our responsibility to see and honor this journey, however difficult and challenging it may be for some families. Coping with a child's diagnosis of autism can be likened to coping with the various stages of grief (Kübler-Ross, 1969), and subsequently denial is a hallmark experience for some parents. Working against this resistance can be a challenging space for therapists. On reflection, some of the greatest learnings and achievements in my career have been in helping parents step outside of the denial phase and move toward the more enlightening stage of acceptance.

Traditional models of therapy should not be ignored but rather integrated into the SST framework. Incorporating evidence-based practice, including Cognitive Behavior Therapy, Mindfulness, Acceptance and Commitment Therapy, Family Systems, and Positive Psychology within SST can only add value and validation to this practice. Focusing on the here and now and what could be done rather than ruminating on the diagnosis itself enables parents to harness control and identify individual and family strengths sooner, therefore leading to earlier intervention, access to support, and improved well-being.

Note

1 The author acknowledges the financial support of the Cooperative Research Centre for Living with Autism (Autism CRC), established and supported under the Australian Government's Cooperative Research Centres Program. She also acknowledges the support of her research supervisors, Professor Cheryl Dissanayake and Dr. Josephine Barbaro, of the Olga Tennison Autism Research Centre at La Trobe University. Most importantly, she expresses her sincere gratitude to all the families who continue to share their stories and experiences following their child's diagnosis of autism.

References

Abbott, M., Bernard, P., & Forge, J. (2012). Communicating a diagnosis of autism spectrum disorder – A qualitative study of parents' experiences. *Clinical Child Psychology and Psychiatry, 18*(3), 370–382. doi:10.1177/1359104512455813.

Campbell, C. (1993). Strategies for reducing parent resistance to consultation in the schools. *Elementary School Guidance and Counseling, 28*(2), 83–91.

Crane, L., Chester, J.W., Goddard, L., Henry, L.A., & Hill, E.L. (2016). Experiences of autism diagnosis: A survey of over 1000 parents in the United Kingdom. *Autism, 20*(2), 153–162.

Feinberg, E., Augustyn, M., Fitzgerald, E., Sandler, J., Ferreira-Cesar Suarez, Z., Chen, N., ... Silverstein, M. (2014). Improving maternal mental health after a child's diagnosis of autism spectrum disorder: Results from a randomized clinical trial. *Journal of American Medical Association Pediatrics, 168*(1), 40–46. doi:10.1001/jamapediatrics.2013.3445.

Hoyt, M.F., Bobele, M., Slive, A., Young, J., & Talmon, M. (Eds.). (2018). *Single-Session Therapy by Walk-In or Appointment: Administrative, Clinical, and Supervisory Aspects of One-at-a-Time Services.* New York: Routledge.

Hoyt, M.F., & Rosenbaum, R. (2018). Some ways to end at SST. In M.F. Hoyt et al. (Eds.), *Single-Session Therapy by Walk-In or Appointmnt* (pp. 318–323). New York: Routledge.

Hoyt, M.F., & Talmon, M. (Eds.). (2014). *Capturing the Moment: Single Session Therapy and Walk-In Services.* Bethel, CT: Crown House Publishing.

Hymmen, P., Stalker, C.A., & Cait, C.-A. (2013). The case for single-session therapy: Does the empirical evidence support the increased prevalence of this service delivery model? *Journal of Mental Health, 22*(1), 60–71. doi:10.3109/09638237.2012.670880.

Johnson, D.C., Harrison, B.C., Burnett, M.F., & Emerson, P. (2003). Deterrents to participation in parenting education. *Family and Consumer Sciences Research Journal, 31*(4), 403–424. doi:10.1177/1077727x03031004004.

Kübler-Ross, E. (1969). *On Death and Dying: What the Dying Have to Teach Doctors, Nurses, Clergy and Their Own Families.* New York: Routledge.

Mackay, R. (2003). Family resilience and good child outcomes: An overview of the research literature. *Social Policy Journal of New Zealand, 20*, 98–118.

McGarry, J., McNicholas, F., Buckley, H., Kelly, B.D., Atkin, L., & Ross, N. (2008). The clinical effectiveness of a brief consultation and advisory approach compared to treatment as usual in child and adolescent mental health services. *Clinical Child Psychology and Psychiatry, 13*(3), 365–376. doi:10.1177/1359104508090600.

McGrew, J.H., & Keyes, M.L. (2014). Caregiver stress during the first year after diagnosis of an autism spectrum disorder. *Research in Autism Spectrum Disorders, 8*, 1373–1385.

Perkins, R. (2006). The effectiveness of one session of therapy using a single-session therapy approach for children and adolescents with mental health problems. *Psychology and Psychotherapy: Theory, Research and Practice, 79*, 215–227.

Perkins, R., & Scarlett, G. (2008). The effectiveness of single session therapy in child and adolescent mental health. Part 2: An 18-month follow-up study. *Psychology and Psychotherapy: Theory, Research and Practice, 81*(2), 143–156. doi:10.1348/147608308x280995

Phelps, K.W., Hodgson, J.L., McCammon, S.L., & Lamson, A.L. (2009). Caring for an individual with autism disorder: A qualitative analysis. *Journal of Intellectual & Developmental Disability, 34*(1), 27–35. doi:10.1080/13668250802690930.

Rabba, A.S., Dissanayake, C., & Barbaro, J. (2019). Parents' experiences of an early autism diagnosis: Insights into their needs. *Research in Autism Spectrum Disorders, 66*, 101415. https://doi.org/10.1016/j.rasd.2019.101415.

Rabba, A.S., Dissanayake, C., & Barbaro, J. (2020). Distress, understanding, and acceptance: Measuring the impact of an autism diagnosis. Manuscript submitted for publication.

Ryan, C., & O'Connor, S. (2017). Single session psychology clinic for parents of children with Autism Spectrum Disorder: A feasibility study. *Journal of Child and Family Studies, 26*(6), 1614–1621. doi:10.1007/s10826-017-0681-0.

Sommers-Flanagan, J. (2007). Single-session consultations for parents: A preliminary investigation. *The Family Journal, 15*(1), 24–29. doi:10.1177/1066480706294045.

Stuart, M., & McGrew, J.H. (2009). Caregiver burden after receiving a diagnosis of an autism spectrum disorder. *Research in Autism Spectrum Disorders, 3*, 86–97.

Talmon, M. (2012). When less is more: Lessons from 25 years of attempting to maximize the effect of each (and often only) therapeutic encounter. *Australian and New Zealand Journal of Family Therapy, 33*(1), 6–14.

The Bouverie Centre, La Trobe University (2020). Web page summary of Single Session Therapy. Retrieved from https://www.bouverie.org.au/support-for-services/our-specialist-areas/specialist-area-single-session-therapy-sst-alternativ ely-referred-to-as-sin.

Walsh, F. (2002). A family resilience framework: Innovative practice applications. *Family Relations, 51*(2), 130–137. doi:10.1111/j.1741-3729.2002.00130.x.

Woodgate, R.L., Ateah, C., & Secco, L. (2008). Living in a world of our own: The experience of parents who have a child with autism. *Qualitative Health Research, 18*(8), 1075–1083. doi:10.1177/1049732308320112.

Young, J., & Rycroft, P. (1997). Single-session therapy: Capturing the moment. *Psychotherapy in Australia, 4*(1), 18–23.

18 Single Session Approaches with Infants: A Collaborative Single Session Model

Rosalie Birkin

The practice of Single Session Work has become embedded in mental health services in Australia (Le Gros, Wyder, & Brunelli, 2019). Single Session Work has also become a more common method of infant mental health service delivery in this country. For many years now, I have been providing single sessions for infants; that is, newborns to three-year-old. This has been mostly within a mental health agency but also in private practice.

For me, the impetus for providing services in this way began 40 years ago when I was first employed within a community mental health service. I was a member of a multidisciplinary team that was charged with the task of exploring alternative ways of delivering child mental health services to those in most need. Together we developed a model of mental health consultation that was referred to as the Victorian Model (Luntz, 1999). Its roots lay in the innovative work of the psychiatrist, Gerald Caplan, who created an alternative model of providing services, which became known as Caplanian Mental Health Consultation (Caplan, Caplan, & Erchul, 1994). Caplan's model involves consulting directly with professionals about their clients, rather than consulting with the clients themselves. It was created in 1949 as a means of meeting the overwhelming need for mental health care for thousands of adolescents who had recently migrated from post-Holocaust Europe to the newly created State of Israel (Caplan et al., 1994).

The Victorian model includes three levels: *Primary Consultation*, where the client is seen by the consultant; *Secondary Consultation*, where the client is discussed with the consultant; and *Tertiary Consultation*, where discussion focuses on program and agency operation (Luntz, 1999).

Primary Consultation can be thought of as a Single Session approach in that it involves a planned meeting with the referring professional (most often at their place of work) in order to gather information immediately prior to the clinical session; and then a follow-up with that professional immediately following the clinical encounter for further discussion. This discussion ordinarily involves thinking together about how the referring professional could best help the person in their care, drawing on the knowledge and skills of the consultant who conducted the clinical session, and the knowledge and skills of the referring professional. In this approach, it is the referring professional who continues providing services to the client (e.g., classroom teaching) while incorporating what has been gained from the consultant. The consultant's involvement is essentially a single session.

In the late 1990s, I established a Multidisciplinary Infant Mental Health Team providing a comprehensive range of services: direct clinical services, mental health consultation services, community development, research, education, and training of professionals. Amongst the clinical services offered were single sessions for infants. Single sessions became the predominant mode of delivering clinical services, and these approaches were very much valued by those within the Multidisciplinary Infant Mental Health Team, and by local health/welfare professionals.

Why Single Sessions for Infants?

There are several reasons for providing single sessions for infants:

- Assessment and/or therapy or recommendations can be provided within a single contact
- Services can be provided in a timely manner; on the day of contact, or within days or weeks, in contrast to the problems related to accessing mental health services in Australia including "long waiting lists, restrictive intake criteria, or complicated intake procedures" (Young, Weir, & Rycroft, 2012, p. 85)
- Working this way means that more infants and their families are able to receive tertiary mental health services
- Single session approaches are resource efficient
- Those infants and families who may not have had the opportunity to access tertiary services for a variety of reasons (e.g., transport difficulties or work commitments) can be provided with tertiary mental health care
- Intervening early in the life of a child means that there is potential to change the child's developmental trajectory and improve the quality of their life. As Thomson Salo and Paul (2007, p. 249) have written: "The longer negative experiences remain unmodified the greater the likelihood that there will be changes in the brain which may mean that therapeutic work cannot ameliorate the early deprivation."

Types of Single Session Approaches for Infants

There are different types of single session approaches that I have found useful in the delivery of infant mental health services. These include:

- Single sessions with one or more infant mental health clinicians at the child and youth mental health facility
- Single sessions with one or more infant mental health clinicians at the infant's home or daycare center
- One-way screen single sessions involving the infant mental health multidisciplinary team and sometimes the primary-care professional already working with the family
- Collaborative Single Sessions involving the primary health or welfare professional, usually at their facility (e.g., a maternal and child health center), or at the infant's home.

Space permits me to focus only on one of these approaches: the Collaborative Single Session Model. This will be followed by a clinical vignette that provides an example of how the model works in practice.

The Collaborative Single Session Model

The Collaborative Single Session Model involves working with the infant and their family, alongside the referring health/welfare professional. These Collaborative Single Sessions aim to provide a brief assessment and therapeutic interventions and/or recommendations for further assessment or treatment. As with Primary Consultation, these sessions are usually held at that professional's center or in the infant's own environment, whether that be the infant's home, childcare center, child health center, or somewhere else – but always with the referring health/welfare professional present.

Caplan's model of Mental Health Consultation that I referred to earlier operates within non-hierarchical relationships: this is considered the cornerstone of the model (Caplan et al., 1994). Similarly, non-hierarchical structures are a fundamental principle of this Collaborative Single Session Model. The professional who engages the mental health clinician brings with them experience and professional expertise that is different from that of the mental health clinician, and it is important for their differences to be acknowledged and valued in this single session approach.

The ordinary practice of the Multidisciplinary Infant Mental Health Team at the mental health service involves two mental health clinicians of different disciplines working alongside the referring professional. The professions of the infant mental health clinicians on the team include psychiatry, clinical psychology, mental health nursing, social work, occupational therapy, and speech pathology. In my private practice, the Collaborative Single Session Model usually involves just the referring professional and myself. Maternal and child health nurses and health professionals working at community health centers have been the most frequent referrers for Collaborative Single Sessions.

Structure of the Collaborative Single Session Model

Ordinarily, the total time set aside for a Collaborative Single Session is 90 minutes: 15 minutes of discussion just with the referring professional; followed by 60 minutes with the referring professional, infant, and their family; and then another 15 minutes discussing the clinical material and the process of the session with the referring professional, after the infant and family have left the facility.

In recognition that this will be a single session, in those first 15 minutes a discussion is had about what the referring professional hopes to gain from the contact. Information is gathered about the infant and their family, including the referring professional's understanding of what the parents most want from the session. We also think together about what the areas of focus for the session will be, keeping in mind that this may change during the session. Clinical decisions are made together about how to arrange the room and what toys and equipment are needed, where those items will be positioned, and sometimes, what needs to be removed from the room.

Decisions also are made about roles that will be adopted when seeing the infant and their family, including which professional will lead the session, who will engage mostly with the infant during the session, and who will engage mostly with the parents. Decisions are sometimes made about which person will raise specific issues or explore specific areas. These decisions are made on the basis of clinical expertise, experience with the model, professional discipline, and relationship with the family, among other factors. Because it is not possible to predict exactly how the session will flow, there is usually an agreement reached that the arrangement made may need to change during the session.

After the referring professional has invited the family into the consulting room and introductions are made, including introducing professionals to the infant, we all talk about the session and what the family hopes to gain from this encounter. One of the professionals may then take the lead at this point to explain the proposed plan for the session, making adjustments in response to the parents' comments and questions. While it is made clear that this is a single session, the possibility of future professional contact is also discussed at the beginning of the session. Information is ordinarily gathered then from parents to assist with better understanding of the infant and their circumstances. The professional who takes this role may be the referring health/welfare worker, or one of the infant mental health clinicians. Following that, one or both parents are ordinarily asked to play/engage with the infant as they would at home. One of the professionals present may subsequently engage separately with the infant to gain more information about the infant's capacities, or to attend to some area of concern (e.g., poor eye contact, limited verbal expression, or delayed play skills).

As the session progresses, the infant mental health clinicians and the referring professional may speak with parents about their observations; highlight child/parent interactions – especially when there have been positive interactions; ask about what the parents have observed or what they have noticed has been helpful (e.g., commenting on what has helped the child regulate their emotions); maybe enquire about the child's communication bids; wondering out loud what might be understood by the infant's behavior; making comments that may evoke thoughts in the minds of the parents to help them to make links with their own experience. When possible, opportunities may be taken to model how to observe and wonder about their child.

Throughout the session the professionals observe, listen, and reflect their thoughts. They may comment or enquire about the child's physical health, development, mental health, relationships, attachment, and general well-being. The focus of the discussion is on assisting parents to better understand the child's development and well-being, and to help them develop ideas of how they can better meet the needs of the infant.

There may be psychoeducation offered depending on the circumstances. Sometimes specific strategies for behavior management, or ideas to promote areas of development, are offered and discussed. There may be recommendations made for referral elsewhere. These strategies, ideas, and recommendations may be offered by any one of the professionals present. Sometimes the infant mental health clinicians may recommend that it is best that the child is referred to an Infant Mental Health Service for a more comprehensive assessment or ongoing therapy. Some recommendations also may relate to the health/welfare needs of the parents.

After the family leaves the facility, 15 minutes are reserved to meet with the referring health/welfare professional to discuss the session in terms of process, observations, interventions, and recommendations. Further thoughts from the infant mental health clinicians about the infant and their family may be provided to the referring professional at this point; thoughts that may have been unhelpful to speak about with the family. For example, the infant may have presented with some signs of autism, but not enough information to be clear that there is a need for a formal autism diagnostic assessment. To raise the possibility of such a diagnosis in these circumstances could be very distressing for parents, and it could be unnecessary. Ongoing observation and monitoring of the health and development of the infant is something that the referring professional can do in their work with the infant and the family following the single session. If the appropriateness of an autism diagnostic assessment becomes clearer sometime later, this can be raised by the referring professional with the parents then[1].

Other information discussed with the referring professional may relate to areas of concern or to services that the referring professional person may need to keep in mind, or to information that may be helpful if similar presentations arise in the course of the professional's work. Likewise, the referring professional may also share information that is helpful for the infant mental health clinicians.

With regard to reporting, sometimes just spoken feedback is given to parents. Sometimes brief notes are provided to the parents about what has been observed, discussed, or recommended. This may be just a paragraph or just a few points noted. Sometimes written reports are prepared subsequent to the single session. Sometimes reports are very detailed and may extend to five pages. That is more likely to be the case if there are developmental concerns, and especially if there are concerns about autism. Reports may be provided directly to the parents, or they are sent to the referring professional, who will then offer that report on to the parents. That may happen in a subsequent session held by the referring professional with the parents, where there is also an opportunity to discuss the material.

Advantages of the Collaborative Single Session Model

This model has advantages in addition to those listed earlier:

- Using this approach can mean that the anxiety aroused in attending another facility is avoided, especially if that facility is a mental health clinic
- Because the health/welfare professional already known to the family is also present for the session, this may help them engage more easily in the process
- It offers the possibility of a significant therapeutic impact and potential for change
- It can reduce the perception of stigma often associated in accessing mental health services
- The referring health/welfare professional can use the knowledge and skills gained in the session in their future contact with that family
- The referring health/welfare professional can use the knowledge and skills gained in the session with others within their care
- If the family has a good experience within the single session, this may change what might have been negative perceptions of mental health services, and may mean that there is less concern and a greater likelihood that they would access mental health services in the future if such services are needed
- If the mental health clinician is from a mental health service and a local record of the contact is kept, then if the family or person present at the service in the future, that record could prove helpful.

Similarities to Other Single Session Approaches

A single session/one-at-a-time approach, while customized to fit each client and context, is also generally characterized by the unfolding of a series of steps or stages (e.g., see Hoyt & Talmon, 2014) that help to organize the beginning, middle, and end of the meeting in order to make the most of the session. Following the overall understanding that it will be a one-off, complete-unto-itself meeting, there is development of an alliance; the identification of specific goals for the session; then engagement in processes to achieve the goals; then some checking to see if the goals have been met; then discussion of next steps and follow-up; then leave-taking. Most of these steps apply to this collaborative single session approach with infants. With this approach, however, the development of an alliance also needs to occur between the professionals prior to meeting the family.

The following clinical example illustrates these stages as we move through the single session consultation.

Clinical Example

A four-month-old infant, Rebecca, had been referred to me by a maternal and child health nurse from a local health center. Rebecca was her parents' first child. The nurse was concerned that Rebecca wasn't making eye contact and rarely smiling. Rebecca's mother was being treated by her general practitioner for post-natal depression. Jane had told the nurse that she felt "defeated" and was not enjoying her baby. The nurse wondered if Rebecca's symptoms might be related to autism or might indicate an attachment problem.

Development of an Alliance with the Professional and Setting Initial Goals

I arrived at the health center about 15 minutes before the family arrived to meet with the nurse so that we could think about the planned single session. She was able to tell me a little more about the parenting couple; the family background; Jane's experience of the pregnancy, birth, and motherhood; and Rebecca's development. She said that Rebecca's father worked night shifts and was not often available to share the parenting load during Rebecca's waking hours. Their families lived overseas. Some friends lived nearby, but more recently, contact even with them had only been via telephone. The nurse added that to date Rebecca's development seemed to be progressing normally. The nurse and I discussed what we thought was important to explore in the session with mother and baby, and how we would assess Rebecca's mental health and well-being.

Establishing the Framework of a Single Session

We met Jane and Rebecca in the waiting room and the nurse invited them into her consulting room. Rebecca was in a stroller, but not appearing interested in the new environment, and not bothering to look in our direction, even after our offering welcoming hellos and smiles. I explained to Jane that this was a once-off session but that if we all thought that more time with the nurse, or with me, or someone else would be helpful, we could talk about that at the end of the session.

Development of an Alliance with the Family and Setting Goals

Jane was clearly depressed. She told us of her worries about Rebecca, and her hope that we might be able to help her baby. She lifted Rebecca from the stroller and held her up in front of her face, as mothers sometimes do. Rebecca immediately turned her head away. Jane became clearly distressed by Rebecca's response.

Engagement in the Process to Achieve Goals

Jane talked about feeling rejected by Rebecca and her overwhelming thoughts of being a "bad mother." She worried that she had harmed her baby because she wasn't being the happy mother that "Rebecca deserved." We reflected on how awful it must be to have these experiences and thoughts, and how much harder this would make parenting. As Jane held her baby on her lap, Rebecca just sat quietly and made no attempt to look at us or to explore the room with her eyes. She showed little expression on her face.

We talked with Jane about her situation, including her isolation from family, and we reflected on how difficult it must be to care for a baby in such circumstances. I asked if I could hold Rebecca, and Jane agreed.

After a time, and quite a bit of effort, I was able to engage Rebecca's eye contact and, not long after that, received a smile. It became clearer as the session progressed that Rebecca was otherwise developing normally, and that perhaps her turning away from her mother's gaze was related specifically to their relationship, and not to Rebecca's development. Perhaps Rebecca's gaze-aversion was related to Rebecca not wanting to see her mother's sad face, and experience that sadness? Perhaps this was also a protective measure to avoid finding that her mother's attention was focused elsewhere? Jane had noticed my attempts to engage Rebecca and expressed relief that Rebecca had been responsive. Maybe this meant to Jane that Rebecca wasn't damaged irreparably after all.

Later in the session as Jane's mood lifted, she tried out the strategies I had employed to engage Rebecca. Jane expressed surprise and delight when Rebecca's eyes met her gaze. Jane asked about what else she might do to engage Rebecca, and we offered a range of ideas: presenting interesting and noisy toys to attract her interest, and then raising these toys to eye level so that Rebecca would meet her mother's gaze; also peek-a-boo games and bubble games to gain her interest and shared enjoyment (*more possible solutions*).

After wondering out loud about Rebecca's turning away, we gently offered our thoughts as outlined earlier. These were presented in a way that was met with acceptance and appreciation from Jane, but also sadness.

As the session progressed, Jane seemed to be enjoying her baby more, and Rebecca seemed more alive. When discussing toys, Jane was able to offer her own ideas of Rebecca having a favorite toy with her when they go out together, and this might be a way to help Rebecca with transitions. The nurse and I both enthusiastically endorsed this idea.

Time was also spent thinking together about Jane's situation: why she was feeling as she was and what additional help might be needed.

Review, Follow-Up, Feedback, and Goodbyes

After reviewing the session together, Jane was given a brief feedback form to complete and return to the nurse. We then said our goodbyes, and the nurse reminded Jane of their scheduled session the next week.

Review of Goals with the Professional

The nurse and I met for another 15 minutes to review the session. The nurse said that she felt more assured about Rebecca's development and well-being and felt more hopeful for both mother and baby.

It was our impression that Jane found this Single Session Collaborative approach helpful for Rebecca and herself, and that was consistent with the feedback she gave to the nurse at her next scheduled visit to the health center.

Conclusion

When working with infants, there are various single session approaches that can be applied. I have mentioned some of those that I have found helpful. In this chapter, I have focused on one of these approaches: the Collaborative Single Session Model, and I have illustrated this model by way of a clinical vignette to more clearly explain how it works in practice. As noted earlier, working together with the referring professional in a non-hierarchical structure is an essential principle of this model, and one I have found very valuable. One must also respect and value the knowledge and experience of all family members in order for this single session model to have a significant therapeutic impact.

It is a very rewarding way of working!

Note

1 *Editors' note:* For a discussion of single session counseling post autism diagnosis, see Rabba, Chapter 17 this volume.

References

Caplan, G., Caplan, R.B., & Erchul, W.P. (1994). Caplanian mental health consultation: Historical background and current status. *Consulting Psychology Journal: Practice and Research, 46*(4), 2–12.

Hoyt, M.F., & Talmon, M. (2014). The temporal structure of brief therapy: Some questions often associated with different phases of sessions and treatments. In M.F. Hoyt & M. Talmon (Eds.), *Capturing the Moment: Single-Session Therapy and Walk-In Services* (pp. 517–522). Bethel, CT: Crown House Publishing.

Le Gros, J., Wyder, M., & Brunelli, V. (2019). Single session work: Implementing brief intervention as routine practice in an acute care mental health assessment service. *Australasian Psychiatry, 27*(1), 21–24.

Luntz, J.J. (1999). What is mental health consultation? *Children Australia, 24*(3), 28–33.

Thomson Salo, F., & Paul, C. (Eds.). (2007). *The Baby as Subject: New Directions in Infant-Parent Therapy from the Royal Children's Hospital.* Melbourne, Australia: Royal Children's Hospital.

Young, J., Weir, S., & Rycroft, P. (2012). Implementing single session therapy. *Australian and New Zealand Journal of Family Therapy, 33*(1), 84–97.

19 Single Session Therapy for People with a New HIV Diagnosis: Achieving a Positive Result

Kieran O'Loughlin

This chapter examines an application of Single Session Therapy (SST) to counseling people newly diagnosed with the Human Immunodeficiency Virus (HIV) at Thorne Harbour Health (previously the Victorian AIDS Council), an Australian community-based, government-funded health agency in Melbourne.

The implementation of SST is presented from the perspective of the author who was a senior staff member of the counseling service at Thorne Harbour Health. The chapter begins with a brief overview of HIV testing and treatment in Australia, and then describes the established pathway from HIV testing conducted in healthcare settings (including the use of pre- and post-test discussions) to post-test counseling, before moving on to an analysis of the adoption of SST with newly diagnosed HIV positive clients at Thorne Harbour Health. Two key questions for the adoption of SST in the agency were whether or not (1) the initial SST session can incorporate a full assessment and still be therapeutic, and (2) its effective use would require training in both the general single session mindset *and* the specific issues likely to arise in counseling newly diagnosed HIV-positive clients.

HIV Testing

Since the late 1980s in Australia, HIV testing has been widely available on a voluntary basis. It consists of a blood test that detects the presence of HIV antibodies as evidence of an individual's exposure to the virus. Where such antibodies are present the person is diagnosed to be "HIV positive," or if not, "HIV negative." Until the late 1990s, in the absence of effective medical treatments, an HIV positive test result was very often a death sentence as the virus would gradually destroy the person's immune system leaving them vulnerable to the range of opportunistic infections that defined AIDS (Acquired Immune Deficiency Syndrome). However, the advent of new antiretroviral therapies (ART) in the late 1990s has changed a new HIV diagnosis into a chronic but manageable condition similar to diabetes for the majority of cases. This significant medical development has helped to promote the value of testing as a key strategy in effective HIV treatment and prevention (Johnson, 2019). In addition, regular adherence to ART enables many people living with HIV to reach the established threshold for a suppressed viral load at which point any risk of them transmitting the virus to other people is effectively eliminated.

Increasing the availability of testing (including follow-up contact tracing where appropriate) and treatment have become the cornerstones of the strategies used by Australian federal and state governments to limit the transmission of HIV over the last decade. The Kirby Institute (2018) reports that in 2017 there were an estimated 27,545 people living with HIV (PLHIV) in Australia. Of those, an estimated 89% had been diagnosed through HIV testing, leaving only 11% who had not been tested and were therefore unaware of their HIV positive status. Of the 21,560 people (87% of those diagnosed) receiving ART, 20,412 (95% of those on ART) had suppressed viral load. This corresponds to 74% of all PLHIV in Australia having a suppressed load in 2017.

Pre- and Post-HIV Test Discussions

Given the potentially serious health implications of contracting HIV, an established practice for the last 30 years in Australia and other Western countries has been for the medical or trained peer health worker to engage the person presenting for HIV testing in brief pre- and post-test discussions (Bor, Miller, & Goldman, 1992; Department of Health, Housing & Community Services, 1992; Johnson & Lenton, 2017; Miller & Bor, 1989). These discussions enable the person presenting for testing to firstly, give informed consent at the end of the pre-test discussion; and, secondly, better understand the psychosocial and other personal implications of their test result, whether positive or negative in the post-test discussion.

Accredited competency-based training programs have been gradually developed in Australia to enable health workers conducting the testing to effectively carry out these discussions. Their content and direction have undergone a number of changes over the last three decades, particularly in response to the availability of ART for both the treatment and prevention of the HIV virus. During the 1980s and 1990s in the absence of effective medical treatment, the focus of these discussions was largely restricted to behavioral change interventions to encourage newly diagnosed people not to expose their sexual partners and/or people with whom they shared needles to the virus. This has evolved now into a practice whose main aim is to link these people into treatment and care (Johnson, 2019; Johnson & Lenton, 2017). Post-test discussions in particular provide an important precursor and bridge for the vast majority of clients presenting for the initial counseling assessment sessions in which SST was eventually adopted at Thorne Harbour Health.

It is noteworthy at this point to underscore that both the pre- and post-test discussions are conducted in a manner close to the spirit of SST, that is, the "non-therapist" healthcare worker, who administers the HIV test, making the most of each discussion as if they may be the only "counseling" event the person presenting for testing may attend. There is no guarantee that the person will seek follow-up counseling at Thorne Harbour Health (or another appropriate service provider) so the healthcare worker naturally adopts an SST mindset to ensure the most relevant issues – including but not limited to the elements listed above – for the newly diagnosed person are covered in one or possibly two 40-minute post-test discussion sessions.

Incorporating SST Practice into an HIV Community-Based Counseling Service

Thorne Harbour Health (previously the Victorian AIDS Council and renamed in 2018) was established in 1984 by activists with the dual mission of providing HIV prevention and support, and improving the health of gay men (the most at-risk population) in general. Counseling services are provided by both paid staff and volunteer counselors. Newly diagnosed HIV-positive clients who are referred to counseling at the agency have historically been fast-tracked into the service's comprehensive psychosocial assessment, which typically lasts 60–90 minutes and is conducted by a paid staff counselor. Prior to the advent of ART in the late 1990s, most of these clients would have then been prioritized for immediate entry into ongoing or intermittent long-term counseling.

By 2014, with many HIV positive people now living fuller and longer lives by virtue of increased, low-cost access to ART, the agency's counseling service had clearly identified through entry and exit feedback that many clients were not seeking long-term counseling to deal with consequences of a new diagnosis. In 2015, the author (in the role of senior clinician, charged with training and capacity building) initiated an investigation into the viability of adopting a single session therapy approach for these clients as one possible counseling option alongside the usual other two established options of 6–12 sessions and more than 12 sessions. The author subsequently undertook formal training in SST at The Bouverie Centre to support him in the development of this new option. This would require staff counselors conducting their initial assessments to make the most of the opportunity to provide counseling to newly diagnosed HIV-positive clients who may or may not choose to return for follow-up sessions. The agency's management eventually supported the trialing of this approach on the grounds of its potential to better meet the immediate counseling needs of these clients. The author was then asked to conduct a short training session for all staff counselors in the use of the SST model as an approach to incorporating counseling into their client assessments. The SST model, with its emphasis on making the most of each session and approaching the session as if it may be the last, was also envisaged as being applicable to any further counseling sessions clients chose to undertake. Furthermore, it was emphasized during the training that counselors were able to adapt their preferred modalities to the SST model since it is an approach to service delivery rather than a therapeutic model *per se* (Young, Weir, & Rycroft, 2012; Young, 2018).

The standard assessment used by counseling services comprised a comprehensive psychosocial evaluation of each client irrespective of HIV status. These assessments were undertaken face-to-face with each new client by a staff counselor soon after the client's initial contact with the agency. The incorporation of SST into this initial client assessment for newly HIV diagnosed clients (henceforth referred to as the "assessment counseling session") was trialed in 2016. The two key questions examined in the trial evaluation were whether or not (1) the initial SST session could incorporate a full assessment and still be therapeutic, and (2) its effective use would require training in both the general single session mindset *and* the specific issues likely to arise in counseling newly diagnosed HIV-positive clients.

Clients were advised at the outset that this first session would include an assessment and some initial counseling. Counselors were instructed to begin the session by saying something along these lines:

> Thanks for coming in today. I will need to ask you for some information and complete a number of forms as part of your assessment. But I would also like you to able to use this as a counseling session. So, I will ask you some other follow-up questions to allow you to expand on answers as we continue. Also, feel free to ask me any questions or raise any other concerns you might have about your health or counseling.

In gathering the necessary client assessment data, counselors were instructed to look for counseling opportunities in clients' responses to the specific questions relating to their HIV diagnosis. For example, the assessment question "When were you diagnosed?" was typically followed up by further ones such as "What was that experience like for you?" and "How well have you been coping since then?" The next assessment question, "Where were you given your test result?" was followed up by other ones such as "Did you have the opportunity to discuss any issues of immediate concern to you about your result straight after that?" and "Would you like to talk about any of those or other concerns you might have here today?" As a follow-up to the standard assessment question, "Who has or might be able to support you at this time"? the counselor was instructed to ask a question about whether and to whom the client had disclosed their HIV status, such as "Have you already told them or would you like to tell them about your HIV diagnosis?" Counselors were also asked to check clients' understanding of their diagnosis and the treatments available to them by asking questions such as:

- "Do you understand what your test result of HIV-positive means?"
- "Are you aware of the treatments that are available to you and how they work?"
- "Have you started or are you thinking about starting the medications soon? Do you understand how they will improve your health and reduce the risk of you transmitting the virus to other people?"

At the end of the session the counselor asked questions such as:

- "So has the counseling work we have done together today been useful to you?"
- "How might you use what we have been discussing after the session?" and
- "Is this enough counseling for the time being?"

If the client indicated they would like to have further counseling the counselor asked, "Would you like to make a time for another counseling session now or contact us when you are ready?"

The trial was carefully monitored over the next 12 months using completed intake forms and case notes from the initial sessions, and interviews with counselors and clients after these and any subsequent sessions. It was evaluated by the author at the end of 2017. The documentation and interview data gathered from fourteen cases were analyzed as part of this process. Of these cases, seven assessment counseling sessions were conducted by three different counselors who had undertaken the pre- and post-test discussion training and the other seven by five different counselors who had not done so.

From the perspectives of the 14 clients, successful use of the SST approach was unanimously found to involve the counselor efficiently and purposefully reviewing then extending the client's previous post-test discussion(s) with the healthcare worker who had tested and delivered their positive result to them within a post-test discussion. As illustrated above, the counselor began the assessment counseling session by asking clients about their experience of their post-test discussion and then honing in on firstly, the aspects of their positive status that clients indicated they wish to explore; and, secondly, any gaps (as perceived by them and/or the counselor) in their knowledge about the virus and treatment options, especially ART and its role in their health management and transmission prevention. The issues that clients most commonly wished to follow up in this initial session included processing the emotional impact of their diagnosis, exploring to whom they might disclose their positive status and determining their psychosocial support needs at this point in time, including whether they wished to undertake further counseling sessions. The gaps in most clients' knowledge about the virus identified by them and/or their counselor related typically to the significance of their current viral load as indicated by their follow-up blood tests, the nature and role of ART medications in reducing their viral load, the optimal time for commencement of these treatments, and the importance of daily adherence to them both for their own health and transmission prevention. This is probably unsurprising given that, as indicated previously, the post-test discussions focused on the immediate non-medical and psychosocial needs of the newly diagnosed person.

From the counselor perspective, successful use of the SST approach in the assessment counseling session underscored the importance of undertaking the pre- and post-test discussion program. The three counselors who had undertaken this training considered they had conducted a successful session when they reviewed and extended the client's post-test discussion focusing particularly on helping them process their diagnosis at an emotional level, then exploring issues around client disclosure and determining their current psychosocial needs. These counselors also thought the session had been successful if they were able to add to the client's medical knowledge about the nature of HIV and their current viral load. They also considered that it was crucial for the client to grasp the critical importance of early uptake of and daily adherence to ART medications in reducing their viral load in terms of disease and transmission prevention.

The five counselors who had not undertaken the pre- and post-test discussion training considered they had delivered a successful assessment counseling session mainly if the client was able to begin processing their diagnosis at an emotional level, then identify who they might disclose their status to and determine the psychosocial supports they required at this point in time, including whether they wished to undertake further counseling sessions. However, none of these counselors believed they had a serious role to play in building the client's medical knowledge about the virus, and the function and importance of ART for treating it and transmission prevention. Six of the seven clients who attended the sessions with these counselors commented negatively on their counselor's lack of attention to help building their medical understanding of HIV and ART. The remaining client was so traumatized by his diagnosis that he was still trying to process it at an emotional level throughout the two counseling sessions he attended and indicated that he would seek follow-up medical advice from a doctor about treatment. However, even this client suggested it would have been useful if the counselor had been able to provide very basic medical knowledge about the virus and ART to reduce his anxiety and panic, and to provide a bridge to subsequent consultations with the doctor.

The use of the SST approach in the assessment counseling session was therefore found to be successful only when counselors had a sound knowledge of both the psychosocial and biomedical dimensions of HIV care and management. In particular, counselors who had successfully completed formal training in pre- and post-HIV test discussions were far more competent in quickly identifying and adapting to meet the immediate (and potentially ongoing) counseling needs of their newly diagnosed clients using the single session model of service delivery. That is to say, both the brevity and content of the discussions they had learnt to use in their training constituted excellent preparation for an SST approach. However, it was also clear that this training needed to be supplemented by additional professional development about medical aspects in treatment and its impact on transmission prevention. As a result of the trial evaluation, only counselors who had undertaken this training program were allocated to future initial assessment counseling sessions for newly diagnosed HIV-positive clients.

Conclusion

There were two key findings emerging from the trial of the SST approach in this specialized community healthcare context. The first was that the initial SST session could incorporate a full assessment and still be therapeutic. The second was that the effective use of SST requires careful training in *both* its general single session mindset *and* the specific issues likely to arise in counseling, particularly in more specialized health contexts.

References

Bor, R., Miller, R., & Goldman, E. (1992). *Theory and Practice of HIV Counselling: A Systemic Approach*. London: Cassell.

Department of Health, Housing & Community Services. (1992). *National Counselling Guidelines HIV/AIDS*. Canberra: Commonwealth of Australia.

Johnson, J. (2019). Normalising HIV testing in a changing epidemic. *HIV Australia*. Retrieved from https://www.afao.org.au/publications/hiv-australia/hiv-australia-2019/.

Johnson, J., & Lenton, E. (2017). *HIV and Hepatitis Pre and Post Test Discussion in Victoria Consultation Report*. Melbourne: Australian Research Centre in Sex, Health & Society.

Kirby Institute. (2018). *HIV in Australia: Annual Surveillance Short Report*. Sydney: Kirby Institute, University of New South Wales.

Miller, R., & Bor, R. (1989). *AIDS: A Guide to Clinical Counselling.* London: Science Press.

Young, J. (2018). Single session therapy: The misunderstood gift that keeps on giving. In M.F. Hoyt, M. Bobele, A. Slive, J. Young, & M. Talmon (Eds.), *Single-Session Therapy by Walk-In or Appointment: Clinical, Supervisory, and Administrative Aspects* (pp. 40–58). New York: Routledge.

Young, J., Weir, S., & Rycroft, P. (2012). Implementing single session therapy. *Australian and New Zealand Journal of Family Therapy, 33*(1), 84–97.

Section V
Applications in Cross-Cultural/ Non-Western Contexts

20 Following the River's Flow: A Conversation About Single Session Approaches with Aboriginal Families

Alison Elliott, James Dokona, and Henry von Doussa

Alison Elliott and James Dokona are Indigenous family counselors from The Bouverie Centre. In keeping with the centrality of oral traditions in both their cultures, James and Alison talked with Henry von Doussa from The Bouverie Centre about using single session approaches with Aboriginal families in the state of Victoria, Australia.

Alison Elliott's main passion and commitment is to her family. She is a mum of seven and step-mum of five children. Alison has family connections to Wiradjuri Country (Dubbo, New South Wales, Australia) and has Anglo Celtic, Polish, and Danish heritage. She grew up on Dharug Country around the Hawkesbury River in Sydney, New South Wales, so has strong connections to the land there as well.

James Dokona originally hails from Papua New Guinea. He is forever indebted culturally and spiritually to Motu Koita of Papua region. His hope in continuing work with the First Peoples of Australia is to understand the subtle nuances of the similarities and unique differences of culture to his own. James feels it is a privilege and an honor to work with people from a different culture and he uses a cultural lens to formulate solution-focused questions in single session environments.

Henry von Doussa is a researcher at The Bouverie Centre. Born in Australia, his ancestors came from England and Germany. He has worked with Alison and James to support and promote their single session work with Indigenous families. Henry's questions will be indicated with Q.

Q: To start off with, what are some of your ideas around brief therapy and why you think it's a good fit for Indigenous families?

Alison: When the idea came to use a single session framework for working with our mobs[1] I was actually quite skeptical – how was it going to work, especially with trauma-saturated stories and thinking that it's going to take a long time because I believed that lots of safety and trust needs to be built up over time. But as I sat with families and just trusted the process and the conversation, I slowly understood that it felt a better fit, and – it was a relief not having to do big assessments or intakes and just meeting someone with where they're at today. For me, therapy is believing always that someone, somewhere in the system is wanting a change. Whether it's a larger system wanting the change, like Child Protection forcing the family to change behaviors or someone within the family system – someone's wanting a change.

Decolonizing

Alison: Brief therapy fits in with building hope that change can happen. It feels really good to be shifting my initial skepticism. Just listening and actually making it about what the family want to talk about, is a decolonizing approach. It's reconciling all that past imposition of a worker/therapist wanting to direct the session: "We're going to talk about this because this is the priority," instead of actually just meeting the person and saying: "What would you like to get out of today?" – "What's the biggest thing for you today?" I think it's really respecting the person and family.

James: When I meet with the family I see the conversation is like a river running: you never know which way it's going to go. The challenge with some other frameworks is the idea of interviewing the family to develop a hypothesis as to what's happening. And I feel that in doing this, already the balance of power has gone towards the worker/therapist. The SST model doesn't do that. You go in and you see the family where they are and explore how they've been managing and what they want to get out of the conversation.

Alison: If the family comes up with a small solution for something that's immediate, it builds hope that change is possible. It's common that families have seen loads of different services or programs that have locked them into six weeks or eight weeks or ten weeks, having this [single session] is like an immediate sense of, "I can do something about that." So, this shorter approach may be refreshing and can then motivate the next bit of change.

Q: Say more, it's so interesting. It sounds like you're both saying perhaps single session has value in its immediacy.

Alison: It feels more ethical and comes to valuing how precious time is. In this single session framework, it really comes back to, "We've got this amount of time, how can it be most useful to you?" And if they can see a small possibility of shifting, even within the session, of how they've thought about what's going on today, then I see that as motivating.

Dadirri

I did want to talk about listening and taking in information because to me it talks to *Dadirri*[2] – that sense of, if you listen deeply without coming up with something as the worker or the therapist, that gives agency straight away to the client because it's giving space for a possible different way of thinking. If you've always been disempowered, where someone's been telling you what to do next (which is colonization in its essence), then it feels like somebody's thought that they know better than you. Listening deeply helps us to pause and really get to what's most important right now and allows nature's timing. Life's the teacher, we're not going to be in their life all the time, that kind of thing is good to keep in mind too. *Dadirri* fits well within a single session framework as the very concept and way of being is to trust, wait for the right time for things and to develop a deeper awareness of when to act and when not to, when to speak and when to be silent. And to be comfortable with not knowing the answers.

Oral Traditions

Q: And you've talked before in our previous meetings about oral traditions and single session fitting well, that's the same sort of thing?

Alison: Absolutely. Even the process of us being interviewed for this chapter speaks to respecting a different way of being able to communicate the information – to be filling out forms or writing a lot of stuff can be a real block because it's still a colonizing way of getting information. Writing definitely has its place, but the process of valuing listening and speaking, receiving information that way and giving information that way talks to the way we learnt and reflected. It is culturally safer.

James: In terms of the conversation with the family, it's totally family led, client led. I just ask one question – then from that first question we don't know where it's going to end up, so similar to that river I was talking about.

Hope

My question elicits that: "What are your best hopes from us meeting today?" I just ask that one question and it's *that question* that starts it all – the way that I view any individual, couple or family who go to therapy is like they are asking for help – and in that, hope is implicit. Any person that walked in the door has come because they have hope.

Containment, Choice, and Control

I usually use the hour, so, I say, "From now until two o'clock, what do you hope from us meeting today?" That kind of sets the time limit and it's contained already just by me using the clock, and I love using this with kids, too, because kids like to predict how long this is going to go for, because often that's their first question, "How long do I need to sit here for?"

Alison: Having a timeframe also talks to trauma-informed practice, which is to create the choice and control but also *containment*. If things have felt chaotic and the family may not have a sense of time – like things have been going on forever, to be able to say, "We're not going to have to talk about this for hours, we've just got this small window of time," can be a relief – especially if you've been to lots of services and have to retell your story over and over, like many Aboriginal families have.

Q: Say more about being with the family, what do you do in a session? How does the session start?

James: I start fresh every time in a session. So how I would normally start fresh with a session is my usual follow-up question: "What's been better since I saw you last? It's been a fortnight now since I saw you" and their usual response is: "No, nothing's been better," which gives me something to work with and then I stay with that, "So you're saying to me that for that whole fortnight you haven't noticed anything different, any changes?" So, I ask questions like this and then nine times out of ten: "Oh yeah," and they'll come up with something they'll notice that has changed and that little change sparks off everything else and we can start the session from there.[3]

It's all fresh again and they might want to talk about some other issue today and I just think well, it's not my place to go back to the last session. If I had said to them, "Remember in the last session we said that you were going to do this" the problem with that is if you ask that and they didn't do it then shame comes up and then all those sort of things. So that's why I don't ask those questions.

Q: What other practical ideas do you have for people who might not already be using the SST model? What might they take from what you and James do?

Alison: When you feel involved you begin to feel respected. If you've never been involved in the decision making, if it's all been done to you or as a directive, even different family members like young children, if they've never felt involved, they've always just sat in the corner in sessions. By asking every person what they want to get out of the time we have together, it's involving everybody in the solutions, and that sense of choice and control being taken before and now we're giving choice and the control even of what you do in the session. "This is how you're wanting to talk; this is what you're wanting to say, or this is how you're wanting to express it – I will not change it unless you change it."

White Man's Language

James: Jargon is not something I use because I just don't think that it's helpful. So, it is the client's language. Always.

Alison: I think that principle speaks to the *Dadirri* where it says, "We've learnt to speak white man's language, we've listened to what he had to say, and this learning, and listening has to go both ways." It's the most respectful way to begin the healing from colonization where we were told what to think and what to say and what to believe. If you use their language choices, and then if they're wanting to shift and go, "Oh, I don't want to say it like that anymore," great, it's their choice, it's not us trying to direct it.

Permission Seeking

James: What I've noticed is the importance of permission seeking. It's crucial. Always, always ask, "Is it okay if I put this here? Is it okay if we do this?" You attend to the slightest thing.

Q: What would be a slight thing you might attend to?

Alison: It could be moving the chair. Anything, ask permission because it's their space, it's not yours. They might've come to you and use this little room; but it's their space for that time and everything is about permission. To me that's been the most healing in the space because trauma and abuse has been a lack of permission, a lack of respect, a lack of asking. Someone's come in and abused your space, they've abused your body or whatever it is, your family, and the minute that you start to go, "Is it okay?" and you just – you can see people relax.

James: The thing that comes to mind is as the worker/therapist I go in with a blank slate. That's the frame that I go in with, with no preconceived ideas. Viewing the family as resourceful, like really abundant.

Q: When you say "resourceful family," how does that look? What questions do you ask or what do you focus on?

James: For instance, if they've been in the same job for ten years saying stuff like "Have you always been that committed?" and usually people say "Oh yeah, I never viewed myself as making a commitment but now you say that."

"How have you been managing? With all this happening how have you been managing?" and usually they'll say, "I don't know." But you keep asking them the same question and it's, "Oh yeah, I suppose I did manage that."

Alison: Yeah, because that's the other thing – if people haven't ever been given choice, given permission, been asked to articulate something positive about themselves, it can feel like the more that you stay on it the more uncomfortable it is to try and come up with something. But giving them that sense of, we're going to work together on this to name how you did it, instead of avoiding it and going onto the next thing because of the difficulty of looking at yourself. Trauma takes away your sense of self – you become self-focused in that it's all about your survival, but your capacity to reflect on yourself in all the chaos is the hardest work. So with James staying with them and going, "No, we're going to stay with this, how did you actually do this?" it gives that chance of a little breakthrough in, "Actually I did do something," and it's a breakthrough into them self-reflecting.

Session Structure

Alison: The other thing for me is reflecting in front of the family. This is a powerful part of the session, when you can actually just get them not to feel that you've written notes up about them or you've talked to colleagues or you've debriefed to your co-worker/co-therapist. It's in front of them – it's actually a relief for both the family and the worker/therapist if you do it in front of them and you can gauge how they receive it. It's much better than trying to write it up and guess things after the session.

Building Trust

James: One of the prompts I always ask in reflection is, "Alison, we've just met this family, what are your first thoughts, first impressions?"

And it sometimes invites within that single session framework something little, something else they might want to add. It's almost like they've been given an opportunity to watch a little bit and then go, "I never noticed that" or, "There's just this other bit" and it ends in a really nice – that's why that sense of containment, it's ended in such a nice, positive way.

So, in summary, desired outcome, resource talk, preferred future, and then we do feedback at the end. That's the structure that I have in my head, but I don't move from the desired outcome because if you don't establish that, you don't have a place to start from. They give you that.

Q: It looks to me as an outsider that you do an enormous amount of instant trust building or something to give you the confidence to do that digging around about what the family or individual really wants. How do you do that?

Alison: I just wanted to go back to those five principles that The Bouverie Centre (2013) uses, which are safety, trust, choice, collaboration, and empowerment. So, I feel like the processes that we've already talked about with the choice, collaboration, empowerment, through using their language, asking permission, working together on solutions, and not coming across as an expert.

The safety and trust process for me is also in sharing. I could ask, "Would it be useful if I told you some of my story?" because a lot of the time you've got to help build that trust by showing that you're not going to ask anything of them that you're not prepared to answer if they asked you. So that we can model it, if I feel like I need to cry, I'll cry. Even vulnerability, to me, builds that sense of safety. It could be viewed as unprofessional, but it could also be viewed as a level of safety in it.

The way I view our role is like midwives. Midwives cannot take away pain, take away the journey, or do the work for the other person. They have to just be with and support. "What would be most helpful if I was to sit here with you? Do you want me to just listen, do you want me to go get you a cup of tea?" You're really getting the person to come up with what they're wanting and you're going to be there for them and build trust through commitment to being with them through it, "I'm going to stay with you, through this window."

It's two-way learning. We need the old ancient university and then we need the modern university stuff. But they've got to sit side by side; one can't be over the top of the other. Your qualifications and all your training and like you're saying ways of working, when you come into the space it has to initially just be put aside and decide when/if it may be useful. It's good to acknowledge that there's both knowledges here, which is like the SST approach with families, it's their knowledge and your knowledge at work together.

Q: From the modern university, do you give people information about the neurology of the brain or the stuff we hear a lot about in trauma recovery?

Having a Yarn[4]

Alison: It used to happen but I haven't found it to happen as much in single session. I think people have Google, people have the oracle, if people really want to know stuff. So again, it comes back to, "Is this the most useful use of their time?" Of course, if that is what the family wants and feel most useful, I would still go with that.

So the whole sense of doing it in the session: just having a yarn, getting the priority, getting them to choose, getting them to focus on what they want, what's changed – even in the session from having that conversation – all of that, then if they want some specific information, I can provide it as well after the session.

Q: One thing we haven't talked about in the practical "how to" is the way you use the whiteboard and I think that's been quite important from what I understand.

Using the Whiteboard to Elicit a Yarn

Alison: Yeah, well we put up their best hopes – so each family member if you've got multiple family members, multiple perspectives – you're kind of getting the priority and normalizing in a way that there's so many different people, and what they hoped to get out, to capture that and giving choice to each one with what color marker they choose, taking turns to put up what their main hope is. So the board is used as a real sense of that there's a map to help us all. Everybody's included, even the dog. If we need to after a session, you could draw up a genogram from the notes on the board, but we do not draw it as such with the family as it's their space and their map. All their hopes are mapped, then you gather the resources, and from gathering the resources you can then weave it into the questions you get a little sense of there's already been change.

Q: Are you documenting the resources on the board as well?

Alison: With permission each time, which is what I was saying, attending to language, we're going to put this or they can write it. There's always choice. Kids might want to draw sometimes. There's lots of ways of using the board in getting the map of what's going on and getting the resources of what they like to do together or what they do for fun.

James: And the beauty about that, Alison, is like, at the end when we ask them, "Do you want to take a picture of it?" and they love that because THEY'VE just taken their session home – because it's not like we're the keeper of their information.

Vulnerability

Yeah. When it's with Alison we were just like hosting a family sitting in the lounge, and we're just sitting there, just having a conversation with them, and that's what it felt like, was just like we're just having a yarn. Of course, it's a structured yarn but it just – and we just butt in whenever, no rules. It was fluid.

Alison: It's a nice way of saying that I interrupt him sometimes.

James: No, no because I would do the same as well.

Alison: Which the family does at home.

James: Yeah. Exactly, and it was so relaxed.

Q: But the difference is that at home the family don't have an hour to contain it, so how wonderful that you have that frame around it.

James: Also, when we were reflecting one time and so Alison and I were talking about this family and their story was hard, and you can't fake that. If your emotions come up, then that is life.

Q: Your emotions as a therapist came up?

James: It's about coming back to that river. Emotions, we're 90% water, if we're not influenced by that then what are you, a robot? I got influenced by this courageous story and just in reflecting. It changed me too.

Q: Can you talk more about vulnerability?

Alison: There's a conditioning around being professional, there's this glitch in the matrix, it's in all our psyches. We think that if we're vulnerable we're going to lose control, we're going to actually make it more unsafe, we're going to possibly do more harm than good for the client and the family that's there in front of us, when in fact showing the vulnerability enhances the safety. It's the complete opposite to what we've been conditioned to think. Showing your tears, that's real emotion, which is a vulnerability, you're opening up to really being present – I'm trusting you as a perfect stranger just as much as I'm asking you to trust me. I'm trusting you with saying, "Your story has changed me forever. I'm so inspired that I'm in tears." That's what you're feeding back to that person.

If you don't actually bring yourself in, how can you expect others to? It's just learning to allow the water, allow the emotions, as scary as it is, to remind yourself that it's not unprofessional, it's not coming undone, it's actually the opposite. Everyone's feeling – it's probably the hardest work, to begin to feel and express.

Notes

1 "Mob" has multiple meanings from describing direct family connections ("You are part of my mob") to describing language groups and nation or country that you are connected with. It is used to refer to what Aboriginal people feel most connected to, "their mob."
2 *Dadirri* is a word that belongs to the language of the Ngangikurrungur peoples of Daly River in the Northern Territory. The activity or practice of *Dadirri* is a way of cultivating a deep level of mind awareness, listening to self and others. It has its equivalent word and meaning in many other Indigenous groups across the continent of Australia. Miriam-Rose Ungumerr-Bauman, a member of the Ngangikurungur People spoke about this way of life at a presentation she gave in Tasmania in 1988. It is her words and explanation that we refer to in this discussion.
3 Here we acknowledge the influence of solution-focused brief therapy (de Shazer & Berg) on asking about hope and pursuing small positive changes.
4 A "yarn" literally comes from spinning a ball of yarn. It is not pure like a strand of cotton or thread, it is a collection of fibres used to weave or knit, so when you have a "yarn" there is no single thread to follow, it is a collection of stories that we form together in the moment. It is constructed as we talk together.

Suggested Reading

Grieves, V. (2009). *Aboriginal Spirituality: Aboriginal Philosophy: The Basis of Aboriginal Social and Emotional Wellbeing.* Discussion paper No. 9. Darwin, NT, Australia: Cooperative Research Centre for Aboriginal Health.
Moloney, B. (2014). A Black and White model for teaching family therapy: Empowerment by degree. *Australian and New Zealand Journal of Family Therapy, 35,* 261–276.
Pakes, K., & Roy-Chowdhury, S. (2007). Culturally sensitive therapy? Examining the practice of cross-cultural family therapy. *Journal of Family Therapy, 29,* 267–283.
Purdie, N., Dudgeon, P., & Walker, R. (2010). *Working Together: Aboriginal and Torres Strait Islander Mental Health and Wellbeing Principles and Practice.* Canberra, ACT: Commonwealth of Australia.
The Bouverie Centre (2013). *Trauma-Informed Guidelines for Family Sensitive Practice in Adult Health Services.* Melbourne, VIC, Australia: The Bouverie Centre.

21 Hope in Remote Places: Single Session Therapy in Indigenous Communities in Canada

Sophia Sorensen

The thick smoke burned the inside of my nostrils and invaded further, infiltrating new territory as it snaked down my throat and into my lungs. The moist heat stung my face and beads of sweat formed quickly on my scalp. I struggled to quell the urge to move and interrupt the cluster of sweat before it rolled rhythmically down the southern path of my spine. Cloaked in damp darkness, minor movements borne of increasing discomfort of my fellow inhabitants, crouched, side by side, sweaty limb against limb in this sweltering cave, echoed. The intensity of the smoke, the heat, the energy emanating from the sheer physical closeness of bodies – all of it dominated my senses – then the chanting of the medicine man began – a low, deep growl in an unfamiliar language.

My journey from the predictable constructs of a traditional therapeutic practice to sitting on the earthen floor of a cedar and stone sweat lodge in a small Indigenous community on Flores Island, the westernmost part of Canada, was long and meandering.

In 2014, I was managing a program at Victoria Immigrant and Refugee Society, providing mental health and psychosocial supports to aid the transition for immigrants and refugees new to Canada. Subsidized through a federal contract, the work was highly structured – meeting with clients on a regular, scheduled basis over the course of 12 months in a formal office setting, and the presenting issues related to adapting to life in a new country were predictable. Simultaneously, my spouse was commuting on a bi-weekly basis to his job in Houston, Texas, and ultimately, we were presented with an opportunity to relocate for one year to Houston.

In preparation for relocation, considerable time was invested in investigating potential opportunities for learning, experience, and contribution. Of the many options, the Houston Galveston Institute (HGI) was most appealing, based on the collaborative approach to systems therapy and practice of single session therapy (SST) – both concepts then new to me. Contact was initiated and evolved through a series of conversations over several months with the Director of

Programs, Adriana Gil-Wilkerson. Once in Houston, I was welcomed by Adriana and Executive Director Dr. Sue Levin, who were both generous in sharing details of their organizational approach, role in the broader Houston community, and intimacies of the therapeutic process.

HGI was the center of an orbit of diversely and uniquely talented practitioners (counselors and social workers), academics and authors from across the globe. Many were drawn to the organization with a similar sense of curiosity about SST, and the collaborative style of practice (see Levin, Gil-Wilkerson, & Rapini De Yatim, 2018).

My training and participation at HGI was unorthodox and unreservedly immersive; as I was learning about SST and collaborative therapy, I was invited to immediately participate as part of reflecting teams, provide service during "drop-in" counseling hours, and co-counsel with an organic complement of practitioners. In terms of broader community connections, HGI hosted and coordinated a myriad of community/peer meetings with a diverse cross-section of practitioners.

HGI supported a manner of professional evolution which was simultaneously intentional, subtle and sophisticated. I learned about the intellectual aspects of collaborative therapy in general, and SST in specific, through discussions with Sue, Adriana, other peers and exposure to the work of Dr. Harlene Anderson (e.g., 1997, 2007; Anderson & Goolishian, 1992); I learned the practical aspects of application through witnessing and participating "in the moment" with clients during each session, and was enthralled with the notion of clients "co-creating" the experience and the potential for alternative interpretations of life experiences.

While at HGI, I observed that individuals were frequently in crisis and were attending counseling at the exact moment it was *most needed* because of the accessibility of a walk-in/single session service, and availability on a weekend. Clients were drawn to the single session approach since it meant there was no requirement to commit to a longer-term process, something that clients from very modest backgrounds would not be able to support. The sessions seemed to be *more focused* in terms of the client's ability to more immediately dive into presenting issues, and clients demonstrated a high level of satisfaction (which HGI measured through post-session evaluations).

After returning to Canada, I was able to employ SST as part of the BC (British Columbia) Provincial Disaster Psychosocial Team, albeit only sporadically when deployed to emergency situations in BC and Alberta. It was several years before an opportunity to employ SST in a revolutionary manner emerged.

The First Nations Journey to Transform Mental Health

The last 10 years has been a journey to transform how health and wellness services were delivered to First Nations communities in British Columbia. In 2011, BC First Nations completed negotiations with the Canadian government to assume responsibility for the delivery of health programs and services. This is the mandate for the first and only organization wholly responsible for First Nations health in the country, the First Nations Health Authority (FNHA).

The First Nations perspective on Health and Wellness is holistic and includes a recognition of the ancestral teachings of First Nations. The approach is centered on a "wheel of wellness," which is the lens through which FNHA works, and is rooted in the teaching and cultures of BC First Nations.

Underpinning all health services (including mental health) is an attitude of cultural safety, defined as a life-long process of self-reflection, understanding of one's own biases and adherence to the goal of maintaining mutually respectful relationships. Practitioners are expected to "adopt a humble, self-reflective clinical practice that positions them as respectful and curious partners when providing care, rather than as a figure of higher knowledge and authority" (First Nations Health Authority, n.d.).

The FNHA is divided into five geographic regions in British Columbia (the Interior, Fraser, Vancouver Coastal, Vancouver Island, and the Northern Region), with collaboration and priority setting for health done within each region, at the level of family groups (and sub-level of communities within each family), each with unique cultural, language, and spiritual aspects.

As a Crisis Counselor on Vancouver Island, my role involved offering mental health support and psychoeducation to 53 First Nations and three distinct tribal regions including the Nuu-chah-nulth, Kwakwaka'wakw, and Coast Salish families. Vancouver Island Nations constitute 20% of the provincial First Nations total population and 6% of the national First Nations total population. The dynamics of each are highly diverse and dispersed across urban, suburban, and rural and remote communities. In addition to the Crisis Counselor role, the FNHA regional Mental Health team includes social workers focused on designing, delivering, and coordinating psychoeducation workshops.

Single Session Counseling in First Nation Communities

The architecture of the FNHA counseling delivery system is anchored in the dual pillars of being "nation-based" and "community-driven"; in action, this means that Indigenous ways of being in the world primarily influence *how* work is done, and all services are *driven by the unique needs* of each community, rather than a traditional unilateral delivery model of government-dictated universal health care.

At the ground level and during the delivery of crisis counseling services, this philosophy was practically translated into the following protocols:

1. Crisis counseling services were always *requested by the leadership* of a specific Indigenous community; services were never presumptive.
2. Counseling services were *always delivered on traditional lands*, in the Indigenous community. Once activated, my role was to travel to the client, which could take from 2 to 24 hours. Out of respect for Elders and previous Indigenous generations, I traveled by traditional modes of transportation. In practice, one trip could include a four-hour car drive, overnight in a small community, and one or two boat rides on the second travel day.
3. Once in community, my *first task was to connect with leadership*. This tended to involve locating the Administration Office or Health Office, and participating in a meeting (similar to critical incident debriefing), led by the Elected Chief or Administrator, and attended by the Health Centre Director (for larger communities) and an assortment of staff members, and occasionally, a Royal Canadian Mounted Police (RCMP) officer. In small communities some of the individuals present at the debriefing were also related to the person at the center of the crisis. The purpose of the meeting was to share the context of the crisis, status of impacted community members, and plans for responding (including communications about the event, contacting family members who lived outside the community, plans for traditional ceremonies, formal inquiries, etc.).
4. As part of this conversation, *the group would determine action items*, including location of counseling space and the days, times, and duration of counseling; requests for other traditional and/or spiritual supports (which sometimes could include both cultural healers and Christian representatives); plans for mourning or funeral events; ways of communicating to family members who lived outside of community and helping them travel back to the community; and arranging financial assistance for the immediate family.

Once in community and oriented to an office (usually in the Health Centre or Administration building), my focus shifted to offering counseling support. The logistics of the delivery of counseling service was consistent in each community and included promotion of the counseling service by word of mouth and social media by community members. All sessions were "walk-in" and there was no intake paper-work (informed consent and limits of confidentiality were communicated orally). There was no time limit on each session; the client determined when the session was completed (sessions tended to last

40 minutes to two hours). Although not part of the intentional design of the service, in consultation with my clinical supervisor, we determined the best approach with this client group was not to take notes during the sessions. Although I am of *Métis*[1] ancestry, I present as Caucasian, and with a long history of colonialism, abundance of residential school survivors and high level of mistrust of Caucasian medical practitioners, taking notes during a session could potentially be a triggering behavior. Finally, outreach counseling was provided if I was asked to provide support at individual homes or other buildings, and as a further demonstration of cultural humility and respect, I always attended community events (funerals and mourning ceremonies) or traditional ceremonies if invited.

This new SST service delivered in community was sometimes accompanied by a parallel service delivered through a collaborative relationship with Tsow-Tun Lelum (TTLL), an organization that coordinates an outreach healing program comprising 30 traditional healers. Although there is now considerable literature supporting this approach, it is a rare occurrence. To my knowledge, this is the first time that the two complementary paths of services supporting both traditional cultural healing and Western-style therapy have been deployed concurrently.

In the situations when we were both deployed (FNHA and TTLL), we met in community and were usually situated in the same building while delivering our distinct services. During many deployments over time, a familiar, organic manner of work emerged and there was often a natural flow of information and clients. Clients sometimes participated in a traditional healing ceremony (i.e., chanting, blessing, cleansing) and then proceeded to a counseling session; at other times, the order was reversed. Occasionally, I was privileged to be invited to witness traditional healing work.

Vignette: Single Session Therapy in a Nuu-Chah-Nulth Community

It was a cold December morning when I was asked to respond in the aftermath of an accidental death of a young man in a small community on traditional territories in an extremely remote area of the West Coast of northern Vancouver Island.

Logistically, it was a four-hour drive from my office to the nearest town of Tofino, where I spent the night. At 7 a.m. the next morning, I met a water taxi at the public dock and after a one-hour boat ride (see Figure 21.1), reached the destination. For the duration, I would be living in the community, staying in a small, old bunkhouse left over from forestry logging crews in the 1980s.

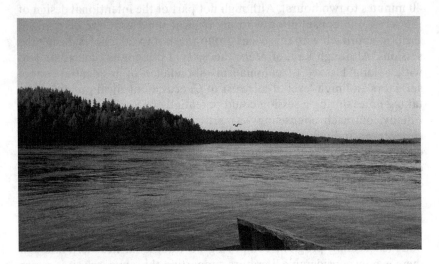

Figure 21.1 The "Door" to My Office.

I was directed to the Band Administrator and after attending a critical incident debriefing, and within an hour, was oriented to an office in a small health center. Health Centre staff and residents communicated about my presence by social media and within hours of landing in the region, clients were arriving. TTLL healers arrived later that day and set up their spiritual healing room.

Actual Experience of Single Session Thinking and Practice

The man who appeared to be in his late 40s arrived at the office door. I invited him inside and returned to my seat. He said he'd rather stand, and probably would not stay very long. He commented that over the years he had seen visiting counselors before[2] but that counseling "never worked," and from this comment, I surmised his expectations of the session were low. He inquired about the need to fill out forms, and pre-emptively added that his reading and writing weren't very good. He also inquired as to who would know that he had come to see me and whom I reported back to about the session.

He told me that he had a lot to say and that he was very angry. He told me that his anger often scared people and over the years, some counselors had kicked him out of the office or refused to see him a second time. After about five minutes of speaking in a quick and mildly agitated manner while pacing in the tiny office, he dragged the guest chair a further few feet away from me and sat down.

His story began with a recounting of the recent fatal accident, one that he witnessed, and that had claimed the life of his cousin. A broad version of his story tumbled out: considerable loss and trauma, a long, evolving history of addictions and complex damaged and dysfunctional relationships. The client had been born in the community and except for short periods of time, lived his entire life in this remote place. He did not work, was unmarried, and had several children by different partners. During the course of his lengthy revelations, there were noticeable changes. The anger dissipated, the tempo of his speech slowed, the volume of his voice dropped, he settled more deeply into his chair, and he appeared calmer. When he concluded this first unburdening, we rested in shared moments of silence and I felt a profound and gentle shift in the energy in the room. Moving forward, his thoughts and words were different and targeted at inquiry and he was focused on "why?" He asked, "Why did all these bad things happen to me?" and "Why have so many people around me died?" and "Why am I still alive?" At one point, he cried.

This shift presented an opportunity to identify and extricate the life factors that had been beyond his control, and the intrinsic resources that had helped him survive. Setting aside the overwhelming, unanswerable questions about "*Why?*" we moved to consider "*How?*" – as in, "*How* did you survive? *How* did you make the right decisions that helped you cope with each situation? *How* did you know who to turn to for support? *How* did you know when to ask for help?" Together, we explored the miracle of his survival and the personal strengths, coping strategies, and positive choices that had helped him. Many of these were intrinsically connected to his culture and community; traditional medicine, relationships with community members, rituals and ceremonies, and spiritual practices.

The session results included an uncovering of client internal strengths and abilities, an appreciation and awareness of some past positive choices and an understanding of the importance of traditional Indigenous practices to the client's well-being. The session ended (after approximately 80 minutes) when the client informed me he had said everything he felt like saying. Energetically, his mood was more positive, he smiled (for the first time during the session), and thanked me as he left.

The Community Context

Entering a remote Indigenous community following a tragedy means stepping into a complex reality; details of events were shared freely amongst community members of all ages (including children) and there was tremendous engagement and speculation on social media. In this situation, as in many, there were several witnesses (including family members) to the fatal event and the deceased, who was a new father, left a partner and two children, as well as his parents and parents-in-law, all of whom lived in community. There was a very high level of intergenerational trauma and individuals had many prior experiences of loss and grief, including an ongoing situation involving a man who had gone missing from a neighboring island (where he had been isolated as part of a traditional Indigenous vision quest healing process).

Other characteristics of the community included a high level of geographic isolation (only accessible by water taxi or float plane), high level of addiction and, as with the client described above, an unsatisfying, disrupted, and often negative history with counselors.

My Lens While in Community

As influenced by cultural awareness and humility training and Indigenous Trauma Informed Therapy, as well as the broader FNHA context, I approached this community with the following intentions:

- Seek first to understand the context of the crisis event
- Connect with anyone who is open to connecting
- Seek ways to connect with Health Centre staff
- Identify family and friends impacted
- Determine how best to be of service and respond reflexively as needs evolve
- Maintain awareness that informal conversations can be therapeutic
- If invited, be open to participate in traditional ceremonies
- Consistently generate awareness about availability of counseling
- Work in collaboration with TTLL cultural healers.

Challenges to Delivering Service

There were layers of challenges to respond to the call for service. I was an obvious outsider, non-Indigenous. Though *Métis*, I present as a European settler. Further, as a female, perceived as an "educated professional" – I elicited a range of responses, many of them based in mistrust.

This specific situation possessed the additional challenges encountered in any crisis involving a fatality; a range of individual experiences with loss and grief. Many of the emotional responses were predictable: shock, disbelief, anger. For many individuals, this "new" loss triggered a complicated cascade of previous losses and grief, as well as a deeper, underlying sense of hopelessness and helplessness.

I counseled in this community for five days and during most of that time, I was present in the designated counseling office and met with clients. The ad hoc prevailing "referral process" often ran through families, and I saw several members of several families; clients were also referred to me by the TTLL healers. In addition, I was asked by the Tribal Chief to provide counseling and "be present" at the homes of the two families directly impacted by the loss, which I did for several hours, accompanied by the TTLL healers.

Considerations for Practitioners Intending to Deliver SST to Indigenous Populations

There is tremendous diversity within Indigenous communities in Canada in terms of language, beliefs, practices, and culture, and it is important to maintain this awareness of uniqueness when approaching this population, as well as the existence and impacts of intergenerational trauma from the legacy of colonization and residential schools. Related to this context is the existence of a high level of mistrust of most individuals (particularly non-Indigenous) from outside the community, and mental health practitioners in particular, sometimes based on previously disappointing and disjointed experiences with counselors. Indigenous community members often experience higher levels of active addiction, tremendous difficulty accessing ongoing treatment and recovery supports, and many live with pre-existing diagnosed and/or undiagnosed mental health issues. In some small communities, there may be a fear of potential lateral violence[3] for accessing a counselor.

The SST approach is extremely well-suited for working with Indigenous clients for many reasons. "Walk-in service," something learned at HGI, helped to remove that barrier and supported a spontaneous desire to connect with a counselor, something most clients have not experienced. Additionally, both I and my clients were aware that one meeting, in the setting and the circumstances, was going to be the reality, so there was a kind of congruence between how the counseling was provided and client needs. I also sensed that the client's anticipation of only one session translated to a sense of freedom from the expectations that may accompany an ongoing counseling relationship. In addition, I believe that my unique adaptations, allowing the client to determine the session length, avoidance of note-taking within the session, willingness to meet clients outside of the office setting, and attendance and participation at traditional ceremonies and meals helped to increase client comfort and trust, and to create a positive experience. Finally, and perhaps most importantly, Indigenous clients often have experienced long periods of a lack of respect and lack of positive endorsement. For this reason, approaching this client group with the mindset that *clients are the experts in their own lives* is especially empowering and sometimes a rare, almost radically empowering experience. By extension, allowing clients the space to share whatever they want to share, for as long as they want to speak and in the location that best suits them, reinforces a sense of importance, attention, and worth.

The Hope in Serving Remote Indigenous Communities

The circumstances that I encountered while delivering SST were prompted by crisis and inherently involved chaos. The permanent community circumstances were often dire; defined by severe economic, social, and prevalent health issues. Despite this, I encountered precious experiences of what I define as "hope" in the therapeutic, foundational context: an energetic connection between two human beings. At the broadest level, delivering this service felt connected to the worldwide momentum for reconciliation, and because my own Indigenous family history had been historically suppressed and discouraged due to shame and fear, this work represented tremendous personal value to me.

It was the ability to honor traditional lands and ways of being on the land through delivering services locally, shifting counseling services to align with client values and culture through the use of SST and collaborating with Indigenous partners with an open heart that led me to the rare invitation – on that cold winter day on Flores Island – to enter that cedar and stone sweat lodge and celebrate the creation of a unique healing process.

Notes

1 *Métis* refers to a person of mixed European and Indigenous ancestry and is one of three accepted Aboriginal Peoples in Canada.
2 This Indigenous community, like many remote communities, previously and for many years, had a contract in place for once a month visits from a counselor, with the individual counselor often changing from month to month.
3 Lateral violence can happen when individuals have endured oppression and suppressed feelings such as anger, shame, and rage; these feelings can manifest in behaviors such as jealousy, resentment, blame, and bitterness. According to Jane Middleton-Moz (1999, p. 116), "When a powerful oppressor has directed oppression against a group for a period of time, members of the oppressed group feel powerless to fight back and they eventually turn their anger against each other."

References

Anderson, H. (1997). *Conversation, Language, and Possibilities: A Postmodern Therapy*. New York: Basic Books.
Anderson, H. (2007). The heart and spirit of collaborative therapy: The philosophical stance – "A way of being" in relationship and conversation. In H. Anderson & D. Gehart (Eds.), *Collaborative Therapy: Relationships and Conversations That Make a Difference* (pp. 43–59). New York: Routledge.
Anderson, H., & Goolishian, H. (1992). The client is the expert: A not-knowing approach to therapy. In S. McNamee & K.J. Gergen (Eds.), *Therapy as Social Construction* (pp. 25–39). Newbury Park, CA: SAGE.
First Nations Health Authority. (n.d.). FNHA's policy statement on cultural safety and humility. https://www.fnha.ca/documents/fnha-policy-statement-cultural-safety-and-humility.pdf

Levin, S.B., Gil-Wilkerson, A., & Rapini De Yatim, S. (2018). Single session walk-ins as a collaborative learning community at the Houston Galveston Institute. In M.F. Hoyt, M. Bobele, A. Slive, J. Young, & M. Talmon (Eds.), *Single-Session Therapy by Walk-In or Appointment: Administrative, Clinical, and Supervisory Aspects of One-at-a-Time Services* (pp. 251–259). New York: Routledge.

Middelton-Moz, J. (1999). *Boiling Point: The High Cost of Unhealthy Anger to Individuals and Society*. Deerfield Beach, FL: Health Communications.

22 Single Session Family Consultation Implementation in *Aotearoa* New Zealand: Cultural Considerations

*Bronwyn Dunnachie, Stacey Porter,
and Karin Isherwood*

In 2015, the Ministry of Health in *Aotearoa* New Zealand[1] launched the *Supporting Parents, Healthy Children (SPHC) Guideline.* The *Guideline* was developed to influence mental health and addiction services to enhance their support for parents with dependent children, a population frequently known as "Children of Parents with Mental Illness and/or Addictions" (COPMIA).[2] It is common for specialist adult mental health and addiction service delivery (second tier services) to operate within an individualistic rather than systemic paradigm (Government Inquiry into Mental Health and Addiction, 2018). Underpinning the *Guideline* is a clear message that services across sectors in *Aotearoa* New Zealand are required to improve family/*whānau*[3] service delivery.

The SPHC *Guideline* speaks to a strengths-based process of enhancing family-inclusive practice through a broad range of activity. The activity aims to enable people working in services to partner and work with families in a relational, intentional, and outcomes-focused way that families/*whānau* view as a positive resource. A key initiative supporting the implementation of the *Guideline* has been embedding the practice of Single Session Family Consultation, a model for engaging families in individually oriented services (SSFC: The Bouverie Centre, 2014; also see Chapter 5 of this volume) across sectors. This has required significant consultation to ensure the framework is "fit for purpose" in the *Aotearoa* New Zealand context. This chapter focuses on the consultation process employed to enable the adaption of the SSFC framework for delivery in *Aotearoa* New Zealand.

Aotearoa New Zealand has an unenviable record of health disparity, with disproportionate numbers of indigenous people (Māori) experiencing mental health and/or addiction concerns (Russell, 2018). To date, these services have not kept pace with the identified need to provide specific and appropriately culturally focused interventions (Mental Health Commission, 2012). Traditionally, Māori view health and well-being from a *whānau-hapū-iwi*[4] perspective, which acknowledges every individual's well-being as an interdependent aspect of the extended family, tribal group, and extended tribal alliances to which they belong. Accordingly, best practice requires all service delivery to be *whānau*-inclusive and *whānau*-focused. *Whānau*-centered practice sits at the base of expectation of service delivery to Māori, which is reflected in the recognition of models of care such as *Whānau Ora*[5] (Te Rau Matatini, 2014).

Whānau ora is a broad term with multiple, interpretive meanings, though it is generally accepted to mean family well-being. In 2009, the Taskforce on Whānau-Centred Initiatives presented a report to the *Aotearoa* New Zealand government exploring changes needed to achieve *whānau ora*. In 2010, the New Zealand government launched *Whānau Ora* as an innovative *whānau*-centered approach to supporting *whānau* well-being and development. *Whānau Ora* is focused on achieving *whānau* potential and recognizes the strengths and abilities that exist within *whānau*.[6]

Understanding the importance of the concept of *whānau ora* to the development of the SPHC Guideline, a review of the differences and similarities of *Whānau Ora* and COPMIA was undertaken by the Māori Workforce Development Programme (Te Rau Matatini, 2014). The review found that while both approaches agreed that current individualistic service provision urgently needed to upgrade to *"whānau*-centered" practice, internationally COPMIA service delivery was still focused on nuclear family systems, whereas *whānau ora* was heavily informed by centuries of collectivist cultural practices throughout the Pacific. *Whānau Ora* aspired to wide *whānau* well-being outcomes measured in terms of sustainability, agency, and interdependence, while COPMIA focused on the needs of children and young people as distinct from those of their parents (Te Rau Matatini, 2014). Such scrutiny of the impacts of implementing mainstream concepts within indigenous communities is a key responsibility for groups undertaking change processes in *Aotearoa* New Zealand.

Bringing any intervention or framework to *Aotearoa* New Zealand, especially when associated with working with *whānau* Māori, requires significant partnership development, co-design, and carefully considered consultation to ensure that alignment is possible and acceptable. With this in mind, the implementation of the SSFC framework in New Zealand required significant collaboration and consultation with our cultural partners.

SSFC: Exploring the Potential for Cultural Adaptation in *Aotearoa* New Zealand

The initial planning process involved several meetings with the SPHC project team. This team comprises members from each of the mental health and addictions workforce development programs funded by the

Ministry of Health. Each program represents a specific demographic or health concern. There are programs for adult; infant, child, and youth; Māori; Pasifika peoples;[7] addictions; and gambling harm.[8] The project team had worked together since 2013 to support the development, launch, and implementation of the SPHC Guideline. Having representatives from the Māori and Pasifika peoples' programs on the project team provided opportunities for Māori and Pasifika peoples' worldviews to be represented and carefully considered throughout. Positive and open relationships within the team enabled robust discussion, thought-provoking challenges and enriched project delivery. The relational basis underpinning the functioning of the project team has been reported by "external" groups, including Ministry of Health funders, as enabling an improved level of traction regarding family/*whānau* inclusion in service delivery in *Aotearoa* New Zealand. These program partners have also been the principal conduit for broader consultation with Māori and Pasifika peoples' services and communities, which has been essential in the implementation of SSFC.

Why SSFC? A key initiative supporting the implementation of the *Guideline* has been embedding the practice of Single Session Family Consultation (SSFC; The Bouverie Centre, 2014) across sectors. SSFC is a brief model of family/*whānau* engagement and inclusion that aims to: help the family/*whānau* identify and respond to their needs; clarify how the family/*whānau* will be involved in the individual's care and make the most of the time spent together using Single Session Work (SSW) principles and techniques. There are three stages to the process: *Convening, Conducting the Session*, and *Follow-Up and Next Steps*. SSFC builds on the practitioner skills of working with families by providing a framework which enables a structure that promotes positive engagement and supports meeting the needs of family/*whānau*.

In the process of planning SPHC implementation, the project team undertook a review of the key family-focused models, interventions, and frameworks available internationally for implementation in *Aotearoa* New Zealand. Considerations included cultural alignment; accessibility with regards to the current level of skill and knowledge capability for working with families; the complexity of the models, interventions, and frameworks (the less complex the better); the anticipated time for implementation to be completed; and costs.

Initial feedback on the cultural suitability of the SSFC model was sought from Māori and Pasifika peoples who had the opportunity to attend a conference presentation led by staff from The Bouverie Centre. Additional feedback came from attendees at SSFC workshops in Auckland and Wellington, which included specific promotion to Māori and Pasifika peoples' workforces. Feedback identified that the framework could work well in the *Aotearoa* New Zealand context, although the resources and language would require cultural consideration and a specific consultation plan.

The Consultation Plan

Acknowledging the importance of a collaboratively designed consultation plan, the project team established a Cultural Advisory Group. The project team extended invitations to people across cultures and ethnicities to join or invite others to participate in the review of the framework, training, and training resources. They were additionally invited to serve as a conduit for further information gathering from their communities and their cultural perspectives. Representatives from Māori, Pasifika peoples, Asian, and European ethnic communities offered time and expertise for an initial process of reviewing material, attending a full-day face-to-face meeting and subsequent online meetings. The establishment of the Terms of Reference, to define the scope of the Cultural Advisory Group, occurred over a two-week period prior to the face-to-face meeting and was crucial to the partnership process. The collective crafting of this document enabled a process of *whanaungatanga* (relationship development), which participants identified as supportive to the group process and enabled focused discussion at the face-to-face meeting. Over one month, the combination of the face-to-face and online discussion enabled a review of the evaluation data from the SSFC-focused events held to that point, in addition to a review of The Bouverie Centre SSFC training content and training resources (promotional material, PowerPoint presentation, video clips, suggested reading materials, and the training evaluation document). The discussion from each meeting, and information shared during all communication with the Cultural Advisory Group, was collected as data for the review process. The project team completed a thematic analysis of the data and shared their findings with the Cultural Advisory Group. Themes from the analysis included:

- Accessing cultural advice (required when working with cultures other than one's own)
- *Kaimahi* (practitioners) connection with their own culture (knowing yourself before working with others)
- Well-being of an individual in the context of well-being of the *whānau* in their community (peoples' well-being being related to the collective)
- *Whānau* support is essential to collective well-being
- Understanding our limits and responsibilities, when working with people from other cultures and ethnicities.

The Cultural Advisory Group further identified that SSFC could be "fit for purpose" in *Aotearoa* New Zealand, but for the framework and associated training to be culturally credible, there needed to be cultural contextualization of the framework, training and training resources.

Cultural Contextualization

The process of cultural contextualization of the SSFC framework, training, and training resources occurred through several meetings with the project team, the cross-culture, ethnically diverse Cultural Advisory Group and input from a Bouverie Centre SSFC trainer, with representatives "testing" the reviewed material with their agencies and communities. The key principles underpinning this process were:

* What is inherently good for *whānau* Māori is good for all families
* The framework, training, and training resources need to be considered from *Te Ao Māori* (Māori perspective characterized by collectivist traditions and systemic relational thinking).

The review had at its foundation several Māori constructs: *Whakapapa, Whānau-centred approach,* and *Mana affirming practice.* While attempts at English translation are inevitably inadequate at capturing a full meaning of these Māori constructs, below is one description for each:

* *Whakapapa* is "the layering of one thing upon another" and in a Māori worldview it provides the structure for explaining how relationships between individuals, *whānau* (extended families), *hapū* (the tribal group), and *iwi* (tribal alliances) are structured. *Whakapapa* is the core of traditional *mātauranga Māori* (Māori knowledge). *Whakapapa* (loosely) means "genealogy" (Lilly, 2016)
* *Whānau* is often translated as "family," but its meaning is more complex. It includes physical, emotional, and spiritual dimensions and is based on *whakapapa*. *Whānau* can be multi-layered, flexible, and dynamic. *Whānau* is based on a Māori and a tribal worldview. It is through the *whānau* that values, histories, and traditions from the ancestors are adapted for the contemporary world (Walker, 2017)
* A *whānau*-centered approach refers to the importance of engaging and including *whānau* as key allies and is the preferred model of service delivery to *whānau* Māori. The well-being of a child will likely require a *whānau*-wide response. This is where the *whānau ora* approach provides valuable insight and examples of best practice to guide our work. Research shows that the sense of belonging is a strong protective factor for *tamariki*[9] (Walsh, Joyce, Maloney, & Vaithianathan, 2019). An example of a *whānau*-centered approach would be a service that involves *whānau* in all aspects of delivery from planning to review. Additionally, referral pathways and funding streams are *whānau* focused
* *"Mana*-enhancing practice refers to practice underpinned by an understanding of the significance of historical relationships, especially within the context of *Te Tiriti o Waitangi* (The Treaty of

Waitangi; see www.treaty2u.govt.nz); the role of narratives in constructing and maintaining cultural identity; and concepts of Māori well-being. *Mana*-affirming practice can be achieved by engaging with people through listening, understanding and respecting cultural difference; valuing the contribution of *whakapapa* and cultural narratives to restorative healing processes through the generations; reaffirming the ability and capacities of *whānau* to engage in self-determination and providing support to do so; and that the cultural wisdom embedded in Māori ideological and philosophical beliefs can generate solutions or resolutions to Māori welfare concerns" (Ruwhiu, 2009, p. 118).

Contextualization of the Resources

To enhance the training, the project team and The Bouverie Centre developed two pre-face-to-face training e-modules which formed Part One of the training; the face-to-face training formed Part Two. The first e-module includes a focus on partnering/working with *whānau Māori* and material from The Bouverie Centre. (The material developed by The Bouverie Centre was reviewed for alignment by the Cultural Advisory Group during production.) The second module focuses on the inclusion of *tamariki* in the SSFC process, further aligning SSFC with the Supporting Parents, Healthy Children Guideline implementation.

The Development of Trainers

In order to extend the reach of the SSFC training and have single session family consultations available throughout *Aotearoa* New Zealand, the people who had attended The Bouverie Centre SSFC training and had implemented SSFC into their practice, were invited to attend a two-day Train-the-Trainer workshop in Wellington. Twenty-five trainees attended the two-day training, which was delivered by Bouverie staff in collaboration with the project team.

The workshop was held on a *marae* (Māori place of gathering) in Wellington. This provided an opportunity for trainees to consider the training content and resources for "fit" within the cultural context. As the training was hosted by Te Hauora O Ora Toa[10] on Takapuwāhia Marae, trainees were treated to an immersive experience in Māori protocol. This included *pōwhiri* (*marae* welcome and tour), *karakia* (spiritual ritual), *waiata* (expression through song), and a *whakawātea* ceremony to close our work. This training focused on the experience of SSFC for families from a range of cultures and ethnicities. The group of 25 trainees included Māori, Pasifika peoples, and Europeans from various countries. Feedback from the trainees on both the alignment of the framework for culturally and ethnically diverse families, and the revised training resources for training delivery included the following:

- Consensus that the SSFC framework and the training resources could be used in their current state providing that contextualization would continue as an ongoing process
- SSFC would receive greater acceptance if the framework was re-named *whānau-hui* (family meeting), as the concept of *single session* may have negative connotations for families from cultures where a principle for working through family issues is "it takes as long as it takes," especially when elders are speaking. Taking this into account, SSFC facilitators may schedule a *whānau-hui* mid-morning and leave the rest of the day free so the *hui* can unfold as it needs to
- Trainers should promote discussion during SSFC workshops on the delivery of the framework to diverse populations. This could include questions such as "How would this work for Māori and Pasifika peoples' families?"
- Trainees should be prepared for larger family groups attending sessions. Māori and Pasifika peoples' families may invite members from the broader *whānau* to be included in the meetings at any point. We have heard reports where facilitators accommodated 20 plus *whānau* members at the family *hui*
- Some people felt that they could not connect to the Australian context and asked that the videos be reshot using a New Zealand family and include children. The production of New Zealand video clips should occur as soon as possible as trainers predicted a potentially indifferent reaction to the Australian resources.

Feedback from Testing the Resources: Messages from Māori Providers

Further testing of the framework and the training resources occurred through visits and discussion between the Māori cultural advisor on the project team and *kaupapa* Māori service[11] leads. Their feedback was that the single session model is a *"tool trainees could acquire in a few days, which would enable them to facilitate valuable conversations that* whānau *otherwise would not have."* For example, when services do not include family-in-treatment planning, *whānau* Māori may assume it is because that is the *Pākehā*[12] way of working and will not feel comfortable attending a session uninvited. When *whānau* are asked to attend and their needs are identified, they feel respected and part of the process.

Māori service providers in the Midlands Region (central North Island, *Aotearoa* New Zealand) considered the irony of receiving advice from Western institutions on a conventional feature and strength of traditional Māori and Pasifika peoples' practice, while others signaled mistrust based on the limited reference to Australian Aboriginal and other Indigenous communities in the original SSFC materials developed in Australia. Overall, Māori feedback appreciated the simple structure and practical strategies throughout the single session process and identified synergies but questioned why an indigenous *Aotearoa* New Zealand framework was not promoted instead of, or as well as, the single session framework.

In response, care was taken in future presentations to provide the *whakapapa* (history) of single session work; its origin and development here, and potential application in *Aotearoa* for the benefit of *whānau*. Equipping practitioners new to working with more than one client or their *tamariki* (children) with a clear structure for *whānau* to engage in deliberate and intentional discussions about their concerns provided by the SSFC model, was expected to contribute to positive outcomes aligned to *whānau ora*. In preparing everyone for the *whānau* meeting, the convening stage of SSFC allows for initial sharing and gathering of vital information needed to *manaaki* (care for and support) *whānau* through those discussions and initiate the *whakawhanaunga* (relationship building) process. Both processes are considered by Māori to be essential elements in genuine *whānau* engagement and potentially aligned to the *whakamoemiti* (prepare and protect), *whakatau* (establish relations), and *whakapuaki* (identify issues) phases of the Pōwhiri Poutama Framework (Huata, 2011). This is an example of therapeutic engagement taken from the traditional *pōwhiri* ceremony of welcoming visitors to engage in dialogue.

Before meeting with Māori *whānau*, clinicians are asked to consider their capacity for *mana* enhancing and *mana* protecting practices and employ these when engaging with Māori. Convening an SSFC with Māori *whānau* may include these additions to the protocol:

- Understanding the service users' and their *whanau*'s traditional needs
- Accommodating speaking in their own language
- Making space to explore their *whakapapa* and the ancestral narratives
- Finding out who carries most influence in the family and whether it is appropriate to directly approach them
- Convening with the *whānau* in person, rather than on the phone
- Expecting to include *tamariki* and *mokopuna*[13]
- Holding the SSFC in the *whānau* home or on their *marae*
- Opening and closing the SSFC with *karakia*[14]
- Providing appropriate *manaakitanga*.[15]

Effective work with Māori *whānau* is possible when practitioners use the tenets of *whānau*-centered best practice and respond appropriately to the needs of the *whānau* and respect their traditional practices.

Relevant literature on existing indigenous models for *whānau* engagement was reviewed and collated to deepen the cultural understanding of participants. Presentations were developed utilizing three culturally endorsed practice concepts to integrate key themes raised by the Cultural

Advisory Group, and further contributors in the implementation of single session work around the country.

- *Whakapapa* is implicated in the indigenous *whānau* experience of intergenerational transmission of and healing from trauma. It requires facilitators to consider longitudinal *whānau* knowledge, roles and responsibilities, to work with them effectively (Pihama et al., 2014)
- *Whānau Ora* approach provides indicators to measure holistic wellbeing for *whānau*, individual practice and service delivery. It requires facilitators to realize *whānau* aspirations for a sustainable future (Ruwhiu, 2009)
- *Manaaki* (Mana Enhancing and Protecting Practice; Huriwai & Baker, 2016) describes cultural best practice during engagement that intentionally does no harm to the *mana* and dignity of *whānau*, while prospecting for opportunities to affirm and strengthen *whānau* agency.

Māori identified multiple elements present in any engagement with *whānau* – the *tangata whaiora* (service user) and *whānau* bicultural experience, the individual practitioner's cultural competency, and the organizational capacity to respond to *whānau* cultural need. This highlighted the need for services to seek local support and cultural advice, set quality improvement expectations in policy and procedure, and support self-reflective practice with emphasis on understanding one's own cultural practice before engaging safely with another's.

Māori-advised adherence to these conditions requires facilitators to recognize *whānau* as potential allies and experts in their *whānau* context and experience. This practice would more likely result in a wellness plan that accounted for the cultural reality and aspirations of individuals, and the *whānau* system with whom they coexist. This was captured in the phrase "let the *whānau* train the practitioner."

Where Are We Up To?

Contextualization is an ongoing process as the feedback continues to shape the cultural focus of the training content and resources. The project team coordinates meetings with the (now) 50 SSFC trainers bi-monthly and has set up systems to receive feedback, and regularly reviews and amends the training material. The video clips have been re-shot in *Aotearoa* New Zealand, partnering with an ethnically diverse group to "act" as the *whānau*. While positively received, feedback is that the *whānau* in the videos portray a nuclear "urban" family, limiting the opportunity for trainees to experience a larger *whānau* likely to be encountered in real practice. The training material is largely consistent with The Bouverie Centre's resources apart from the *te reo* Māori language additions. Feedback regarding the development of the cultural module as part of the e-training has been very positive, and this material has been re-purposed many times for inclusion in other initiatives (e.g., Werry Workforce Whāraurau's *Foundations in Mental Health* and *CEP*[16] blended learning packages) where a cultural viewpoint has been required.

In essence, our attempts at cultural contextualization of the Single Session Family Consultation (SSFC) framework for *Aotearoa* New Zealand have been broadly acclaimed with invaluable frank and helpful feedback from Māori and Pasifika peoples' communities. To all those who have offered their wisdom in this process, *ka mihi ake* ("thank you"), *kia haere tonu ā tatou pai* ("may our good work continue").

Notes

1 *Aotearoa* is a Māori name for New Zealand, literally "land of the long white cloud." The country is often referred to by both names. Consistent with our bicultural approach, both English and Māori terms will be used throughout.
2 *Aotearoa* New Zealand adopted COPMIA from Australia and added "Addictions" to fit with national policy.
3 *Whānau* is the Māori word for "family," typically extending beyond the nuclear situation and bound in kinship defined by the *whānau* themselves.
4 Māori terms for extended family (*"whānau"*), tribal group (*"hapū"*), and extended tribal alliances (*"iwi"*).
5 *Whānau Ora* is an *Aotearoa* New Zealand government *whānau*-centered initiative to improve *whānau* well-being.
6 See www.tpk.govt.nz/en/whakamahia/whanau-ora.
7 Pasifika peoples refers to people from all Pacific Islands.
8 *Editors' note:* For a discussion of single session counseling with those affected by gambling, see Cohen, Daley, and Northe, Chapter 28.
9 *Tamariki* is the Māori word for "children."
10 Tribal *Whānau Ora* provider.
11 *Kaupapa* Māori services are delivered from a cultural perspective and may use traditional methods of healing.
12 This term is used to denote a non-Māori New Zealander.
13 *Mokopuna* is the Māori word for "grandchildren."
14 *Karakia* are Māori incantations and prayers, used to invoke spiritual guidance and protection and ensure a good outcome for the gathering.
15 *Manaakitanga* is the Māori word for "hospitality" (e.g., food and drink).
16 *Foundations in Mental Health* and *CEP* (Co-Existing Problems) e-learnings are freely available (with sign-up) at https://www.goodfellowunit.org/.

References

Government Inquiry into Mental Health and Addiction. (2018). https://www.mentalhealth.inquiry.govt.nz/inquiry-report/he-ara-oranga/

Huata, P. (2011). Unpacking the Pōwhiri Poutama. Workshop sponsored by Waikato Institute of Technology. Hamilton, NZ.

Huriwai, T., & Baker, M. (2016). *Manaaki: Mana Enhancing and Mana Protecting Practice.* Wellington, NZ: Te Rau Matatini.

Lilly, S. (2016). Whakapapa: Genealogical information seeking in an indigenous context. *Proceedings of the Association of Information Science and Technology, 52,* 1–8.

Mental Health Commission. (2012). *Blueprint II: How Things Need to Be.* Wellington, NZ: Mental Health Commission.

Ministry of Health. (2015). *Supporting Parents, Healthy Children.* Wellington, NZ: Ministry of Health.

Pihama, L., Reynolds, P., Smith, C., Reid, J., Tuhiwai Smith, L., & Te Nana, R. (2014). Positioning historical trauma theory within Aotearoa New Zealand. *AlterNative: An International Journal of Indigenous Peoples, 10*(3), 248–262. https://doi.org./10.1177/117718011401000304

Russell, L. (2018). *Te Oranga Hinengaro: Report on Māori Mental Wellbeing Results from the New Zealand Mental Health Monitor & Health and Lifestyles Survey.* Wellington, NZ: Health Promotion Agency/Te Hiringa Hauora.

Ruwhiu, L. (2009). Indigenous issues in Aotearoa New Zealand. In M. Connolly, M. Harms, & L. Harms (Eds.), *Social Work: Context and Practice* (pp. 107–120). Melbourne, Australia: Oxford University Press.

Te Rau Matatini. (2014). *Whānau Ora and COPMIA: The Interface Literature Review.* Wellington, NZ: Te Rau Matatini.

The Bouverie Centre (2014). *Single Session Family Consultation Practice Manual* (version 2). Melbourne, Australia: The Bouverie Centre, La Trobe University.

Walker, T. (2017). "Whānau – Māori and family – Contemporary understandings of whānau." *Te Ara – The Encyclopedia of New Zealand.* http://www.TeAra. govt.nz/en/whanau-maori-and-family/page-1 (accessed 18 October 2019).

Walsh, M.C., Joyce, S., Maloney, T., & Vaithianathan, R. (2019). *Protective Factors of Children and Families at Highest Risk of Adverse Childhood Experiences: An Analysis of Children and Families in Growing Up in New Zealand Data Who "Beat the Odds."* Wellington, NZ: Ministry of Social Development.

23 Single Session Team Family Therapy (SSTFT) in China: A Seven-Step Protocol for Adapting Western Methods in Eastern Contexts

John K. Miller, Dai Xing, Hu Yaorui, and Xu Yilin

> *The man who moves a mountain begins by carrying away small stones.*
> – Confucius (551–479 BCE)

In 2009 the lead author, a U.S. professor of family therapy, developed a year-long single session therapy service in Beijing as part of a Fulbright grant. At the time, Western-based family therapy was becoming popular among the early therapy providers in China yet there were few therapy services or training/supervision institutions available and many barriers to providing care. One of these barriers included the fact that the general Chinese population did not commonly know what the concept of "therapy" was or how it might be useful and for which problems. In fact, there was not an immediately translatable word for the concept of "therapy" in the Chinese language at the time. Over the past few years the Chinese therapy community has adopted the Chinese term for "family treatment" (*Jiātíng liáofǎ*) to express the concept of family therapy. The term we have adopted to reflect the one-time nature of the meeting is "single session and brief" (*Dān jié jiǎnjiè*).

The service was developed in collaboration with a pioneering group of Chinese faculty and doctoral students at the Institute for Developmental Psychology at Beijing Normal University. It was advertised to the public through flyers as a two-hour single consultation opportunity for common family problems, to be conducted in Mandarin by the Chinese doctoral students under the live supervision of the Chinese faculty supervisors and the lead author. A team of Chinese doctoral student therapists also observed and offered feedback. A translator was always present to assist in communication between the clients and the lead author. The services were offered free-of-charge to the community, with the faculty supervisors watching all sessions from a video observation room. Clients were seen by appointment. Each client was surveyed after their single session consultation to inquire about how they felt about the experience, what did they think was most helpful about the session, did they think it was sufficient to address their concern, would this experience make it more likely they would seek therapy in the future, and what type of therapy service they would prefer (e.g., expert-based, non-expert/collaborative, directive, non-directive, humanistic, individual, family, etc.)? The data revealed that those surveyed would prefer an expert-based, family-focused, structured, brief, directive, intervention-rich, and team-based service (Miller, 2014). The Chinese faculty supervisors felt this was consistent with Chinese cultural values regarding the general population's views of health services.

Since 2016, the lead author has organized a group of 20 Chinese family therapists through the *Sino-American Family Therapy Institute* (SAFTI) in Shanghai to further develop the implementation of single session consultations to fit with Chinese cultural expectations. The SAFTI is a post-degree training organization founded in 2005 to further intercultural exchange between Western and Eastern scholars and therapists. This second generation of Chinese single session family therapists followed a seven-step protocol developed by the lead author. Each Chinese client family is seen over a three-hour period with a team observing. The original 2009 protocol was for two hours, but we decided to add an extra hour to provide an opportunity for an appreciative inquiry interview (Step 6) and the post-session supervisory discussion (Step 7). Each of the 20 therapists takes turns bringing a family for the Single Session Team Family Therapy (SSTFT), with the other therapists serving as the observing/reflecting team. The lead author supervises all the cases.

The group has been conducting SSTFT consultations continuously since 2016. The goals of the service are twofold. Firstly, we hope to provide a high-quality consultation service that fits with the already noted Chinese cultural values of expert-based, brief, directive, family oriented, etc. So far, all those who utilized the service (about 48 families) reported that it was useful and helpful in addressing their problems. Secondly, the service strives to provide an opportunity for the participating Chinese therapists to receive live clinical supervision in an environment with few other supervisory opportunities.

The Seven-Step Single Session Team Family Therapy (SSTFT) Protocol

Each three-hour session is apportioned into seven steps.

Step 1: The Pre-Session Briefing with the Team

During the first 30 minutes, the lead therapist for the case provides a standardized briefing for the team before the family arrives. The briefing includes who is in the family and the nature of the problem, treatment history, attempted solutions, a genogram, supervision goals, and what the therapist is seeking from the consultation for the family.

Step 2: The Family Session

The therapist then meets the family. The structure of the process, including the use of reflecting observers, is explained and the family's consent is obtained. For the next 45 minutes the lead therapist conducts the first part of the session with the family. The therapist asks typical single session therapy questions (Miller & Slive, 2004), such as:

- "How would each of you describe the problem today and what would you like to get out of the session?"
- "How would we know that this session had been useful to you?"
- "What have you tried in the past that helped?"
- What are some things you haven't yet tried, but that you think might help?"
- "If the problem disappeared tomorrow, what other problems might you have?"

The team's task during this part of the session is to generate as many ideas as possible in four areas of inquiry. These include:

1. Compliments, commendations, and validations for the family
2. Other questions to ask the family
3. Alternative stories (reframes) that could be used to describe the situation
4. Interventions.

Step 3: Team Break and Construction of a Team Message

During this step, the family takes a break in another room while the lead therapist meets with the team and supervisor for about 30 minutes. Each member of the team shares their thoughts with the therapist regarding the four areas of inquiry. The lead therapist selects five team members to take in to meet with the family to share their feedback. During Step 3, the lead therapist may alter a team member's message to best fit with what they think the family needs (we have termed this "tailoring the message"). Additionally, the lead therapist may suggest that a team member come up with a suggestion that they think would be useful (we have termed this a "plant"). The supervisor serves as a member of the team that goes into the therapy room to meet the family during Step 4.

Step 4: Team Metalogue in the Presence of the Family

The family is brought back into the therapy room to meet with the five team members, the supervisor, and the therapist, who will offer their reflections on the four areas of inquiry. The family sits at one side of the room, while the team, supervisor, and lead therapist sit at another. After introductions, the supervisor usually gives the following message directly to the family:

> We have talked with your therapist about ideas we have for you to take home tonight. We tried to think of as many things as we could. These five team members represent the entire team that was observing. I'm the supervisor. We have no secrets from you, and we want you to know everything we are thinking. To help facilitate this, we want to have a condensed version of the conversation we just had with your therapist in front of you and have you overhear us. It will perhaps sound odd, but we will talk about you as if you are not in the room to preserve the tone of the original conversation. We ask you to pretend there is an invisible wall between you and us. We will pretend that you can see and hear us, but that we cannot see or hear you. We had to take our best guess about what is happening based on what we heard tonight. We ask that you lower your expectations about our feedback, as all we know is what we heard in the last 45 minutes. Hopefully, some things will be useful, but some things might be off target. If so, please feel free to let your therapist know after we leave. We will talk for about 30 minutes and then leave. We advise you to take notes on what stood out for you and talk about it with the therapist after we leave. Do you have any questions about this idea? Is it ok with you for us to proceed?

The supervisor waves his hand to indicate "the wall" is up once the family is ready to begin. Each team member takes turns talking to the therapist about their feedback in the four areas of inquiry. The team's emphasis is to focus on the process (metalogue) instead of merely the content of the family situation. Our hope is that team metalogue guides the family to "second-order thinking" (thinking that is up one level of abstraction, getting at the process of how things happen instead of simply the "what is happening," or content). The idea of a metalogue was introduced by Gregory Bateson (1972), relating to a discussion of a problem in such a way that the structure of the conversation matches elements of the problem. The development of the use of the team in this way was influenced by the work of Tom Andersen (1987). This "invisible wall" strategy was modified from a technique developed by Wendel Ray at the Mental Research Institute (MRI) (Ray, Keeney, Parker, & Pascal, 1992). Step 4 usually takes about 30 minutes.

Step 5: Post-Team Metalogue (or Reflection) about Family Reaction, and Intervention Construction

During this step, the supervisor lowers the imaginary "invisible wall," thanks the family for coming in, and the team and supervisor leave the therapy room. The team and supervisor return to the observation room, and the lead therapist then asks each family member what they noticed from the team's comments. The therapist uses the information from the family's reaction to the team's comments to construct a final message to the family and interventions to take home. The therapist then leaves the family in the therapy room and returns to the observation room. Step 5 usually takes about 15 minutes.

Step 6: Appreciative Inquiry Interview with Family

At the beginning of Step 6, the supervisor returns to the therapy room to ask the family a few questions about their experience with the therapist. The following is a typical explanation provided by the supervisor to the family:

> If you don't mind, I would like to take a few minutes to ask you a few questions about your experience with your therapist. These questions don't have anything to do with your case, but are focused on feedback you have for your therapist. I am your therapist's supervisor, and we are always working on improving things so we can provide our clients the best service possible. With this in mind, your feedback is very important to us. Your therapist is observing our conversation from the observation room, and I'm sure will be very interested in your thoughts. Is it OK with you that I begin?

The three questions asked of the family focus on what they appreciate, and include:

1. What are characteristics of your therapist that you appreciate?
2. What are the things that your therapist did that helped with your problem?
3. What advice would you give your therapist?

This approach is modified from Cooperrider and Srivastva's (1987) work on "appreciative inquiry" (AI). Instead of criticism and problem solving, it is a strengths-based and positively focused way to gather feedback and promote meaningful change. This part of the interview helps the family to see themselves not only as people with a problem seeking help from "experts," but also as people who are experts themselves in helping the therapist and the team become better in their work. The fact that the therapist's supervisor is the one conducting the AI interview reflects a hierarchy that fits with Chinese culture. Chinese culture tends to revere teachers as holding a special place in society. As opposed to typical Western values, Chinese cultural values tend to have a more established and clearly delineated hierarchical structure regarding these roles. We find it useful and demystifying for the clients to see this hierarchical structure by meeting with the supervisor in this way. Also, the AI discussion with the supervisor encourages the second-order type thinking we described in the metalogue discussion of Step 4 (e.g., asking the clients to think about how the therapy is going, versus the content of the therapy itself). At the conclusion of the interview the clients are thanked for their feedback and depart the therapy offices.

It is possible for families to return, but we have not had that happen yet. The therapists choose which family to bring. The therapists brief the family on what to expect. They describe it as a one-time consultation opportunity. The team method and setup are explained and consent gained before the session. We encourage the therapists to follow up with the families with regard to the outcome of the SSTFT.

Step 7: Post-Session Supervisory Discussion with the Lead Therapist and the Team

During this final step, the supervisor returns to the observation room to discuss the clients' feedback about the lead therapist, the lead therapist's thoughts about the session, and any final supervisory feedback to the lead therapist and the team. The advice the family provides to the therapist is usually productive, and often involves encouragement from the family for the therapist to push them more or take more direct action in their interventions. This step usually takes about 15 minutes.

Case Example

The following composite illustration describes a family seen using this seven-step protocol.

Excessive Spending of an Adult Son

Middle-aged, middle-class parents and their 28-year-old son consulted the team in relation to the son's excessive spending, which had led to tremendous loans and family conflict. This family had been meeting regularly with their Chinese therapist, who brought them to the team for the SSTFT consultation. The son was the family's only child, and all three lived in the same apartment. The mother was a full-time homemaker, while the husband was an executive at a successful company. The family reported that the problem began when the son graduated college and began dating. He was new to dating and showed his affection for the women he went out with by purchasing expensive gifts with loans he would take out, yet was unable to repay. The son had just experienced his first break-up with a girlfriend and was distraught, which led to the parents' discovery of his excessive debts.

The parents explained that they felt the problem was probably related to their failure when he was young to prepare him for adult relationships and responsibilities. The father confessed that he did not think he was there enough for the son when he was growing up because of his focus on success in his work, aimed to provide a lifestyle that previous generations were not able to enjoy. Like many families in China, the previous generations experienced extreme financial hardship so the new opportunities of his generation were difficult to resist. The mother relayed that she felt her contribution to the problem was that she was too permissive with her son when he was growing up, partially to counter the husband's absence, and perhaps to deal with her own loneliness. The son agreed that he felt unprepared for life after high school, and did not discipline himself enough in college because he was so relieved with the relatively pressure-free life college provided.

During the metalogue, the team complimented the family for their self-reflection and insights about each of their possible contributions to the problem, as well as their ability to be vulnerable as individuals during the discussion. They reflected on the situation many families in China are faced with regarding the rapid economic advancement of the society, and that everybody can be doing what they think is the right thing to do but problems can still emerge without anyone being at fault. Our focus on trying to positively frame each family member's actions fits with our sense of the Chinese cultural emphasis on "saving face" (*mian zi*). We have found that no matter how technically sophisticated the feedback or intervention, it will rarely be accepted by Chinese families if it is delivered in such a way that the clients lose face.

One team member offered the idea that this problem might provide an opportunity to sort some things out in the family. Another team member asked what the family would talk about at home if the problem of the son's loans and relationships were off the table. Did they have other topics to discuss that were not focused on the son, or was this their only conversational topic? Another team member commented on how everyone in the family seemed to be motivated by concern for the others, and that as they go about making changes they should be careful not to lose this valuable quality of the family. Next, the team discussed how they noticed a pattern in the way that each of them showed this concern for others. The father showed his concern for his family by working hard so that he could provide money for them, and perhaps the son had subconsciously learned this lesson about how to show concern to others. If this was true, one thing they might try is to develop other ways to show concern within the family.

Once the team left the room, the family discussed how the feedback had brought a profound impact on them to hear so many therapists' opinions. The mother seemed to be greatly relieved that she was not being blamed for the problem and began to discuss with growing confidence her feeling that there must be a solution. She discussed how she now regarded the mistakes of the past as a learning experience for the family. For instance, she talked about how she was more prone to find faults rather than praise and approve of her son, and she should change this. The father discussed his realization that his son was already 28 years old, but he had been supervising him as if he were only 18. The son discussed his realization that he only knew the one way to show affection and resolved to develop new ways. The therapist conducted a follow-up interview with the family three months after the SSTFT session. The son had moved into his own apartment with a roommate. The parents had helped the son repay his loans this one time, but committed themselves to stop meddling in his daily life. The son had gotten a new job, and was taking his time to re-enter dating relationships.

Conclusion

We have found that one advantage of this method lies in the ability of the team to capitalize on the "wisdom of the crowd," a concept proposed by the English social scientist Sir Francis Galton in 1907 that demonstrated that the group as a whole is often wiser than any one individual in the group. This idea is very consistent with Chinese culture's focus on communal collaboration and collectivism as an ancient core value. In our experience, this method of team consultation matches the Chinese tendency to "gather around" a problem in an effort to solve it as a group. This is congruent with other reflecting team methods utilized in Western contexts (Andersen, 1991; Friedman, 1995; White, 1995). We have also incorporated this concept of working together as a group in our learning/ teaching culture with student therapists at the *Sino-American Family Therapy Institute* (SAFTI). We have termed this a "collaborative, cohort model" where we encourage collaboration over competition. To cultivate the culture of the team cohort, therapists join the team at the same time and commit to work together with the SSTFT consultations for a minimum 12-month period. In this way, we hope not only to provide something useful for the families we see, but also to learn how to be better therapists by watching one another conduct therapy sessions.

In closing, we would like to emphasize how using this seven-step protocol has also provided a valuable opportunity for a rich two-way exchange of ideas between Eastern and Western therapists. Western therapists who have participated in the team over the years have all commented on how much they have learned about Chinese families, and the variety of new and creative ways the Chinese therapists address problems. Given that the majority of the world's population lives within about a 3000-mile radius of Shanghai, there is much to learn about how these "majority world" families live and work (Miller, Platt, & Conroy, 2018). As Confucius tells us in the epigraph at the beginning of this chapter, big changes often originate from small actions. This is consistent with our understanding of the practice of single session therapy throughout the world.

References

Andersen, T. (1987). The reflecting team: Dialogue and meta-dialogue in clinical work. *Family Process, 26*(4), 415–528.

Andersen, T. (Ed.). (1991). *The Reflecting Team: Dialogues and Dialogues about the Dialogues*. New York: Norton.

Bateson, B. (1972). *Steps to an Ecology of Mind*. New York: Chandler Publishing/ Ballantine Books.

Cooperrider, D.L., & Srivastva, S. (1987). Appreciative inquiry in organizational life. In R.W. Woodman & W.A. Pasmore (Eds.), *Research in Organizational Change and Development* (Vol. 1, pp. 129–169). Stamford, CT: JAI Press.

Friedman, S. (Ed.). (1995). *The Reflecting Team in Action: Collaborative Practice in Family Therapy*. New York: Guilford Press.

Galton, F. (1907). Vox populi. *Nature, 75*, 450–451.

Hoyt, M.F., & Talmon, M. (2014). The temporal structure of brief therapy: Some questions often associated with different phases of sessions and treatment. In M.F. Hoyt & M. Talmon (Eds.), *Capturing the Moment: Single-Session Therapy and Walk-In Services* (pp. 517–522). Bethel, CT: Crown House Publishing.

Miller, J.K. (2008). Walk-in single-session team therapy: A study of client satisfaction. *Journal of Systemic Therapies, 27*(3), 78–94.

Miller, J.K. (2011). Single-session intervention in the wake of Hurricane Katrina: Strategies for disaster mental health counseling. In A. Slive & M. Bobele (Eds.), *When One Hour Is All You Have: Effective Therapy for Walk-In Clients* (pp. 185–202). Phoenix, AZ: Zeig, Tucker, & Theisen.

Miller, J.K. (2014). Single session therapy in China. In M.F. Hoyt & M. Talmon (Eds.), *Capturing the Moment: Single Session Therapy and Walk-In Services* (pp. 195–214). Bethel, CT: Crown House Publishing.

Miller, J.K. (2018). Single session social work in China. In Z. Fang (Ed.), *Fudan University Social Work Teaching Case Collection* (Vol. 1, pp. 129–148). Fudan, China: Fudan University Publishing House.

Miller, J.K., Platt, J.J., & Conroy, K.M. (2018). Single-session therapy in the majority world: Addressing the challenge of service delivery in Cambodia and the implications for other global contexts. In M.F. Hoyt, M. Bobele, A. Slive, J. Young, & M. Talmon (Eds.), *Single-Session Therapy by Walk-In or Appointment: Administrative, Clinical, and Supervisory Aspects of One-at-a-Time Services* (pp. 116–134). New York: Routledge.

Miller, J.K., & Slive, A. (2004). Breaking down the barriers to clinical service delivery: Walk-in family therapy. *Journal of Marital and Family Therapy, 30*(1), 95–103.

Ray, W., Keeney, B., Parker, K., & Pascal, D. (1992). The invisible wall: A method for breaking a relational impasse. *Louisiana Journal of Counseling and Development, 3*(1), 32–34.

White, M. (1995). Reflecting team as definitional ceremony. In *Re-Authoring Lives: Interviews & Essays* (pp. 172–198). Adelaide, S.A., Australia: Dulwich Centre Publications.

24 Single Session Ericksonian Strategic Hypnotherapy for Disasters in Mexico

Rafael Núñez and Jorge Abia

We started studying and using hypnotherapy in Mexico in 1988 during our clinical training. We got interested as a result of the needs of our patient population and because many cases in the history of this discipline had been single session interventions. Indeed, one of the earliest case reports (Gavin-Jones & Handford, 2016) was that of the work of Franz Anton Mesmer in 1777, about a young woman who allegedly was born blind and recovered vision through hypnosis in a single session. One of the first important systematic published reports was by James Esdaile (1846), a civil assistant surgeon working in Bengal, India, whose use of hypnotic anaesthesia during surgery diminished mortality rates from 50% to 5%. These antecedents encouraged us, and we began doing research to answer what appeared to us a main question: *What is understood in Spanish-speaking Mexican patients while in hypnotic trance?*[1] (Abia & Núñez, 2014). We went on working with single session interventions with adults, adolescents, children, families, couples, and groups in a 10-session format, and also with a single session format (Abia & Núñez, 2012). In 1996, Núñez presented his work with a single session to quit smoking. The results encouraged us to go on working in this way and to further acknowledge the therapeutic effect of single session hypnotherapy.

Hypnosis is an alternative state of consciousness which nowadays is very well known from an experimental neuro-psycho-physiological perspective (Erickson, 1980; Haley, 1985; Yapko, 2018). It is one of the 12 different consciousness states that the human brain and body may be in (Ardila, 1980; Abia & Núñez, 2014). Hypnosis in therapy helps lower pain to functional levels, saves time, and improves the results of patients' efforts. This state of mind happens spontaneously in many social or personal activities, and has been described to be useful in health disciplines since the year 3000 B.C.

After more than three decades, various research results and most of all our patients – our best teachers – have clarified for us how to intervene with only one hypnotherapy session with individuals, couples, families, groups, and big groups. Doing follow-ups with persons who have gone through these experiences has allowed study, identification of mistakes, and correction in strategic thinking oriented towards helpful possibilities and achieving specific clinical goals in single session therapy – efficient results which are very frequently needed in our country.

We see single session hypnotherapy occupying a particular niche within the array of more traditional therapeutic services. Our work deals with developing and testing specific techniques for clear-cut goals. Sometimes one session is all that is possible – and all that is needed. It has been useful in a range of situations that include handling crises, improving habit control in certain patients, emotional stabilization and catharsis, suicide prevention, bodily responses to medical emergencies, and disaster intervention. All of these are oriented to improve functionality, learning, self-observation, treatment compliance, and acknowledgment of needing help. In this panorama we have developed an Ericksonian Strategic Model that has been very suitable for crisis interventions during disasters.

Our Ericksonian Strategic Model

Based on clinical research (Abia & Núñez, 2012, 2014; Núñez, 2002; Núñez & Abia, 2001, 2005, 2009, 2012), the model has the following basic elements:

1. Give understandable information to potential patients, prior to beginning, about what hypnosis is, as a state of consciousness, its spontaneous presence in daily life and its application to health disciplines as hypnotherapy.
2. Define a therapeutic relationship as collaboration to address objectives defined by the person who seeks consultation and is advised by the health professional in the framework of human rights and with informed consent.
3. Explain the concept of the unconscious mind as the source of experiences and learnings that are not consciously noticed.
4. Explain the logic of the unconscious mind, different from the dominant social logic, and define it as individual, subjective, metaphorical, with opposites not being exclusive but instead complementary.
5. Define the strategic therapeutic work relationship based on a goal or goals. In each session, ask about the problem to be solved, defining the solution according to the criteria of the person who seeks consultation, and asking how the consultant would know that she or he is taking effective steps towards therapy goals.
6. Define an estimated number of sessions (between 1 and 10). At the end of therapy, make an evaluation of the achievement of goals and arrange follow up if the person who consults so wishes.

In our experience, the number of patients in a single session group hypnotherapy session has varied from 2 to 500, reaching a total of 4321 persons during a five-day crisis intervention for a single disaster, in which groups of up to 200 people were treated by 12 hypnotherapists. We have found the main implementation aids in this field to be paradoxically also the main factors that create obstacles, and come from two sources: (1) the need for carefully defining interventions from a framework that includes epistemology, philosophy, theory, and practice in a logical manner that allows learning from criticisms, approaching them as opportunities to correct design, methods, and application; and (2) the prejudices and misunderstandings that patients may have about hypnosis, for example, as a method for having a "black-out" experience with spectacular changes easily achieved, the risk of losing control and being in the hands of the hypnotherapist, or even a way of having a spiritual experience and maybe having a channel to communicate with extra-terrestrial entities (we're not kidding!) – these are the most usual preconceptions of hypnosis as a near-magic method.

What we have been doing is to be very clear about what hypnosis is as a scientifically known state of mind, and what it is not; and how it could it be useful for particular problems. Before proceeding to do hypnosis and hypnotherapy, we explain to patients precisely every point of what hypnosis and hypnotherapy are. At our Erickson Institute in Mexico City, we also offer a weekly free presentation to inform people that all that is needed is to share control with the hypnotherapist as the health professional listens to the patient's wishes and needs. The main referral source of patients is word-of-mouth recommendation. In the single (or first) session, goals and length of treatment are set with the patient, ranging from single session hypnotherapy to 10 sessions of hypnotherapy. If the intervention is not due to a disaster or any kind of crisis, we usually offer 5 or 10 hypnotherapy sessions.

For Milton Erickson, *resistance* is a protector of hypnotic trances, since it prevents us from destabilizing the unconscious mind in an effort to help the patient; and at the same time *resistance* is an ally for the hypnotherapist because by pointing out where not to go, the patient indicates the route by which he or she can accompany the therapist in the construction of solutions for his or her difficulties. "One always tries to use everything that the patient brings to the consultation. If resistance is what you carry, let us appreciate that resistance" (Erickson, in Erickson & Rossi, 1981, p. 16).

When working with those who have suffered disasters, we allow the resistance to participate and show us the way to direct change. "The resistances that are part of the problem can be used by enhancing them, whereby, and under guidance, the patient is allowed to discover new modes of behavior favorable to recovery" (Erickson, 1980, Vol. 4, p. 48). For example, the patient is often reluctant to speak directly about the trauma in the event of a disaster, so a metaphor is proposed in order to elaborate the trauma.

Since the intervention is carried out by hypnotherapists certified by the National Autonomous University of Mexico (UNAM) of the Health Division of the Mexican Navy, duly uniformed, the population seeks to participate in the service offered. The Mexican Navy has a program called *"Plan Marina,"* whose mission is to assist the civilian population in cases and areas of disaster or emergency (http://www.semar.gob.mx/planmarina/). To this program, it was possible to add the use of the single session with hypnotherapy to reduce the consequences of traumatic stress.

Example: Single Session Group Hypnotherapy After the 2017 Mexico Earthquake

In September 2017, two terrible earthquakes struck Mexico, wrecking more than 180,000 buildings, injuring thousands, and killing more than 500 people (Milenio, 2017). We were called to supervise our hypnotherapy students, as well as psychologists and physicians of the Mexican Navy. Arriving to support isolated Indigenous communities in rural areas in the State of Oaxaca in Navy helicopters and airplanes because the roads were destroyed, we observed social and family disorganization. People were sleeping outside because of fear of more earthquakes, there were nervous breakdowns, some people were refusing to eat, and most were having trouble sleeping. Twelve hypnotherapists cared for groups from 20 people to just over 200 people in village public squares, a few days after the earthquake occurred. The ethics of hypnosis requires reporting that an exercise with hypnosis is going to be applied, with the recipients voluntarily agreeing to participate. All participants were informed that the exercise would last 30 minutes, plus 10 minutes to take the tests before and after, to measure the results of the intervention. They were also told that it would be a unique session to support them so that they could better organize themselves as a community, reduce nervous breakdowns, and improve sleep.

While explaining the framework and the purpose of the hypnotherapeutic exercise, all the persons in the group received modeling clay and a 20-centimeter piece of string. They were asked and shown how to fashion a pendulum attached to the string, or they received pendulums already made by other persons in the community.[2] Persons that received ones already made were asked to remodel the pendulum they received, to make it a personal pendulum. The Navy personnel brought the modeling clay and strings, along with paper and pencils that were used during the hypnotic trance to draw the internal reality of the problem and also the internal reality of the solution, the hypnotic automatic drawing to be done by the unconscious mind. This technique (pendulum and writing) was used to "hook" the unconscious mind in the healing process during and after the hypnotic trance.

Most of the people were in states of acute stress. Crisis intervention counseling was done within open communal spaces; most people sat on the dirt floor or in chairs when possible. Ambient noises and voices were present along with pets coming around and children talking and some playing during the hypnotic trance – stimuli that were used to deepen the hypnotic experience.

Once the people were assembled and prepared, when the hypnotherapist had the group's attention, she or he began:

> In this hypnotic exercise you are going to handle this pendulum that you already modelled. Please take your pendulum with your thumb and index finger, place your elbow in a comfortable position, maybe upon your leg, so you can see the pendulum comfortably.

> Stare at the pendulum and come into contact with your breathing ... feel how you take in air from outside that is renewing you healthily, and feel how the air inside you is coming out, finally taking out all that you no longer need ... stare at the pendulum ... your unconscious mind is going to be communicating with you through this tool that is the pendulum ...

> ... And as you go further into this experience, you now begin, automatically guided by your Unconscious Mind, automatically drawing – a very nice, very nice drawing, you are automatically drawing, drawing that picture in which you are promising your life, taking care of it forever ... today better than yesterday and tomorrow better than today ... healthily enjoying, automatically learning, healthily enjoying taking care of your life ... healthily enjoying taking care of it, automatically learning, healthily enjoying taking care of your life ...

The hypnotherapist went on, speaking and pausing to allow people to absorb and process. After approximately 30 minutes, they concluded:

> ... that promise to take care of your life remains with you, which you can always redraw. It accompanies you forever, life has changed ... from today it improves healthily, you learning some things automatically and other things by reflecting. And you share that promise to take care of your life with all members of your family, with all the women in your family, with all the men in your family, with all the girls in your family and all the boys in your family. The only thing that can happen is that this promise to take care of your life healthily, reminding you that you enjoy being you, yourself, everyday enjoying

your life better healthily, the only thing that can happen is that it brings you healthy wellbeing ... We are preparing to finish the exercise ... your attention is turning again to this world that surrounds you, full of opportunities to continue rebuilding your life healthily, rebuilding your life healthily, enjoying and learning, rebuilding your life healthily, protected, learning automatically.

When everything is ready to finish this exercise, take a deep breath, a lot of air, then softly stretch your body, as if you were waking up from a pleasant dream, and go on opening your eyes, returning to a usual state of very pleasant consciousness ... To finish we applaud ourselves.

For the measurement of results, we administered the Hospital Standardized Anxiety and Depression Scale (Zigmond & Snaith, 1983; Pascual, Barranco, Alvarenga, Ovando, Velázquez & Martinez, 2002) before and after the intervention, obtaining a statistically significant difference ($p < 0.05$; Levin, 1990) within the group of 4321 people who were affected by the earthquakes and attended the one-session hypnotherapy. People continue to be in touch reporting improvement after Navy personnel left.

Navy personnel also reported physical and emotional fatigue ("burn-out") due to the impact of the disaster and the people affected in different ways according to their ages and family roles. The Navy personnel received the same single session procedure, blending hypnotic suggestions to help relieve exhaustion, insomnia, and acute stress and to improve their force and energy administration, along with emotional stability and balance, reactions to emergencies, and team cooperation (Abia & Núñez, 2012).

We operate from the assumption that the Unconscious Mind is the main agent responsible for trauma management, both psychologically and physiologically. If we manage to intervene in the first six weeks after a trauma, we greatly increase the chances of attenuating the symptoms caused by acute stress due to a disaster. In addition, we also have a self-hypnosis (Spanish-language) audio program that our consultees can access through our website (www.institutoerickson.com.mx), in order to give more support to the intervention in case of disasters.

In strategic Ericksonian hypnotherapy, the use of metaphors facilitates the understanding of the problem and the elaboration of solutions (Núñez, 2002; Núñez & Abia, 2009). Metaphors are designed that are specific for each group or community. Thanks to this, as the following example illustrates, we were able to adapt and intervene in Indigenous communities that do not speak Spanish. Fortunately, we have a Navy lieutenant of the Health Division who was originally from one of those villages, and she supported us as a translator. They are communities where barter is still practiced, in their original language. They privilege the use of the *we* over the *I*, the relationship with nature is through characters similar to gods, the earthquake is because Mother Earth is upset by the damage being done to it, dreams are more important than concrete reality, being unable to sleep means they lose that possibility of communication with otherness. During the hypnotic trance we support the Unconscious Mind to elaborate the emotional part of the trauma. Outside of the trance with the Indigenous spiritual leaders it is requested to organize the pertinent rituals to stabilize the community's relationship with Mother Earth.

Another Example: Single Session Hypnotherapy with Zapotec Villagers

One of the many places where hypnotherapy was provided is 730 kilometers (453 miles) from Mexico City. The village is called Xadani. As mentioned, a colleague from the Navy was originally from there and translated the hypnosis exercises from Spanish into Zapotec. Villagers were summoned by Radio Totopo, the local radio, to attend the group sessions with hypnosis in order to catch up on sleep and speak the language of Mother Earth again and for women to have their clitoris alive. Yes, you read that correctly: Zapotec is a metaphorical language in which "being happy" is expressed as "having the clitoris alive." During the hypnotic trance, when referring to an earthquake, it was translated into Zapotec as *Xu*, which is the onomatopoeic sound that the earth makes when it trembles. And when "well-being" was suggested the "living clitoris" was mentioned. Suggestions were also made to manage insomnia, which was translated as "sleeping better to return to understand our Mother Earth that we have damaged so much."

Conclusion

It is important to continue to preserve other types of psychotherapy that cover as many areas as the diversity of human beings that we are. At the Milton H. Erickson Institute of Mexico City, we have designed a 240-hour training for Health and Education professionals in Group Hypnotherapy endorsed by UNAM (National Autonomous University of Mexico) (Abia & Núñez, 2012), largely to attend to the aftermath we have suffered from the declared war on drug trafficking, which has caused the murder of 250,000 inhabitants of our country in the last 13 years. Our armed forces are overwhelmed by the situation and it becomes essential to have intervention tools for the restoration of peace and to reduce the social decomposition that we suffer. In addition to the failed war against drug trafficking, in Mexico we also have the continuous risk of natural disasters such as earthquakes and hurricanes. Within the Mexican Navy we have more than 120 graduates of the Health Division and more than 3000 graduates in the civilian population, whether they are health or education professionals. The training we offer has the option of applying a single session in cases of intervention in war or disaster or five sessions for group medical hypnotherapy or ten sessions for hypnotherapy in psychotherapy.

A great challenge has been to adapt hypnotherapy interventions to different points of view. Part of the population of Mexico has more acculturation towards a U.S./American style; 70% of the population is in poverty; another part of the population is of Indigenous origin (60 Aboriginal languages are spoken in Mexico today). Since 1988, we have given ourselves the task of adapting interventions to these different circumstances. At our Institute, we have been able to demonstrate to the National Autonomous University of Mexico and to the Mexican Navy the utility of having the option of single session group hypnotherapy in cases of disasters. With more quantitative and qualitative studies, more and more human beings can benefit from the option of a single session intervention.

Notes

1 During the awake state of consciousness, the right brain hemisphere does not understand all language; it needs the left hemisphere cooperation to get into a semantic interpretation. Likewise left brain hemisphere needs right brain hemisphere cooperation to understand the emotional analogic sense of language. During hypnosis there is an increase in activity in the right frontal lobe as well as in the right temporal lobe and right occipital lobe activities. We studied clinically which changes in Spanish are useful for better therapeutic results; for example, changes in word order, words to protect the experience, use of adverbs, simple past or present progressive tense arrangements during a hypnotic intervention. We concluded that there are better ways for communicating with the unconscious mind during hypnosis with Spanish-speaking people. We have been working for more than 30 years testing specific techniques for specific purposes, using this kind of "Hypnotic Spanish."
2 This is an adaptation of what is called Chevreul's Pendulum, named after the 19th-century French scientist, Michel-Eugene Chevreul, who first used it to induce hypnosis. In hypnosis and hypnotherapy pendulums are tools used to focus and at the same time dissociate attention, so persons may have a double attention level – one part looking at the pendulum is oriented inwards through hypnotic suggestions, and the other part of attention stays consciously in touch with the hypnotherapist's suggestions. Making a personal pendulum or re-modeling one to make it personal helps to engender a physical, emotional and perceptual process that nonverbally sends the message of being in control, the same as when the person handles the pendulum by herself or himself. The two maneuvers of making a personal pendulum and then having it used by the person that is going to go into hypnotic trance were designed by Rafael Núñez to help create a safe therapeutic process.

References

Abia, J., & Núñez, R. (2012). *Hipnoterapia Grupal Ericksoniana Estratégica (13 Manuales)*. México City: Editorial de la Sociedad Mexicana de Hipnosis.

Abia, J., & Núñez, R. (2014). *Bases de la Hipnoterapia Ericksoniana Estratégica: Hipnoterapia Ericksoniana Estratégica para Adultos (13 Manuales)*. México City: Editorial de la Sociedad Mexicana de Hipnosis.

Ardila, A. (1980). *Psicología de la Percepción*. México: Trillas.

Erickson, M.H. (1980). *Collected Papers* (vols. 1–4; E.L. Rossi, Ed.). New York: Irvington.

Erickson, M.H., & Rossi, E.L. (1981). *Experiencing Hypnosis*. New York: Irvington.

Esdaile, J. (1846). *Mesmerism in India and Its Practical Application in Surgery and Medicine*. London: Hartford Press.

Gavin-Jones, T., & Handford, S. (2016). *Hypnobirth*. New York: Routledge.

Haley, J. (1985). *Conversations with Milton H. Erickson, M.D* (vols. 1–3). New York: Triangle Press.

Levin, J. (1990). *Fundamentos de Estadística en la Investigación Social*. Mexico City: Editorial Harla.

Milenio. (2017). Destrucción, lo que dejaron los sismos de 2017 (Destruction, what's left from the earthquakes of 2017). https://www.milenio.com/politica/comunidad/19-s-destruccion-lo-que-dejaron-los-sismos-de-2017.

Núñez, R. (1996). *One Session for Quitting Smoking*. Presentation at the 7th European Congress for Hypnosis Budapest, Hungary.

Núñez, R. (2002). *Hipnoludoterapia Familiar: Tesis Que Se Presentó Para Obtener el Título de Maestría en Terapia Familiar en la Universidad de las Américas*. Mexico City. Available at www.institutoerickson.com.mx

Núñez, R. (2014). *¿Para Qué Siento lo Que Siento?* México: Editorial de la Sociedad Mexicana de Hipnosis.

Núñez, R., & Abia, J. (2001). *Revista Virtual: Estados Alternativos de Consciencia (Números 1–7)*. Mexico: Editorial Sociedad Mexicana de Hipnosis. Available at www.institutoerickson.com.mx.

Núñez, R., & Abia, J. (2005). *Estados Alternativos de Consciencia, Revista Electrónica; (Números 1–7)*. Mexico: Editorial de la Sociedad Mexicana de Hipnosis.

Núñez, R., & Abia, J. (2009). *Diplomado de Hipnoterapia Familiar y de Pareja (13 Manuales)*. México: Editorial de la Sociedad Mexicana de Hipnosis.

Núñez, R., & Abia, J. (2012). *Hipnoterapia Ericksoniana en Niños y Adolescentes (13 Manuales)*. México: Editorial de la Sociedad Mexicana de Hipnosis.

Pascual, R.J.S., Barranco, J.G., Alvarenga, J.C.L., Ovando, Á.S., Velázquez, V.V., & Martínez, D.A. (2002). Exactitud y utilidad diagnóstica del Hospital Anxiety and Depression Scale (HAD) en una muestra de sujetos obesos mexicanos. *Revista de Investigación Clínica, 54*(5), 403–409. www.imbiomed.com.mx.

Weitzenhoffer, A. (1989). *The Practice of Hypnotism* (vol. 2). New York: Wiley.

Yapko, M. (2018). *Trancework* (5th ed.). New York: Routledge.

Zigmond, A.S., & Snaith, R.P. (1983). The Hospital Anxiety and Depression Scale. *Acta Psychiatrica Scandinavia, 67*, 361–370.

Section VI

Single Session Thinking and Practice with Families

25 Families at First Sight: Practice Innovations Towards Making Family SST More Friendly and Effective

Tess McGrane and Ron Findlay

In the TV show "Married at First Sight," two people who have never met before marry. They try to open up, be vulnerable, share intimate information, all towards reaching their aims. For clients, Single Session Family Therapy (SSFT) has many similarities. The therapists are (usually) strangers to them. Family members take the daunting risk of opening up and sharing personal information and problems, to try and get help and answers to their problems. In this chapter, we describe steps we are trialing towards making therapy less stressful and more family-friendly and comfortable, more effective and worthwhile. We also discuss our approaches to making our co-therapy work for client families and for colleagues.

Background

headspace[1] is a federally and state-funded nationwide youth-oriented counseling service with centers all over Australia. We will describe the work we do at the Elsternwick and Bentleigh headspace branches in Melbourne's inner southeast. Both branches offer free SSFT. About five SSFT[2] sessions are available per week including one with a reflecting team of three or four clinicians behind a one-way mirror. Each session usually has the same two therapists in the room with the family (except for the reflecting team session, when the therapists rotate). Appointments are usually obtainable within a week or two. Approximately 70% families come once ("at first sight"); 30% go on to attend more sessions (Barbara-May, Denborough, & McGrane, 2018). Any headspace individual counselor is welcome to attend the SSFT of their client.

Tess is a state government-funded coordinator and clinician for the SSFT work at the two centers and does about two or three SSFTs a week. Ron is a private practitioner family therapist consultant who charges fee for service, paid by government rebates, so no cost to families. He does about two SSFTs a week.

Our SSFT Process

A single session format is used, meaning that the first session is treated as if it is also the last (Hopkins, Lee, McGrane, & Barbara-May, 2016; Hoyt, Bobele, Slive, Young, & Talmon, 2018). Sessions are two hours with two co-workers in the room. Co-therapists are diverse in age, experience, qualifications, and models of practice.

Pre-Session. Access (intake) or the young person's individual counselor arranges the SSFT and explains (in person or on the phone) what it is and why an SSFT is recommended. Once the SSFT is booked, an "SST explanation" brochure, consent form, and pre-session questionnaire and information page are emailed to the family.

The Session. There are a number of steps typically addressed in sequence:

- "Meet and Greet." Session process is explained. Family and staff "selfies" taken (optional – discussed below). Email addresses of all family members are obtained in order to email them after-session notes
- Each person is asked to hold off discussing "the problem" and to first describe their activities and interests
- Each person is asked to tell us what they want to work on (problem focus) or achieve (solution focus) from the session. Pre-session questionnaires with this information are reviewed with family
- Co-therapists and family members together prioritize what is to be covered
- The main issues or aims are discussed according to the training and orientation of the co-therapists
- Other mid- or end-of-session options include:

  a. Therapists give advice, tips, or a reflection/feedback to the family, according to their style of training, e.g., compliments, developmental and parenting opinions, interpretations, hypotheses, witnessing.

  b. Therapists talk to each other in front of the family regarding reflections or advice. (In the once-a-week SSFT with a reflecting team and one-way screen, the team and family will swap places for this).

  c. Towards the end the family is asked if there is anything that hasn't been talked about that needs to be raised, which is then discussed.

  d. At the end, each family member is also asked what was good and bad for them about the session and what they might "take away" to think about or try in the future. A brief discussion about what happened in the session that sparked any positive insights may occur.

- Final step is the "what happens next" speech where options for the future are explained (e.g., individual therapy, formal family therapy, another SSFT, a parent education group). We usually ask the family to wait two weeks before booking another SSFT, but we bend this guideline especially if a young person asks for another SST.

Post Session. Co-therapists chat and debrief afterwards if time permits. Notes of the session are composed by one or both workers and emailed to each family member, hopefully within the next 10 days.

Evolving Our SSFT Co-Working Together: "The Whole Is Greater Than the Sum of Its Parts"

Our SSFTs follow an SST format but the two co-therapists decide the therapeutic approach they each follow.

Tess is systemically trained and Ron has a narrative therapy background so we had to work out ways to get along and use the best of our skills. Practicing what we preach, we endeavor to align our different approaches, remaining true to our backgrounds and still be genuinely helpful to the family. Other SSFT clinicians are trained in systemic (mainly) or other approaches, e.g., developmental, attachment, open dialogue, psychodynamic, etc. and have to do something similar.

Sometimes we "tag team" (i.e., take it in turns); sometimes it's "free for all." If one is tired or uninspired, the other will take a bigger part. We might discuss or argue in a session or even take opposing views, although hopefully (usually) in a collegial spirit. We are getting better at stating and explaining to the family what and why we are doing this, our different ways of thinking about things and how sometimes we prefer different techniques and ideas. Sometimes we get it right, often we scrape through. When we debrief after the session, we try to check in with each other that we both had a go, and compliment useful aspects of each other's work.

It works best when we "add to each other" (i.e., build on, within our own models, what the other contributes). For example, if mother and daughter are fighting, Tess might lead the (systemic/family of origin) discussion about the mother's experiences of childhood and how that impacted the mother then and now (Goding, 1992; Rothbaum, Rosen, Tatsuo, & Uchida, 2002) and how her parenting of her daughter is similar or a reaction to it. She might then discuss times when the family finds the problem not so bad and then ask how the family members could increase those times. Tess might also share something about her own experiences as a mum and of having a mum. Ron might then enter the conversation inquiring about the values the mother holds about herself and parenting. He might find externalized (see White, 2007) names from her words for what she calls the problem, and ask about its effects. He might then ask about unique outcomes (when the problem is reduced) and her positive skills and knowledges that are in opposition to the problem. This might then lead into asking all the family members about their positive techniques for managing similar types of problems (narrative/solution) (de Shazer, 1988; White, 2007).

Our Aims and Reforms

We aim to make SSFT more friendly and effective, and have instituted a number of practice reforms.

Aim 1. Be More Family Friendly

Before arriving, families can be anxious about coming to an SSFT, not helped by the fact they are meeting with new workers for the first (and often only) time. The difficult process of discussing personal family problems can be "raw" and stressful, and the session atmosphere can feel "official" or "clinical." So we wondered what might reduce the discomfort and make it all more welcoming and family friendly, especially as we may only get this one go at it. We also thought that the session notes we later sent to them needed to be more personal and less "forensic."

Aim 2. Be More Effective – According to the Families, Not Just Us

Families can go to a lot of trouble to get to the appointment. Hence, they want to get something useful out of the session and they have their own ideas about what would make a session effective. They often tell us explicitly that they want not just a theoretical discussion but hopefully something practical and concrete to "take away," like constructive feedback on what they are doing, and useful tips and steps for a happier family life. When we ask, "If you had to pick one thing to get from this one session" they often nominate "how to communication instead of argue," "feeling listened to" (young people), and "parenting help" (parents). Many say they think this is an SSFT's purpose.

Aim 3. To Reduce Distressful Conflict and Storm-Outs

We don't believe that excessively critical and distressful comments and arguments and storm-outs are friendly or effective. They hurt people and can ruinously suspend or stop a session in its tracks, creating a potential "catastrophic failure" for an SSFT where you may not get another chance.

Practice Reforms to Promote Friendliness and Effectiveness

Reform 1. Selfies

We now seek a family "selfie" photo at the beginning of the session. Consent is asked first and, using staff equipment, they (not us) are invited to take the selfie. Selfies usually generate a smile, and act as an "ice breaker," helping to start the session on a friendly footing with a more light-hearted, informal atmosphere and ambience. Tess and Ron (see Figure 25.1) also take a co-therapists' selfie ("what's good for goose is good for gander") which is pasted into the session notes, along with the family selfie, and emailed to the family so that when the family opens the email they see their own friendly family greet them. As a bonus for us, the selfies help us remember who each family member was after the session when we are writing the notes or if they contact us in the future.

Other staff tend to be hesitant about their own or family selfies or both, often not liking photos of themselves or worrying about not having control of where their photos might go. Families, on the other hand, are usually very accepting of selfie requests, often saying things like "its normal" and "it makes it personal." Most are keen; only about 1 in 10 decline.

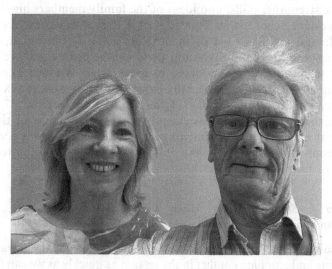

Figure 25.1 Staff Selfie by Ron and Tess. We wanted to show a family's selfie, but privacy and confidentiality considerations wouldn't allow it. Here's a typical one of us.

Reform 2. Using the Clients' Dialogue to Construct Solutions

Another important step in making the single session family friendly and effective is highlighting the positive discoveries, strengths, skills, and ideas of the family members that are brought to light in the session (Epston, 1999; White, 2007; Denborough, 2008). One way to do this is by using samples of family members' own words in developing the descriptions of the problems and the solutions. As an example, while Molly (age 14) was discussing suicidal thoughts, positive thoughts also emerged. To highlight these, Ron asked:

Ron: "What are you finding out about yourself that you like?"
Molly: "I don't like to say. It's like bragging."
Ron: "OK, it feels like bragging but we would like to hear if that's OK?"
Molly: "I'm good at English. When I was three I taught myself to read."

Reform 3. Family-Friendly Letters

We try to use a friendly tone when writing the letter emailed to the family, and deliberately resist an aloof "professional" tone that is not uncommon in mental health services. We favor "I" statements and everyday language. Another important ingredient is including the positive strengths, skills, and ideas of the family members highlighted in the session, recorded (as best we can) in their own words. We might compile and include a list of them (Fox, 2003; Denborough, 2008). Reading (and maybe re-invoking) these can help the family feel supported, respected, and even liked in some ways. We also like to include any "wise quotes," especially from a young person; for example, *"How can I learn from mistakes if you don't let me make any?"* Single session therapy greatly values client evaluation, so the letter they get ends with each person's comments of what they thought was good and bad about the session, plus any "takeaways" that they plan to think about or try.

Reform 4. Stopping Overt Major Verbal Clashes, Excessive Criticism, and "Storm-Outs"

Depending on therapist style and judgment, we are moving towards intervening and stopping conflict in the session as quickly as we can for two reasons. One is the human harm they can cause (see below) and two, if these problems interrupt or stop the session in its tracks, the chance to help the family might be gone forever. Being an SSFT, we may not get a second go.

When to intervene? Opinions vary both in families and clinicians. At one extreme there is "zero tolerance – *intervention is a responsibility*" (especially if it is abusive); at the other extreme, allowing them to go on unhindered to express themselves and then sort it out themselves, i.e., *"non-intervention encourages dialogue."* Ron leans to zero tolerance and Tess will allow a bit. Practically we have found that if we don't intervene quickly, we get more "storm-outs," usually by a young person – and then the session is over, or we lose a lot of time while they get calmed and return – a big spanner [wrench] in the works for any one-and-only session. Prevention is useful, too. If we suspect that a major clash might occur, we state upfront that we seek to prevent or minimize it as we believe it is unproductive or counterproductive.

We might also try "milder" interventions like discreetly (or not) changing the topic, pointing out what is happening, or suggesting an alternative, such as introducing anti-arguing communication skills. Even if deemed necessary, intervening like this rarely feels good for us. Ron worries he overdoes it, Tess that she underdoes it. People usually don't enjoy being interrupted; some are offended. Some family members criticize us for stopping them, others that we didn't stop the criticism soon enough. Another technique might involve inviting the young person (usually) about to storm out under a tirade of parental or sibling critique to sit sheltered behind the one-way screen if we have one and participate from there, or by video-call (e.g., Facetime or Zoom) from another room. One of the therapists can offer to sit with them but we find they often like to be left alone for a while. Or we could ask the "criticizer" to sit out and watch in silence instead.

Short of an outright verbal fight, conversation can still be harmful if it is full of personal criticisms and counter-criticisms (Masland & Hooley 2015; Gottman 1998). As well as hurting, inflaming, and being unproductive or counterproductive, it is often "nothing new." To have an effective SST it helps to be time efficient. Many of the points and interventions above also apply to monologues or dialogues of intense personal criticism. We can talk with families about psychological theories (above) that describe how destructive personal criticism and contempt can be, and then ask if this persuades them to tame it for now. Another option is to talk about "adversarial practices," i.e., arguing about "facts" where no one usually wins but everyone escalates or leaves (Epston, 1988). A third option to try is to raise homespun wisdoms like "Go for the ball not the player," "Don't discipline a child in anger," and even "Does the end justify the means?"

We sometimes try comments such as "How are they reacting now when you're saying that?" and "Do you want to ask them if they see it as educating or preaching?" The idea that educating, explaining, giving solutions and suggestions, even well-meaning ones, is at times experienced as arguing and criticizing is often surprising and salutary to parents in particular. Then, if they agree and want it, we try to help them move away from personal criticism as best we can, and "road test" other ways of talking and problem-solving as a family (discussed below).

We also need to tame our own urges to criticize them for criticizing, balanced by the need to "call it what it is" and not allow it free rein. We always remind ourselves people don't enjoy being interrupted – even if for their own good.

Reform 5. Coaching the Practicing of New Ways of Communicating Live in the SSFT

Most families clearly state they want better communication. Many directly ask for new "positive" communication techniques and specify that for an SSFT they rate this as a high or highest priority. On the flip side, they want less "negative" communication so that they are less likely to escalate into arguments, fights, and conflict. In response, we may often explain and describe well-known, potentially helpful "Communication 101: Talking and Listening Techniques" such as reflecting back, active listening, empathic statements, and "I statements" (Faber & Mazlish, 2000; Rogers & Farson, 1957). headspace staff trained in running "Tuning into Teens" groups for parents (Havighurst, Kehoe, & Harley, 2015) introduce these ideas, too. Asking others their opinion and problem-solving skills also can be raised.

Ron's favorite is "experience questions" that develop a focus on experience rather than facts. Tess's favorite is encouraging her version of reflective feedback, i.e., listen, feedback using their words as best as you can about what they just said, and then ask something like "Did I hear you right?" We usually combine the two favorites.

We may demonstrate anti-arguing communication techniques when talking to each other and to the family, and make it overt and transparent when we are using them. (In session notes sent after the session we include further reading references, but for most busy families these only make the "to-do list" that never gets done.) However, we found a problem: educating and demonstrating are great but are premised on follow-up sessions to review how the family practice went with them at home. SST work, a one and maybe only session, requires we do it differently. So we invite them to practice the techniques with each other in the room, with our coaching, before they go home, then discuss, review, and re-practice before the SSFT ends. (We tend to start with questions about experience because questions about facts often invite disputation.)

Then a second hurdle particular to SSFT presented itself. We found it took family members too long for them to craft questions and we ran out of time. So we modified the coaching by having us providing the first actual questions for them to test ("Try asking this question ..."), experience, and evaluate, until they get the swing of it. For example:

Molly:	"I want to know more about my father."
Mum:	"Tell me something you'd like to know."
Molly:	"I know nothing!"
	[Molly angry faced, getting defensive, Mum angry face, too, both on the attack and close to full-on arguing.]
Tess [jumping in and providing the question]:	"You could reassure her or disagree with her or you could ask her this experience question – 'What's it like to know nothing?'"
Mum [obliging]:	"What's it like to know nothing?"
Molly:	"It sucks. You feel like part of you is missing."
Tess:	"You can reflect back what she said and ask, 'Is that right?'"
Mum:	"So it's like part of you is missing, am I hearing you?"
Tess:	"I suggest, ask her another experience question, 'What it's like to feel that?'"
Mum:	"What's it like to feel part of you is missing?"
Molly:	"I don't know myself coz I don't know that part."
	[Molly and Mum's angry faces are now gone. Molly now has a sad face but a reaching-out-to-Mum one, Mum an empathic face reaching toward Molly. Now they can also discuss important facts without arguing.]
Molly:	"Did he have siblings?"
Mum:	"A brother who I was friends with at the time. That's how I met him."
	[Mum then went on to describe her years with Molly's father, how they met, how they got together, their life together, how it fell apart, and their eventual breakup. All very meaningful for Molly to hear.]

We ask families their experience and evaluation of the coaching with "tailor-made" questions. Common feedback is that it is emotionally confronting, but worth it. Young people usually say it was easier to talk and they felt heard. All agreed that when doing the coached conversation, arguments were avoided, at least with the "coaches" present, and all hoped that could also work at home. Most families reported it's the best part, making the single session helpful and worthwhile.

Interestingly, families or young people we see later for any reason, usually say they had forgotten the actual techniques practiced in the session but not the positive effect. They reported that the actual experience of talking to each other differently in the single session lasted and inspired them (with varying degrees of success) to find their own ways of achieving the same.

Making Family SST More Friendly and Effective

The innovations we have outlined here are all intended to help make the most of what for many youth and families will be their first and often only therapy encounter. Objective research on these family-friendly practices is a next step.

Notes

1 *Editors' note:* headspace is branded in lowercase to appeal to youth (for a discussion of the impact of SST implementation in headspace centres around Australia, see Fuzzard, Chapter 12 this volume).
2 *Editors' note:* Providing a single family session for ongoing individual clients is also called *Single Session Family Consultation* (see Terminology section in Chapter 1).

References

Barbara-May, R., Denborough, P., & McGrane, T. (2018). Development of a single-session family program at Child and Youth Mental-Health Services, Southern Melbourne. In M.F. Hoyt, M. Bobele, A. Slive, J. Young, & M. Talmon (Eds.), *Single-Session Therapy by Walk-In or Appointment: Administrative, Clinical, and Supervisory Aspects of One-at-a-Time Services* (pp. 104–115). New York: Routledge.

Denborough, D. (2008). *Collective Narrative Practice.* Adelaide, SA, Australia: Dulwich Centre Publications.

de Shazer, S. (1988). *Clues: Investigating Solutions in Brief Therapy.* New York: Norton.

Epston, D. (1988). Internalised other questioning with couples: The New Zealand version. *Catching Up with David Epston* (pp. 61–68). Adelaide, SA, Australia: Dulwich Centre Publications.

Epston, D. (1999). Co-research: The making of an alternative knowledge. In P. Moss (Ed.), *Narrative Therapy & Community Work: A Conference Collection* (pp. 137–157). Adelaide, SA, Australia: Dulwich Centre Publications.

Faber, A., & Mazlish, E. (2000). *How to Talk So Kids Will Listen and Listen So Kids Will Talk.* New York: Avon Books.

Fox, H. (2003). Using therapeutic letters: A review. *International Journal of Narrative Therapy and Community Work, 4*, 26–36.

Goding, G. (1992). *The History and Principles of Family Therapy.* Melbourne, Australia: The Victorian Association of Family Therapists.

Gottman, J. (1998). *Raising an Emotionally Intelligent Child.* New York: Simon & Schuster.

Havighurst, S., Kehoe, C., & Harley, A. (2015). Tuning into teens: Improving parental responses to anger and reducing youth externalizing behavior problems. *Journal of Adolescence, 42*, 148–158.

Hopkins, L., Lee, S., McGrane, T., & Barbara-May, R. (2016). Single session family therapy in youth mental health: Can it help? *Australasian Psychiatry, 25*(4), 108–111.

Hoyt, M.F., Bobele, M., Slive, A., Young, J. & Talmon, M. (Eds.). (2018). *Single Session Therapy by Walk-In or Appointment: Administrative, Clinical, and Supervisory Aspects of One-at-a-Time Services.* New York: Routledge.

Masland, S.R., & Hooley, J.M. (2015). Perceived criticism: A research update for clinical practitioners. *Clinical Psychology: Science and Practice, 22*(3), 211–222.

Rogers, C.R., & Farson, R.E. (1957). *Active Listening.* Chicago, IL: University of Chicago Press.

Rothbaum, F., Rosen, K., Tatsuo, U., & Uchida, N. (2002). Family systems theory, attachment theory, and culture. *Family Process, 41*(3), 328–350.

White, M. (2007). *Maps of Narrative Practice.* New York: Norton.

26 Embedding the "Family Oriented Collaboration Utilising Strengths" (FOCUS) Clinic in a Child and Youth Mental Health Service and University Partnership

Helen Mildred, Lia Hunter,
Belinda Goldsworthy, and Peter Brann

For over 20 years there has been a strong collaborative training and research relationship between the Post Graduate Clinical Psychology Program within Deakin University School of Psychology, and Eastern Health Mental Health Program – a publicly funded tertiary health service comprising four hospitals and associated community clinics situated in the Eastern Metropolitan Region (EMR) of Melbourne, Australia.

In 2011, Deakin University and Eastern Health (EH) deepened the partnership by embedding the University's Clinical Psychology Training Clinic (required for post-graduate course accreditation), within Eastern Health's Child and Youth Mental Health Service (EHCYMHS). EHCYMHS targets services to those children and young people affected by the most serious and significant complex mental health and psychosocial difficulties, who engage in very risky and/or self-damaging behaviors, and for whom previous mental health intervention has not been helpful.

Historically significant demand challenges on publicly funded mental health services lead to most managing lengthy waitlists. The imbalance between supply and demand has continued over recent years, requiring mental health services to investigate new ways of providing meaningful but efficient intervention to clients and their families. A review of routine treatment for over 500 EHCYMHS clients in one year found that almost 50% were judged by clinicians as having finished treatment prematurely (Johnson, Mellor, & Brann, 2009). Talmon (1990) however, found that when contacted, client families who had seemingly dropped out after one session, generally reported that the single session had been sufficient to enact changes they had maintained and extended. In 2010, EHCYMHS noted that a significant proportion of families attended only a few sessions – despite both the acuity and chronicity of their difficulties – and the availability of ongoing work over many months if required. This finding contributed to the creation of the EHCYMHS/Deakin FOCUS Clinic – the acronym representing Family Oriented Collaboration Utilising Strengths. It utilizes a single session framework to provide treatment to children, young people and their families living in the EMR who meet EHCYMHS' eligibility criteria.

Being a training clinic, FOCUS is staffed by Deakin's post-graduate clinical psychology masters and doctoral students – registered provisional psychologists on placement. These trainee psychologists gain real-world training and experience working from a strengths-based stance, with complex and challenging children/young people and their families, as well as with the service systems that support them (e.g., child protection). Clinical accountability, supervision, and trainee evaluation are provided by senior clinical psychologists. Thus, FOCUS can be viewed as having two service recipients: those clients and families we consult, and the trainee psychologists with their clinical learning and development plans.

The Model

Children and young people up to 25 years of age and their families are initially offered a single session with FOCUS. They can access further single sessions (up to six in total), though families often only come for one or two. Trainees focus on one or two goals identified and agreed upon by the young person and their family. As with all single session therapies (SSTs), the aim is to achieve as much as possible in the limited time available. We use a solution-focused brief therapy (SFBT; de Shazer, 1985, 1988) model to empower clients to focus on their strengths. We encourage them to identify and augment their existing knowledge, skills, resources, and values, so that clients can then mobilize these against their difficulties. SFBT has an emerging evidence base – particularly in relation to working with children and adolescents (Bond, Woods, Humphrey, Wymes, & Green, 2013; Perkins, 2006). More specifically, SFBT is effective in helping young people reduce the intensity of negative feelings and make changes in behaviors such as aggression, stealing, and property destruction (Kim & Franklin, 2009; Kim, 2007).

Dilemmas and Resolutions

Most CYMHS have policies, procedures, and required documentation that support the standard practice of longer-term treatment but which present challenges when adopting SST. For example, client risk to self, and risk to and/or from others, is always at the forefront of EHCYMHS work. The SFBT approach, however, tends to steer conversations and questions away from formal problem assessment. Due to the brevity and therapeutic emphasis of SST, when establishing FOCUS, the service's senior management and clinical leadership decided clinical work should rely on information from a variety of sources to inform its work, rather than undertake a full comprehensive biopsychosocial assessment or clinical diagnostic interview. Trainees utilize the information gathered by the intake team from the family, school, and professionals (such as previous psychiatrists or psychologists). They also consider clients' descriptions of their most pressing issues, the risk assessment, clinical impressions, supervision, and clinical review to guide the generation and discussion of ideas with the client and their family as to what could be most helpful (Gee, Mildred, Brann, & Taylor, 2015). Leadership also decided that due to its novice work-force, clients with very high levels of risk (e.g., acute suicidality, psychotic presentations) should be assisted by other teams within EHCYMHS rather than FOCUS. Many such dilemmas were managed in this way during the implementation of FOCUS with the early months supported by consultation from The Bouverie Centre.

Single Session Process at FOCUS

The first session includes the young person, their care system (family, partner, etc.), and two trainees in the room. The family is fully oriented to EHCYMHS, FOCUS and its training function, and the single session model/process including a reflecting team. With client consent, a one-way screen is used by a senior psychologist and three or four other trainees to maximize the clinical thinking and formulating, as well as to provide feedback to the trainee.

Initially, the trainee asks the family to prioritize their concerns regarding the issue they feel is most important. Discussion then concentrates on the strengths, values, and abilities of the client and family, and activities they enjoy. Immediately prior to a 10-minute break, the family waits in the reception area while the trainees undertake a risk assessment with the young person individually (or with the parents present if aged 10–12 years or less) for 10–15 minutes. This risk assessment is fundamental to all EHCYMHS services. If significant risk issues emerge, the trainees, client, and usually the parent(s), together create a safety plan. Parents are always given some feedback regarding risk level, even if there is none.

Following the break, those behind the screen provide the family with reflections regarding their individual and family strengths, achievements, values, etc., and the family is given the opportunity to discuss their experience of these reflections (see Andersen, 1991; Friedman, 1995; and White, 1995 for information regarding reflecting teams). This is almost universally experienced as a powerful and immensely positive process. Young people frequently express profound relief (and in some cases, overt gratitude) that they are not being talked about "as if I am the problem" and that we can "talk about all the good stuff in the family, too." Parents are often moved and almost always appreciative that the team sees them as loving and capable, "trying our best even though things seem so hard." These messages are strikingly contrary to the negative ones they give themselves, each other, and that they receive from the broader community (e.g., other services, society's tendency to blame mothers, etc.).

At the conclusion of the session, tasks are set such as: the client and parents keeping separate "secret" lists of positives. In one family, members were asked to notice a time every day when Jimmy (14 years old with major depression) seemed lighter, happier, or relaxed, and for family members to compare lists after one week.

If the family requests further sessions (which they express at the end of the session or in a follow-up phone call) these tend to commence with a brief discussion of what the family have noticed since the previous session. When the family attends for more than one session, the group often (though not invariably) separates for 30 minutes: one trainee works with the parents and the other, with the young person. For both the parents and the young person, this separate time can be validating, helpful and allow both parties to explore issues without immediately impacting on the other. Parents are often angry and distressed, while young people often require a space to explore new perspectives and their preferred path forward. Both reunite in the last 20 minutes of the session to share reflections, and plan tasks for home. At the conclusion of the final session (if there is more than one session), "strengths letters" are written – one for the parent(s) and one for the young person – combining and summarizing the family's and the clinicians' reflections on skills, attributes, values, and progress (see Epston, 1994; Fox, 2003; Omer & Alon, 1997; Cooper & Ariane, 2018).

FOCUS Evaluation and Feedback

In addition to the very positive feedback we have had from families both spontaneously and written in the formal "Experience of Care" survey, FOCUS has undertaken outcome evaluation with data gathered from the over 200 families and 100 trainees who have attended the clinic in the last seven years. Results show that trainee-, client-, and parent-rated outcome measures completed prior to and post-treatment demonstrate statistically and clinically significant symptom reduction for FOCUS clients. Evaluation of trainees also consistently shows that they gain critical clinical skills, understandings and competencies at FOCUS. Qualitative and quantitative data from both client groups – young people and their families, and trainee psychologists on placement – indicate that the FOCUS Clinic is successful both as a high-quality treatment service and training clinic. A recent study further showed FOCUS to be as effective as treatment as usual when comparing lower acuity CYMHS clients matched by age and initial Health of the nation outcome scale for children and adolescents (HoNOSCA) total score (Wagner, Mildred, Gee, Black, & Brann, 2017).

In addition to the client outcomes and from a training perspective, trainees appreciate both the widening of their perspective beyond psychopathology, and the associated interventions that FOCUS demands of them. They report liking the transparency of the single session model and the overt "permission" to "quickly get down to tin tacks" with clients in a collaborative respectful manner.

FOCUS Single Sessions Promoting Positives

Here are three illustrations from FOCUS sessions of how SST can unite family and clinicians in pursuit of developing new understandings and courses of action.

1. Single Session Frankness

Joel (13 years old) was referred to FOCUS with a two-month history of spontaneous right leg paralysis lasting up to half an hour several times a week. Comprehensive neurological investigation indicated no organic cause and the discharge diagnosis was Somatization Disorder. Joel lived with his six-year-old twin sisters (Chloe and Ella) and his mother Suzie and father Tony (both of whom, it was noted on the referral, suffered depression and anxiety).

When we met the family, Tony was particularly frustrated by the neurological diagnosis that implied a mental rather than physical health issue. Tony was not currently working due to a work accident. Suzie (who worked casually in a cafe) was teary and quiet, deferring to Tony to answer questions. The girls played together happily in the corner, spontaneously offering relevant comments. The young female trainees struggled with Tony dominating and continually steering the conversation away from strengths, towards Joel's condition. The SST framework enabled them to stop the session, and suggest the family suspend judgment regarding the usefulness of the meeting "just for this one session." This reference to SST created an almost bold "nothing to lose" atmosphere. Tony then seemed freer to allow others to speak, which led them (particularly the girls) to venture comments about Tony's "sadness...drinking and temper." When reflections were given to the family regarding their love for Joel and their separate and combined efforts and determination to help him, both parents were teary, which surprised Joel. Despite Joel denying difficulties during the separate risk assessment, Tony admitted his shame and sorrow that he sometimes becomes desperate and enraged, particularly when he has been drinking, and that he shouts a lot. In recent months, he had started to "become physical (increasingly) with Joel, pushing and smacking him." Tony's honesty and courage in discussing these painful feelings and events were acknowledged by the trainees, one of whom supported him to go to another room and phone child protection services. The family was linked with family support and Tony with counseling. In a call a month later the family reported that things were much improved. The intensity of having only one session meant that "everyone spoke up much more frankly than they had thought likely or possible" (Suzie). Joel had not had further paralysis, and Tony said his "mood was improving."

2. **Unity and Creativity in a Systemic Single Session**
Bryce was an eight-year-old boy with high-functioning autism and a jokey personality. Bryce was having almost daily serious "meltdowns," as school termed them, which were sudden and of high intensity with him hitting, kicking, throwing things around the classroom and tipping over tables. The school had reduced his attendance to two hours in the morning and responded to these episodes by removing the other children from the classroom while the principal tried to calm Bryce down. Bob (Bryce's father) would then be called from his work. A single session at the school was offered by a trainee (with a supervisor's support) to Bob, Steve (his 11-year-old brother), the principal, teacher, and welfare aid. Bryce's mother had died of breast cancer when he was five.

The trainee was very curious about everyone's ideas about why and how Bryce became distressed so quickly. The power of single session in this situation was that everyone was joined in earnest against the clock to find the key or pattern to the difficulty, and to generate some strategies. Everyone's wisdom was garnered to identify when the "episodes" were more likely to happen. A chain of events was identified including elements such as: *"If Bryce is late to bed there are difficulties getting up and he doesn't eat breakfast" (Bob)… "Bryce rushing makes getting out of the car into school hard" (Steve)… "Class moving to a music activity makes Bryce non-cooperative" (classroom teacher)… "If I am near Toby [who unbeknownst to anyone called Bryce "weird"] I get upset" (Bryce).* Putting all the elements together was helpful for everyone, particularly Bryce – who had not realized so many things could combine to upset him and that adjusting them could prevent this. Bryce and the people in his world – buoyed by this unique opportunity to meet together – energetically generated ideas about what things could be useful at each potential point of vulnerability. Bryce and his family were delighted that the difficulties were now seen as him being overwhelmed and distressed rather than dangerous, unpredictable, and unmanageable. School staff were able to adapt their prevention and response strategies to match Bryce's internal experience better, which in turn gave Bryce self-responsibility and pride in his success as he slowly increased his time at school.

3. Cumulative Gains from a Series of Single Sessions

Alex, a young woman in her early 20s, lived with her mother June who had separated amicably from Alex's father Joe 10 years ago. Alex recently had completed a diploma in art, and currently was working in aged care. She had a physically disabled younger sister who required extensive daily care from her mother. Alex first attended FOCUS with June, stating that she wanted assistance with her social anxiety, low self-esteem (thinking she is not good enough and should be doing more with her life), and a strong tendency to compare herself negatively with others in social situations. These notions were bemusing to her mother who reported that Alex is a wonderful, warm young woman who is often very passionate in her views, and who has numerous creative talents and achievements especially in the area of photography.

Alex stated that she wanted to meet with a trainee individually without her mother, and that she also thought she wanted the maximum (6) single sessions available, but liked that she could stop before if she wanted. In a phone call to her a week after each session, Alex would decide if, and when, she would return for another session, setting her own pace.

Alex was clear and determined in session – yet reported that she struggled to bring these qualities to bear in her social interactions. At each meeting, Alex tackled different aspects of her low self-esteem, approaching each session as an individual event – like its own bite-size piece of therapy – which then combined to create a fuller, more constructive, and confident sense of herself. In each session, the trainee and Alex talked about how she could identify, attend to, and honor her strength of character and purpose without reverting to the negative views she imagined others had of her. Small experiments were developed to assist her achieve this. For example, Alex challenged herself to have a coffee with a friend and described "really listening to her" rather than being distracted by negative thoughts.

At the final session, Alex spoke of "feeling more capable and less insecure," which she stated she "didn't think she would say at all" when she first attended the Clinic. She spoke of feeling more confident with others, more positive and proud of herself, with a reduction in self-criticism and increased self-kindness.

Conclusion and Learnings

These examples from our work illustrate the power and flexibility of SST. In Joel's situation, the family was able to grasp that this was possibly *the only conversation* they would have together about difficulties they wereexperiencing, Hence each family member took risks in speaking about matters unnamed before, and reported experiencing relief and hope as a result. For Bryce, the systemic single session joined everyone in the task of respectfully piecing together the various triggers and circumstances that could lead him to becoming highly overwhelmed. There was a gentle urgency in the time-limited one-off session, which resulted in numerous constructive ideas regarding how to avoid and disrupt the build-up of Bryce's distress. With Alex, in addition to the actual therapy, she enjoyed deciding *if*, *when*, and *what* to discuss in each session – which fits with her desire as a young adult to relinquish constraining thoughts and beliefs about herself.

In conclusion, while it is not argued that all CYMHS work should be single session, FOCUS demonstrates that people with complex and enduring mental health and psychosocial difficulties can have significant positive experiences and outcomes from a single session framework – even when provided by a trainee psychologist! More is not always more, nor is it always required. To give the last words to trainees:

Esther: *Working with this single session model taught me the therapeutic power of focusing on the exceptions to the problem-saturated rules, namely, what's going well for the client and their family system, and what strengths, talents, and protective factors can be identified, celebrated, and leveraged to move the client and their family toward a better future, defined in their terms.*

Sam: *The single session model was useful in giving the therapeutic work a clear direction and focus. Although most clients present with several difficulties, the time-limited approach encouraged us to address the most pertinent issues. It also motivated me to make the most of every session, since I knew my time with the client was limited.*

References

Andersen, T. (Ed.). (1991). *The Reflecting Team: Dialogues and Dialogues about the Dialogues*. New York: Norton.

Bond, C., Woods, K., Humphrey, N., Wymes, W., & Green, L. (2013). Practitioner Review: The effectiveness of solution focused brief therapy with children and families: A systematic and critical evaluation of the literature from 1990–2010. *Journal of Child Psychology and Psychiatry, 54*(7), 707–723.

Cooper, S., & Ariane. (2018). Co-crafting take-home document at the walk-in. In M.F. Hoyt, M. Bobele, A. Slive, J. Young, & M. Talmon (Eds.), *Single-Session Therapy by Walk-In or Appointment* (pp. 260–269). New York: Routledge.

de Shazer, S. (1985). *Keys to Solution in Brief Therapy*. New York: Norton.

de Shazer, S. (1988). *Clues: Investigating Solutions in Brief Therapy*. New York: Norton.

Epston, D. (1994). Extending the conversation. *Family Therapy Networker, 18*(6), 30–37, 62–63.

Fox, H. (2003). Using therapeutic documents – A review. *International Journal of Narrative Therapy and Community Work*, *26*(4), 26–36.

Friedman, S. (Ed.). (1995). *The Reflecting Team in Action: Collaborative Practice in Family Therapy*. New York: Guilford Press.

Gee, D., Mildred, H., Brann, P., & Taylor, M., (2015). Brief intervention: A promising framework for child and youth mental health? *Administration and Policy in Mental Health and Mental Health Services*, *4*(2), 121–125.

Johnson, E., Mellor, D., & Brann, P. (2009). Factors associated with dropout and diagnosis in child and adolescent mental health services. *Australian and New Zealand Journal of Psychiatry*, *43*(5), 431–437.

Kim, J.S. (2007). Examining the effectiveness of solution-focused brief therapy: A meta-analysis. *Research on Social Work Practice*, *18*(2), 107–116.

Kim, J.S., & Franklin, C. (2009). Solution-focused brief therapy in schools: A review of the outcome literature. *Children and Youth Services Review*, *31*(4), 464–470.

Omer, H., & Alon, N. (1997). *Constructing Therapeutic Narratives*. Northvale, NJ: Jason Aronson.

Perkins, R. (2006). The effectiveness of one session of therapy using a single session therapy approach for children and adolescent with mental health problems. *Psychology & Psychotherapy: Theory, Research & Practice, 79*(2), 215–227.

Talmon, M. (1990). *Single-Session Therapy: Maximizing the Effect of the First (and Often Only) Therapeutic Encounter*. San Francisco: Jossey-Bass.

Wagner, G.A., Mildred, H., Gee, D., Black, E.B., & Brann, P. (2017, August). Effectiveness of brief intervention and case management for children and adolescents with mental health difficulties. *Children and Youth Services Review, 79*, 362–367.

White, M. (1995). Reflecting team as definitional ceremony. In *Re-Authoring Lives: Interviews & Essays* (pp. 172–198). Adelaide, SA, Australia: Dulwich Centre Publications.

27 Integrating a Single Session Family Therapy Approach in Two Child and Youth Mental Health Services

Myf Murphy and Denise Fry[1]

We work in two different and geographically separate Australian child and youth mental health services – one in Melbourne (Alfred CYMHS), the other in Hobart, Tasmania (known as CAMHS South). The Alfred team serves 0–25-year-olds from urban families, and the CAMHS South team serves 0–18-year-olds from a mix of rural and urban families.

The Alfred team has been providing a single session approach to family work for 10 years. These sessions are offered to families within a week of initial contact, whereas the Hobart team began inviting the majority of new client families to engage in a single session in 2015 (see Westwater, Murphy, Handley, & McGregor, 2020). Both groups incorporate orientation and training into their single sessions, particularly for new staff and for medical staff on rotation. Both groups use a similar process preparing for, conducting, and following up single sessions.

What follows is a summary of the collective experience of these two services, in terms of:

- The impetus for using a single session approach
- The outcomes, and
- Collected reflections and learnings.

The Impetus for SST

Historically, in both services, clinicians had their own caseloads and conducted protracted four-part assessments followed by long-term interventions. As evidence grew about the potential of SST to promote client-centered care and family collaboration, both teams embarked on implementing Single Session Therapy. Growing waitlist was an additional incentive for the Hobart CAMHS.

With the emerging evidence for the single session framework and experience of its utility in other CAMHS settings (Campbell, 1999; Fry, 2012; Hampson, O'Hanlon, Franklin, Pentony, Fridgant & Heins, 1999;

Perkins, 2006; Perkins & Scarlett, 2008) we were hopeful that this was an opportunity to meet the service demands in a more responsive, family-sensitive way. The rationale that underpinned this decision, despite some trepidation, was the undeniable increasing community demand, the growing recognition of the family as expert in their own lives, consistent research outcomes from other CAMHS services, and the inefficiency of the traditional assessment model. Bringing team members out from behind closed doors, where they were focusing on their own individual caseloads and into a more team-based way of working was an added advantage.

The Single Session Process

Children and young people are referred to our services by health providers including: pediatricians, general practitioners, and private practice therapists. Referrals are processed by our intake workers who are senior clinicians. If the referral to the service would benefit from a single session and this is also what the family is wanting they would be allocated. As a Child and Youth Mental Health Service, there are other forms of assessment and treatment available.

The intake clinicians explain the single session process and send written information to the family, describing what to expect. Family members are asked to complete pre-session questionnaires. Wait times for families vary, but in general across both services families are seen within two to four weeks from the initial intake call for a single session. The team allows 2 hours and 15 minutes for the session, inclusive of the pre- and post-team discussions.

Both teams utilize one-way screens with a multidisciplinary reflecting team (as described in Andersen, 1987; Friedman, 1995; White, 1995). Always having sought clients' informed consent, the process used for the session is similar at both locations, with two therapists working together in front of the screen, and a small team behind the screen who provide a reflection for the family. The family and therapists swap places with the reflecting team part-way through the session so the family (and therapists) can witness the reflecting team's observations and thoughts. In general, there is little to no preparation for what is discussed between reflecting team members, so as to provide a genuinely rich "ecology of ideas" (Bogdan, 1984). The reflecting team looks to focus on strengths, exceptions, patterns of interaction, psychoeducation, and will often make recommendations for the family to try.

The session ends with the family and therapists swapping again with the reflecting team so the family can comment on the team's feedback and to discuss possible take-away messages with the therapists. In a particularly efficient innovation at Alfred CYMHS, a member of the reflecting team writes a summary of the session, including therapeutic suggestions in real time, for the family to take home.

Each service uses a pre-session questionnaire, which asks family members to describe the main problem and to rate on a scale ranging from *0 = Not at All* to *10 = Extremely*:

1. How much is the problem interfering in your life?
2. How worried do you feel about the problem?
3. How confident do you feel in managing the problem?

A follow-up phone call appointment is made, usually around two weeks after the session, to speak with family members who attended the session. A post-session questionnaire is used to guide the phone call and to re-ask the rating scale questions that were part of the pre-session questionnaire. These questionnaires were adapted from the training provided by The Bouverie Centre.

Outcomes

For Families

1. **The Alfred Team**

   The number of sessions has moved from approximately 30 sessions a year in 2009, 80 sessions a year in 2013, to our current level of 120 sessions in 2019. In the past year, the majority of families (69%) have attended one session, 4% attended for two sessions, and 1% attended for three sessions. Twenty-six percent of families seen through the single session program were allocated for ongoing generic case management.

2. **The Hobart Team**

   The number of single sessions in Hobart since starting in 2015 has been on average 100 families per year. Our recent local research project conducted in 2018–2019 indicated that over 60% of the families in our study did not feel they needed any further specialist CAMHS input following a single session. At the post-session follow-up throughout the research period, of 89 parent responses, 81% rated their satisfaction highly (at least a 7 on a 0–10 scale). Furthermore, results indicated that family members' level of worry decreased, while parental confidence in managing the presenting issue(s) increased. Young people had a reduction in worry, though a significant increase in confidence was not evident in this cohort. Notably, 100% of responses from siblings indicated satisfaction with the single session process. The sibling group also showed a reduction in worry. Parents' typical comments included:

- *"Felt comfortable. Could talk openly."*
- *"Came out with a few ideas – great!."*
- *"Confirmed we've done all that we can."*
- *"Once we got talking the 'dauntedness' went … all the anguish just went."*
- *"Good to hear the girls open up; got a lot out of it. Nice to discuss and hear others get stuff off their chest."*

And some typical comments of the young people themselves:

- *"Gaining different perspectives on our family situation. Heard opinions from my family that I hadn't thought about."*
- *"Could see it was helpful to my parents."*

And from their siblings:

- *"Having everything out in the open; left with a plan."*
- *"Felt nice to get it out."*
- *"Good to hear other thoughts"*
- *"It got the family talking more."*
- *"Very beneficial. Loved hearing feedback."*

For Staff

1. The Alfred Team
Staff in general have chosen to be a part of the single session teams. There are internal and informal discussions where staff describe liking the framework and approach, as well as the opportunity to be exposed to different clinical styles and levels of experience. Further feedback from staff came via a research project conducted at The Alfred focused on reviewing psychiatric registrars' experience of child and youth mental health and family therapy delivered in the single session format. More than half (9 of 14) who completed the research project reported that taking part in single session family therapy had changed their decision about further training or specialization in this area, with half saying it had positively influenced them to continue in this field. It is interesting to note also that five staff members went on to engage in formal family therapy training.

Some typical comments from the psychiatric registrars:

- *"Allowed me to develop confidence in working with families."*
- *"It made family therapy look more appealing."*
- *"The reflecting team was very powerful."*

- *"It made the change for families and young people visible; seeing changes occur in a short space of time were important and rewarding experiences."*
- *"Participating in this program helped me to see, understand and value the role of the family in caring for the young person. It also exposed me to a strengths-based approach."*

2. The Hobart Team

Since 2015, we have witnessed the team's growing confidence, strengthening professional relationships and mutual learning. There has been a sense of improved CAMHS team morale, a sense of unity, and a knowledge of each others' clinical skill set.

Consistent with a family therapy and reflecting team environment that invites multiple perspectives, it feels that we have increased our therapeutic flexibility with families even further. The initial and ongoing growth and learning together is a commonly reported benefit of working in this way. It is a very powerful opportunity to genuinely collaborate with families, be more family-centered, and make the moment with that family truly count. The Hobart Team was invited to complete an anonymous survey monkey questionnaire about their experience of single session work. Staff members reflected on challenges and gains for themselves in the work, and also on the satisfaction that they received from being able to provide a timely response to families. Some typical responses:

- *"I have been surprised by the powerful nature of one session and the positive response of families to the reflective team; going away feeling more hopeful, more empowered."*
- *"I have strengthened my collaborative skills."*
- *"The increase in team cohesiveness."*
- *"Lots!! I've learned I can be more confident in front of the group; I've learned that I can trust my colleagues; I've learned great phrases or ways of asking questions by watching and listening to colleagues; but mostly it's really consolidated for me how important the family system is in helping the young person."*

For the Agency

1. The Alfred Team

The need for such family-based interventions and their popularity is reflected in the fact that the number of single session family therapy appointments provided has risen dramatically from 2009: there are now three teams meeting weekly to provide single sessions for families.

Having the entire family system involved from the outset – intact, blended, separated, divorced – and being responsive to families when they seek support, has helped the effectiveness of the treatment response. The ability to offer a session to the family within a week of their contacting our service has allowed the treating team to take advantage of the family's motivation and momentum for change.

2. **The Hobart Team**

   Enabling families to be seen closer to the time that they are seeking help is one of the best outcomes of introducing a single session approach for our team. There has been a significant reduction in wait time for families to receive a CAMHS initial face-to-face service (50–60% reduction in waiting time since 2016–2017). However, this does not mean that ongoing work is immediately available – families usually need to wait another few weeks following the single session for ongoing case management with our team or a facilitated referral elsewhere.

Further Reflections

Our two services have been able to establish a single session approach in children and young persons' mental health settings for the families, the young person themselves, the (often forgotten) siblings, AND for staff members and the agency as a whole. It is good to recall that, "It is the family system that continues to manage, support, educate, guide, direct, care for, and love their child, day and night, week in, week out. It is our responsibility and our goal to assist and empower families to use their existing resources to gain a greater sense of stability and confidence" (Fry, 2012, p. 64).

Our experience suggests some lessons to keep in mind:

• Having a mix of experience and qualifications represented in the team has allowed for richness in the work and an opportunity for staff to work alongside each other. This has provided a well-supported learning environment for new entry-level staff to the workforce, as well as to psychiatric registrars in their brief rotational placement.

• Involving intake staff from the beginning has been crucial to successfully implementing the single session family therapy approach just as the set up and preparation for the session itself starts at intake.

• Delineating this as a program in its own right and having a dedicated coordinator and administrative assistance has allowed the program to run smoothly.

• Limiting the amount of paperwork and report writing has been significantly helpful in managing overall workload requirements. At The Alfred, the summary of the session at its completion (which the family receives as well) makes up the clinical file entry. If there are any concerns regarding risk factors they would be captured within this summary. In Hobart, the clinical file entry is written behind the mirror during the session; this is not given to the family. Instead the family and the clinicians use a take-away message pad to document what the family feels is most important to them to leave the session with. *Take-aways* (see bouverie.org.au) enable a copy of what is written to stay with the service and one for the family to take home. Entries include the messages the family wish to record and some useful next steps, contact details, and the follow-up phone call appointment time. The clinicians may introduce ideas to take away if the family doesn't generate these independently.

- Having the entire family present where possible (whether intact or separated, blended, three-generational, whatever ....) has assisted in the effectiveness of the session.

- Promoting the philosophy and practice of single session work across the community of referrers, who may misunderstand the approach and assume that "single session" means only a one-off contact, has been important. All of our written communication to external referrers post-session includes a paragraph on the process of a single session. It is emphasized to the referrers and the family that a single session involves a series of contacts, a collaboration and an opportunity for a team of clinicians from different discipline backgrounds to seize the moment with the family when they need it most. Despite our efforts in this area, there is always more to do to help referrers and other professionals appreciate how it works. The high rates of satisfaction from the families who experience the process helps to sustain the teams' motivation and commitment to this way of working.

- Promoting the benefits for teams of professionals who are open to working in this (sometimes anxiety-provoking) format, has helped embed the service. Clinicians who are new to this way of working and perhaps new to the team have reported anxieties related to working in front of their colleagues, for fear of "getting something wrong" or "missing things." As the team has grown to enjoy the learning from each other and as trust develops, anxieties reduce and the team becomes more of a comfort and growth point for individuals. There is need to attend regularly to team dynamics and processes, and to be open to challenge. Both The Alfred and Hobart teams utilize a session every eight weeks to check in with each other around these points. This time is the length of a usual SSFT session. The single session team members attend and it is facilitated by the team coordinator. Cases may be reviewed for learning opportunities and reflection rather than as a clinical governance process. In addition to these sessions, supervision sessions have been facilitated by external providers from The

Bouverie Centre. This has been an invaluable part of optimizing team functioning, improving team relationships and revising procedures. Support from policymakers in the agency is essential for the program as a whole, as are clinical supports and supervision for individual team members.

• Offering help to families at the time that it is needed increases young people's and families' motivation and momentum for change. This timing has immeasurable benefits for the families and for the professionals working with them.

Working with the family system often enhances outcomes for young people attending mental health services. But not all staff are trained in family therapy, and even when they are, families with a young person in crisis can be daunting to work with. A multi-disciplinary team-based single session approach has positive benefits for clients, staff members, and service provision as a whole. While it might seem resource-intensive to use a whole team to provide service to a single family at any one time, both teams find great value in this for staff training, retention, productivity, and the potency and effect of a team message to the family with multi-disciplinary inputs. We hope that this account from two quite separate services gives some idea of the broad and long-term benefits made available by a single session family approach for children and young people who present with complex mental health challenges.

It is a privilege every single time to sit with a family, to hear their story and then to imagine new possibilities with them. It takes openness, flexibility, and courage for team members to embrace this way of working. Clearly, some of the benefits show in the growth of confidence, the strengthening of professional relationships, and mutual learning. Giving the family a sense of hope – helping them discover some previously undiscovered knowledge – or providing reassurance that the key to change may be actually what they're already doing – these are just some of the simple yet powerful possibilities in a single session.

Note

1 Acknowledgments to the Hobart CAMHS Single Session research team, Dr. Jason Westwater, Christine Handley, and Dr. Lucy McGregor, and the highly skilled clinical team who have embraced single session work.

References

Andersen, T. (1987). The reflecting team: Dialogue and meta-dialogue in clinical work. *Family Process*, 26(4), 415–528.
Bogdan, J.L. (1984). Family organization as an ecology of ideas: An alternative of the reification of family systems. *Family Process*, 23, 375–388.

Campbell, A. (1999). Single session interventions: An example of clinical research in practice. *Australian and New Zealand Journal of Family Therapy, 20*(4), 183–194.

Campbell, A. (2012). Single session approaches to therapy: Time to review. *Australian and New Zealand Journal of Family Therapy, 33,* 15–26.

Friedman, S. (Ed.). (1995). *The Reflecting Team in Action: Collaborative Practice in Family Therapy.* New York: Guilford Press.

Fry, D. (2012). Implementing single session family consultation: A reflective team approach. *Australian and New Zealand Journal of Family Therapy, 33*(1), 54–69.

Hampson, R., O'Hanlon, J. Franklin, A., Pentony, M., Fridgant, L., & Heins, T. (1999). The place of single session family consultations: Five years' experience in Canberra. *Australian and New Zealand Journal of Family Therapy, 20*(4), 195–200.

Perkins, R. (2006). The effectiveness of one session of therapy using a single-session therapy approach for children and adolescents with mental health problems. *Psychology and Psychotherapy: Theory, Research and Practice, 79*(2), 215–227.

Perkins, R., & Scarlett, G. (2008). The effectiveness of single session therapy in child and adolescent mental health. Part 2: An 18-month follow up study. *Psychology and Psychotherapy, 81*(2), 143–156.

Westwater, J.J., Murphy, M., Handley, C., & McGregor, L. (2020). A mixed methods exploration of single session family therapy in a child and adolescent mental health service in Tasmania, Australia. *Australian and New Zealand Journal of Family Therapy, 41*(3), 258–270.

White, M. (1995). Reflecting team as definitional ceremony. In *Re-Authoring Lives: Interviews & Essays* (pp. 172–198). Adelaide, S.A., Australia: Dulwich Centre Publications.

28 Single Session Therapy with Those Affected by Gambling: Listening to Clients and Their Therapeutic Counselors

Bonita Cohen, Gretta Daley, and Vicky Northe

Australians, per capita, are the highest spenders on gambling in the world (H2 Gambling Capital reported in *The Economist*, 2017). In the year 2017 to 2018, AU$24,887 billion was lost by Australians on gambling, a 5% increase on the previous year (Queensland Government Statistician's Office, 2019). As reported by the Victorian Responsible Gambling Foundation (VRGF), the impact of gambling includes financial problems, relationship difficulties, health problems, emotional distress, work or study issues, cultural problems, and criminal activity. Research shows that 85% of gambling harm in Victoria, Australia, occurred with people whose gambling was considered low or moderate risk. This has implications for understanding the burden of disease, as well as for designing suitable treatment approaches for people who may not see themselves as having a problem (Victorian Responsible Gambling Foundation, 2017, www.responsiblegambling.vic.gov.au).

Harm from gambling may be experienced by family, friends, and community, as well as the person gambling. The effects of gambling may be felt long after the gambling has stopped and can exacerbate other stressors (Browne et al., 2016). Gambling issues are very often comorbid with mental health and substance use issues, with gambling behavior often serving as a coping mechanism (Becona, Del Carmen Lorenzo, & Fuentes, 1996; Petry, 2001). Research shows neurobiological overlap between gambling and substance use disorders (Clark et al., 2013). This is reflected in the reclassification of gambling harm from "pathological gambling" under impulse control disorders in *DSM-IV* to "gambling disorder" under substance use disorders in *DSM-5*, a significant shift not only for the gambling field but for understanding of addiction more generally (Clark et al., 2013).

Traditionally, gambling harm is seen as an individual issue with the locus of control in the individual. However, the way gambling products are designed, situated, and marketed has become increasingly sophisticated and pervasive. The product design induces "gambler's fallacy" and an "illusion of control," with aspects including "near misses" and "losses disguised as wins" (Clark et al., 2013). Gambling behavior and concomitant gambling harms occur within broader social contexts and must be considered as a public health issue.

Stigma, Shame, and Loss

Research in Australia has found that despite wide social acceptance of gambling, people with gambling difficulties have self-perceptions of stereotyping, loss of status and discrimination, and they anticipate negative judgments and reactions from others (Hing & Russell, 2017). Stigma regarding gambling harms people's mental health and creates a barrier to self-acknowledgment, disclosure, therapy, and recovery (Hing, Russell, Gainsbury, & Nuske, 2016). Gambling was considered by research participants to be more stigmatized than other conditions including schizophrenia, alcoholism, and depression (Hing, Russell, Nuske, & Gainsbury, 2015).

This research suggests that people who gamble may experience a unique form of stigma, as well as shame, which is very highly correlated with addiction (Brown, 2010). A relationship with an addictive substance or behavior like gambling can temporarily relieve the pain of shame and can feel more comfortable than interacting with a person. Behaviors like gambling, however, can increase feelings of humiliation or shame, becoming a self-perpetuating cycle (Lewis, 2015; Ronald Potter-Effron, 2002).

Many people experiencing gambling harm struggle to be truly open and vulnerable with close family members and friends. Though human contact can offer physiological regulation, closeness – particularly for those experiencing shame – can evoke fear of hurt and abandonment and fear of being found out to be "disgusting" (van der Kolk, 2015). DeYoung (2015, p. 18) explores how shame can seem like an individual issue, a feeling of personal failing ("There's something wrong with me") when it's a relational problem needing a relational focus.

Research with counselors has noted the importance of supporting clients to overcome self-stigmatizing beliefs in order to commence therapeutic work with a relationship of trust and hope in recovery (Hing, Nuske, Gainsbury, Russell, & Breen, 2016). It is important for therapists to incorporate a self-compassion approach with high-shame clients (Gilbert, 2011; Neff, 2015). Compassion for one's own suffering can foster resilience and participation in challenging and rewarding life activities (Hanson & Hanson, 2018).

As we will discuss below, SST at pivotal points along with long-term work can offer a new relational viewpoint, particularly for family members who do not wish to commit to ongoing couple/family therapy. This can be particularly helpful in compassionately approaching issues of stigma and shame.

Mental Health and Gambling Services Working Together

The Victorian Responsible Gambling Foundation (VRGF) funds Gambler's Help (GH) services throughout the state of Victoria, Australia. Gambler's Help Southern (GHS) is a program of Connect Health and Community, a community health center in southeastern Melbourne. GHS is the largest Victorian GH service, covering ten local government areas. GHS has been offering a suite of evidence-based psychotherapeutic interventions for individuals and families with gambling issues since 1995.

In addition to direct GH services, since 2010 the VRGF also funds a specialist service: the Alfred Mental Health and Gambling Harm Service Victoria (AMH&GHSV). AMH&GSV is a program of Alfred Mental and Addiction Health (AMAH), a major Victorian public mental health service. The service was established as a result of finding that 17.6% of people presenting to the crisis or emergency mental-health services of AMAH, with issues of suicidality, acknowledged being affected by gambling harm (Lee et al., 2012). A United Kingdom study examining treatment-seeking gamblers found that approximately 30% of individuals accessing treatment had attempted suicide (Sharman, Murphy, Turner, & Roberts, 2019). AMH&GHSV provide a short-term dual-specialist clinical mental-health and gambling harm service. The program works collaboratively with services to transfer knowledge through shared interventions.

SST has been offered by AGH&MHSV since 2018 and is still in an early stage of development. The program has built on staff experience in delivering SST in other settings and has established a culture of respect, transparency and collaboration. We incorporate SST in a wider systems approach, combining offering clients and families the opportunity for a single therapeutic intervention with a number of professionals from different services sharing their reflections, together with collaborative consultation with the clients' GH therapeutic counselors (TC) who provide the ongoing counseling.

Single Session Therapy

Why We Use SST

Talmon (2018, p. 150) wrote "About 90% of patients, using planned and mutually agreed upon SST, will benefit from such lengths of therapy and will be highly satisfied with the session, as well as having short- and long-term positive outcomes."

We have observed SST to foster a "competency-emphasizing" approach, facilitating therapeutic passion including human connection and the power of love (Hoyt, 2017, 2018, Talmon, 2018). Our approach offers

SST for clients and their ongoing counselors and is both a therapeutic and clinical consultation opportunity. With a number of therapists in the session, we risk being therapist-centered, but in fact the feeling of deep care in the room for the family members very much embodies the power of relational therapy that Carl Rogers (1961) so movingly described. While the content of the session is important, it is also important for clinicians to have right-brain connection including safety cues of prosody, intonation, facial expression, and posture (DeYoung, 2015; Porges, 2011, 2017; Tatkin, 2011). The structure of our SST aims to provide a space for family members to "immobilize without fear" (Porges, 2011, p. 222), to reduce defensiveness and sit in the space with openness.

For GH therapeutic counselors, the experience of witnessing their clients and families in the SST context is often a source of new insights and linkages, later brought into continued ongoing (individual, couple, and family) counseling. A complex aspect of GH counseling is balancing unconditional positive regard for the person gambling with acknowledgment of the impact of harm to affected family and friends. SST sessions can facilitate deepened connection for the person gambling with the way their choices extend beyond themselves, building empathy and starting to repair fractured relationships.

How We Offer and Provide SST

We will first outline the structure of a typical SST session and then elucidate the process further with a case illustration.

All clients referred to the AGH&MHSV have the option for single session therapy. To date, SST has occurred in consultation with clients' existing GH counselors. The single session therapist shares information about the service with clients and referrers, arranges appointments, and ensures logistical details, including scheduling for up to 90 minutes. Clients provide written consent to their ongoing GH counselors in the referral to the AGH&MHSV. Pre-session questionnaires inviting clients' views of their issues and the outcomes they seek are sent to clients and affected others attending with the request to complete and return prior to the session.

Where possible, the session includes two therapists from AGH&MHSV and may include at least one additional therapist in a reflecting team, together with GH TCs. (For more about reflecting teams, see Andersen, 1991; Friedman, 1995; White, 1995.) The reflecting team was originally located in a different room with audiovisual technology to support this or with two groups in the same room. More recently, SST is provided with clients and their affected others meeting together with counselors. SST has also been offered by video conferencing, all participants being in different locations, with positive feedback.

SST on the day is divided into three parts:

1. SST therapists and ongoing GH counselors meet half an hour before the session. They read the pre-session questionnaires and discuss case conceptualization, counselors' goals for the session, clarify the process, and prepare for the session. Reflections are encouraged to include all clients, focusing on what is said and observed in the room.

2. The session begins with everyone being welcomed and introduced. The AGH&MHSV SST therapist requests and facilitates the Outcome Rating Scale (ORS) being completed by the clients at the beginning and the Session Rating Scale (SRS; Miller & Duncan, 2004) at the end for feedback and evaluation. The therapist emphasizes that this meeting will focus on the issues outlined in the pre-session questionnaires, that all voices will be heard and that the discussion will focus on clients' strengths and their solutions. They also describe the reflective aspects of the session, where therapists may take small breaks during the meeting or towards the end, to reflect with one another in front of the group.

   To start the discussion, the therapist invites clients to share their two main issues as identified in their pre-session questionnaires. Therapists elicit the dialogue and check in with clients to ensure that everyone is included and that the conversation is on track. Toward the end of the session, the primary therapist encourages a conversation identifying what has been helpful and what clients may find supportive post session. Therapists sum up key concepts, phrases, and plans that have been made and obtain permission to contact clients after a few weeks to discuss the impact of the SST and to offer a further SST if the clients want this.

3. Therapists meet for about a half hour after the session to debrief, reflect, and review. GH therapeutic counselors are often working with different family members and may not have met the family together before. Discussions occur with an expanded perspective of the client's relationships and family dynamics. GH therapeutic counselors are encouraged to reflect on their hopes and hypotheses prior to and after the session. The AGH&MHSV SST therapist documents and usually sends a therapeutic letter to the clients, which includes key phrases and themes from the session. (For more about the use of therapeutic letters, see Epston, 1994; Omer, 1991; White and Epston, 1990.) The letter is framed in a compassionate way to validate perspectives, hopes, and choices. Clients are contacted by the primary SST therapist a few weeks post session for feedback and a follow-up SST may be arranged. GH therapeutic counselors receive copies of therapeutic letters and updates of any contacts. Follow-up secondary consultation to GH therapeutic counselors is also offered.

SST: An Illustration with Reflections

Participating counselors and clients have reported largely positive as well as challenging experiences. Following is a GHS example that illustrates some of the complexities of our SST service delivery.

Example. Two GHS counselors referred their individual clients, Sally and Peter, for SST together with their teenage daughter, Louise. Sally had moved to Australia from the USA after meeting Peter on holiday in the 1990s. Peter had migrated from Greece as a child with his large extended family. As Sally's work required her to be away from home for long periods, Peter was the primary caregiver to their daughter, Louise, and his family assisted with childcare. Sally had borrowed large amounts of money from Peter and his family for her business. Over time it became clear that she had gambled away this money on electronic gaming machines and the family was in debt as a result. This had occurred previously for Sally and was partly why she had migrated. Upon their financial hardship becoming apparent, Sally took up business opportunities overseas. She kept in contact with Peter and Louise but was away for a few years, where she accrued further business debts. At the time of the SST, Sally had moved back to Australia and had not gambled for some months. She had experienced a deterioration in her mental health, including increased anxiety and depression requiring acute community psychiatric intervention. Sally's mental health had recently stabilized; however, the couple were uncertain how to move forward.

Two AGH&MHSV therapists were with Sally, Peter, and Louise in the room. Two GHS counselors and a third therapist were in the reflecting team in another room using video conferencing.

The session focused on Louise's anger at her mother whom she described as a "liar" who had "betrayed" them. Louise sat between her mother and one therapist. The intensity of her anger and distress was obvious to all in the room. She was crying and glaring at Sally who did not respond to her and appeared to be unmoved. Peter verbally acknowledged their daughter's distress and suggested examples of how Sally might develop a closer relationship with Louise, spoke of her confidence in business but her ambivalence with mothering and household tasks, and her shame associated with her gambling. At this point, the family began to collaborate on ideas of what might help. Throughout the session, Louise expressed distress and frustration regarding her mother's need to be cared for rather than caring for her. At one point, however, she said, "I don't want to hate my mum."

As Louise had moved her seat and slumped down at times during the session, she was partially hidden from the reflecting team. Furthermore, the sound was muffled as the room was warm, requiring a fan. Despite this, all therapists experienced the session as a powerful insight into this family. It was useful to explore the family dynamics in the post-session reflection, including non-verbal body language and facial expressions, attachment styles and shame, which the GH counselors witnessed and would continue to explore in Sally's and Peter's ongoing individual counseling. Secondary consultation continued to be provided by AGH&MHSV to one of the GHS counselors following the session. Sally and Peter did not want a follow-up SST although they requested assistance referring Louise to an adolescent therapy service.

Feedback from the GHS counselors indicated that the SST approach helped to highlight the ways in which this family was stuck, some of which related to the couple's different cultures and values. The counselors reported the session as facilitating each family member's voice, which was then brought back into Sally's and Peter's ongoing GHS individual counseling. Sally demonstrated a significant shift after the SST session in connecting with herself and the needs of her husband and daughter. She maintained abstinence from gambling and continued GHS counseling, exploring relationship challenges and healthy, constructive choices for her life. Though Sally and Peter later separated permanently, they both rated and described their SST and ongoing counseling as beneficial. It was clear that their implementation of a new relational understanding and a softening of defenses greatly supported their functioning as individuals and parents, united in their care for their daughter.

Conclusion

We have found that SST offers opportunities to bring individuals, families, and services together to explore gambling and facilitate conversations of hope and connection. People who gamble and their families frequently experience shame and multi-layered losses. Brown (2010, p. 40) notes how shame that is kept locked up "festers and grows" – but because shame exists between people, it can also be healed between people. SST with families experiencing gambling harm can provide a useful and safe structure to facilitate a relational focus. Including long-term GH therapeutic counselors in our AGH&MHSV SST program provides a flexibility of combined approaches to meet a unique need.

References

Andersen, T. (Ed.) (1991). *The Reflecting Team: Dialogues and Dialogues about the Dialogues*. New York: Norton.

Becona, E., Del Carmen Lorenzo, M., & Fuentes, M.J. (1996). Pathological gambling and depression. *Psychological Reports, 78*(2), 635–640.

Brown, B. (2010). *The Gifts of Imperfection: Let Go of Who You Think You're Supposed to Be and Embrace Who You Are*. Minneapolis, MN: Hazelden.

Browne, M., Langham, E., Rawat, V., Greer, N., Li, E., Rose, J., ... Best, T. (2016). *Assessing Gambling-Related Harm in Victoria: A Public Health Perspective*. North Melbourne, VIC, Australia: Victorian Responsible Gambling Foundation.

Clark, L., Averbeck, B., Payer, D., Sescousse, G., Winstanley, C., & Xue, G. (2013). Pathological choice: The neuroscience of gambling and gambling addiction. *Journal of Neuroscience, 33*(45), 17617–17623.

DeYoung, P.A. (2015). *Understanding and Treating Chronic Shame: A Relational/ Neurobiological Approach*. New York: Routledge.

Epston, D. (1994). Extending the conversation. *Family Therapy Networker, 18*(6), 30–37, 62–63.

Friedman, S. (Ed.) (1995). *The Reflecting Team in Action: Collaborative Practice in Family Therapy*. New York: Guilford Press.

Gilbert, P. (2011). Shame in psychotherapy, and the role of Compassion Focused Therapy. In R.L. Dearing & J.P. Tangney (Eds.), *Shame in the Therapy Hour* (pp. 325–354). Washington, DC: APA Books.

H2 Gambling Capital (2017, February 9). The world's biggest gamblers. *The Economist*, https://www.economist.com/graphic-detail/2017/02/09/the-worlds-biggest-gamblers

Hanson, R., & Hanson, F. (2018). *Resilient: How to Grow an Unshakable Core of Calm, Strength and Happiness*. New York: Harmony Books/Penguin Random House.

Hing, N., Nuske, E., Gainsbury, S., Russell, A., & Breen, H. (2016). How does the stigma of problem gambling influence help-seeking, treatment and recovery? A view from the counseling sector. *International Gambling Studies, 16*(2), 263–280.

Hing, N., & Russell, A. (2017). How anticipated and experienced stigma can contribute to self-stigma: The case of problem gambling. *Frontiers in Psychology, 8*(235), 1–11.

Hing, N., Russell, A., Gainsbury, S., & Nuske, E. (2016). The public stigma of problem gambling: Its nature and relative intensity compared to other health conditions. *Journal of Gambling Studies, 32*, 847–864.

Hing, N., Russell, A., Nuske, E., & Gainsbury, S. (2015). *The Stigma of Problem Gambling: Causes, Characteristics and Consequences*. North Melbourne, VIC, Australia: Victorian Responsible Gambling Foundation.

Hoyt, M.F. (2017). *Brief Therapy and Beyond: Stories, Language, Love, Hope, and Time*. New York: Routledge.

Hoyt, M.F. (2018). Single-session therapy: Stories, structures, themes, cautions and prospects. In M.F. Hoyt, M. Bobele, A. Slive, J. Young, & M. Talmon (Eds.), *Single-Session Therapy by Walk-In or Appointment: Administrative, Clinical and Supervisory Aspects of One-at-a-Time Services* (pp. 155–174). New York: Routledge.

Lee, S., Harrison, K., Field, M., Kennedy, A., Cosic, S., Symons, E., & De Castella, A. (2012). *Victorian Statewide Problem Gambling and Mental Health Partnership: 2010–2012 Final Report*. Melbourne, Australia: Alfred Mental and Addiction Health.

Lewis, M. (2015). *The Biology of Desire: Why Addiction is Not a Disease*. New York: PublicAffairs/Perseus Books.

Miller, S.D., & Duncan, B.L. (2004). *The Outcome and Session Rating Scales: Administration and Scoring Manual*. Chicago, IL: Institute for the Study of Therapeutic Change.

Neff, K. (2015). *Self-Compassion: The Proven Power of Being Kind to Yourself.* New York: HarperCollins.

Omer, H. (1991). Writing a post-scriptum to a badly ended therapy. *Psychotherapy, 28*(3), 484–492.

Petry, N.M. (2001). Substance abuse, pathological gambling, and impulsiveness. *Drug and Alcohol Dependence, 63*(1), 29–38.

Porges, S. W. (2011). *The Polyvagal Theory: Neurophysiological Foundations of Emotions, Attachment, Communication, and Self-Regulation.* New York: Norton.

Porges, S.W. (2017). *The Pocket Guide to the Polyvagal Theory: The Transformative Power of Feeling Safe.* New York: Norton.

Potter-Effron, R. (2002). *Shame, Guilt and Alcoholism* (2nd ed.). New York: Haworth Press.

Queensland Government Statistician's Office. (2019). *Australian Gambling Statistics* (35th ed.) Brisbane, QLD: Queensland Treasury.

Rogers, C. (1961). *On Becoming a Person: A Therapist's View of Psychotherapy.* London: Constable.

Sharman, S., Murphy, R., Turner, J.J., & Roberts, A. (2019). Trends and patterns in UK treatment seeking gamblers: 2000–2015. *Addictive Behaviors, 89*, 51–56.

Talmon, M. (2018). Being a single-session therapist. In M.F. Hoyt, M. Bobele, A. Slive, J. Young, & Talmon (Eds.), *Single-Session Therapy by Walk-In or Appointment: Administrative, Clinical and Supervisory Aspects of One-at-a-Time Services* (pp. 149–154). New York: Routledge.

Tatkin, S. (2011). *Wired for Love.* Oakland, CA: New Harbinger Publications.

van der Kolk, B. (2015). *The Body Keeps the Score: Brain, Mind, and Body in the Healing of Trauma.* New York: Penguin Books.

Victorian Responsible Gambling Foundation. (2017). *Hidden Harm: Low-Risk and Moderate-Risk Gambling.* Background Paper. Retrieved from www.responsiblegambling.vic.gov.au.

White, M. (1995). Reflecting team as definitional ceremony. In *Re-Authoring Lives: Interviews & Essays* (pp. 172–198). Adelaide, S.A., Australia: Dulwich Centre Publications.

White, M., & Epston, D. (1990). *Narrative Means to Therapeutic Ends.* New York: Norton.

29 Single Session Family Consultation with Adults Affected by Eating Disorders

Carmel Fleming

Eating disorders (EDs) such as anorexia nervosa, bulimia nervosa, and binge eating disorder are serious illnesses associated with significant personal and family costs (Fox, Dean, & Whittlesea, 2017). Effective treatments are rare, and outcomes are poor, especially for adults. Due to their biopsychosocial nature, people affected by eating disorders can present with a unique combination of high risk and low awareness. This presents a challenge to treatment acceptance and retention as well as to interpersonal relationships. Families can find themselves ill prepared and oscillating between anxious over-involvement and accommodating reactions when faced with their loved one's deteriorating health. A negative interactional cycle can result that produces further family stress and burden for carers and leads to poor coping (Whitney & Eisler, 2005). Ongoing mental, physical, and social problems can then impact the recovery of both the individual and the family system (Schmidt & Treasure, 2006).

Research has shown that educating and supporting carers can help support treatment and improve outcomes for both adolescents and adults with EDs (Hodsoll et al., 2017; Magill et al., 2016). The inclusion of families in treatment is regarded as a core component of comprehensive care (National Institute for Health and Care Excellence, 2017) and may decrease attrition across care pathways for adults (Waller et al., 2009). Families report problems accessing services, however, and can experience exclusion from treatment programs and negative interactions with professionals (Fox et al., 2017). Although proactive engagement and involvement is routine in child and adolescent EDs, with family-based treatment models considered the first-line approach, treatment for adults remains dominated by individual methods and family inclusion is not typical.

In other mental illnesses, stepped-care approaches, including low-intensity options, have been effective in engaging and supporting families (Mottaghipour & Bickerton, 2005). As a means of connecting with carers early in the clinical pathway, single session therapy with families has been used in Australia for over 20 years (Hampson et al., 1999; Poon, Harvey,

Fuzzard, & O'Hanlon, 2019; also see Chapter 5 of this volume) but remains relatively novel in EDs and untested with adults from this population.

Introducing the Single Session Family Consultation Process

The Queensland Eating Disorder Service (QuEDS) first considered use of Single Session Family Consultation (SSFC), as described in The Bouverie Centre (2016[1]) model, in the context of an investigation into the options to better engage and involve families in an adult outpatient clinic. SFCC entails negotiating with an individual client about how best to bring family members in for a single session-inspired meeting to discuss how the family can best be part of the individual client's ongoing treatment.

Currently no evidence exists in the field as to the necessary, or sufficient, amount of contact or intensity of response required when working with adult families affected by EDs. Family interventions that have been trialed that include both the adult client and their family members require considerable time and attendance commitments (Baucom et al., 2017; Dimitropoulos et al., 2018; Magill et al., 2016; Runfola et al., 2018; Schmidt et al., 2015; Wierenga et al., 2018).

Policy imperatives for carer inclusion at QuEDS and review of a new level of care in the outpatient clinic (a day hospital program) at the service revealed high drop-out levels and a need to activate family support to assist clients remain engaged with the clinic. An accessible and efficient family involvement option that could be used as an adjunct to individual treatment as usual was needed. The intervention also needed to clarify the nature of family involvement with the clinic, assist families to identify and meet their needs during the treatment process, and support clients to transfer treatment goals to the home environment. This latter aim is important in EDs as behaviors like food preparation, approach to mealtimes, and self-care can become severely disrupted. Meeting these requirements in a large, multidisciplinary clinic demanded a flexible process suitable for the diverse family forms seen in a transdiagnostic, adult clinical population. As part of a statewide specialist service with capacity building remit across the region, the family intervention also needed to be scalable and generalizable to other services. As a brief, cost-effective intervention that has an evidence base with other serious adult mental health conditions, SSFC was chosen to trial in the QuEDS outpatient program.

Applying the SSFC Process

The SSFC process as applied at QuEDS contained four points of contact:

1. When the client and their family attended a treatment orientation session where additional information about SSFC was provided
2. The client and their individual treatment key worker met to discuss and confirm the decision to involve family in the treatment program and administer pre-session forms
3. The conjoint family session itself, attended with clients face-to-face and family members or other supports as appropriate, either in-person or by virtual attendance via telephone or video conferencing
4. The follow-up process, carried out with clients in their usual key worker appointments and with carers via a phone call or email two and four weeks after the session by the family worker, was completed. No subsequent contact with the family worker was had unless requested by the client. Additional sessions, as needed, only occurred if a further issue was identified that the client considered suitable for SSFC.

Each conjoint family session followed the broad phases of *convening*, *conducting*, and *concluding* the family work process outlined by The Bouverie Centre model (2016). Convening the SSFC process involved specifically introducing the idea of family involvement and, via individual key worker sessions, getting the client to think about whom to include, discuss any concerns, consider pros and cons of family involvement, clarify goals, and identify any off-limits areas of discussion. Consistent with the voluntary nature of QuEDS treatment, the adult relationships, and the central issue of control for many people affected by EDs, all invitations for family members to attend the service were issued by the client directly.

Conducting the SSFC process included exploration of the presenting issues identified on the pre-session forms and collaboratively identifying, negotiating, and prioritizing participants' needs and concerns; responding to and working on the prioritized areas and apposite issues; and closing the session by summarizing the discussion and deciding on next steps for both the client and their supports. Where appropriate, these were concurrently written up by a facilitator of the session and duplicated for participants on a takeaway sheet.

Concluding the SSFC process encompassed setting the follow-up arrangements between two to four weeks later (via individual key worker appointments for the client, and via a phone call or email from the family worker for carers) and completing a post-session questionnaire as well as responding to any further needs of participants by providing further relevant resources and/or referral to pertinent services as requested. Between one and six months after the intervention, participants were invited to provide feedback on the SSFC process via a service evaluation process. To encourage open feedback, all interviews were conducted by members of the QuEDS service development and research team who were not involved in the therapeutic program.

In addition to this basic structure, adaptations were necessary to maximize the fit of SSFC for adults affected by EDs. Given the low mental health literacy about EDs in the general public, and to help in the transferability of the broader treatment goals of the outpatient program to the home environment, written treatment orientation materials and disorder-specific psychoeducation (Treasure, Smith, & Crane, 2016) were provided. Referral was made to specialist family therapy programs or other family support services where necessary to deal with additional needs not provided by the EDs service. Other adjustments included the use of multimedia delivery methods for the SSFC via video or telephone calls, which allowed remote attendance by carers where necessary as many clients identified support people they did not live with. The concurrent caseload requirements of the multidisciplinary team members meant that a reflecting team was not able to be scheduled during the sessions but client case review meetings enabled other treating staff to provide input prior to the SSFC follow up.

Illustrating the SSFC Process

Examples drawn from three respective cases will be used to demonstrate aspects of convening, conducting, and concluding the SSFC process with adults affected by eating disorders.

Convening the SSFC Process

The Green family attended the ED service when their daughter, Kelly, a medical student aged 20, was assessed for the outpatient day program. Kelly had a one-year duration of atypical anorexia nervosa and, despite currently being in the healthy weight range, had deferred her studies as her calorie restriction and excessive exercise were affecting her attendance. Kelly identified her parents and her live-in partner, Damien, as supportive contacts. Her parents attended the treatment orientation session and were given an SSFC information sheet and psychoeducational material. Kelly took an information pack home for her partner. Kelly then met with her individual key worker and was asked if she would like family members to be involved in any other way. Kelly said her parents wanted to come in and an SSFC was held with Kelly, her parents, key worker, and the QuEDS family worker. Pre-session questionnaires were completed and issues for discussion were identified. Both parents stated they thought Kelly's relationship with her partner (which they felt was generally helpful for Kelly) had deteriorated and needed to be addressed. During the session they were able to support Kelly to identify a way to approach her partner Damien about this. Following this, Kelly invited Damien to an SSFC. Damien stated his main concerns were "Kelly not eating dinner or just not eating a good amount of food" and

"Knowing how to not get angry at her eating disorder behavior." This matched Kelly's experiences of the conflicts around eating and the session then proceeded to examine a solution to these issues.

Comment. When interviewed (separately) about their experiences with the SSFC process, Kelly noted that this graded and collaborative convening of the SSFC with both her parents and with her partner was important. She said that she was initially reluctant to include her loved ones in the ED issue because it had been a source of conflict in the past. Being encouraged by her key worker to consider the benefits of involving others by using a structured and facilitated process she was able to overcome her ambivalence. She stated, "I was nervous to start with, because any time that I'd sat down with Damien before and tried to talk about things, it had ended up in an argument. I think having my key worker there defused anything that would have ended up in an argument." Convening the session in a way that was considerate of Damien's concerns also seemed to have an impact on how he was able to participate in the session as he identified the most helpful aspect of the session was that it was "a no judgement zone where you can feel free to express how you're feeling and just know that whatever you say isn't wrong." The participant-led nature of the SSFC approach and the collaborative agenda-setting technique seemed particularly helpful when, like Kelly and Damien, family members avoided communicating about the ED problem until a conflict occurred, which in turn, encouraged more avoidance of the difficult topic. At follow-up Damien reported that he had begun attending a carers' support group.

Conducting the SSFC Process

Michelle, a 54-year-old legal professional with bulimia nervosa diagnosed eight years prior, attended the QuEDS outpatient program after multiple hospital admissions for medical complications from her binge-purge symptoms. Michelle requested her husband, Jim, attend an SSFC during her individual outpatient treatment. The couple's pre-session forms revealed what initially seemed like divergent concerns. Michelle indicated her main issue was "Managing my expectations of Jim to support me regarding my eating behaviors. How do I know when I'm asking for or expecting too much from Jim as I continually think I am expecting too much and feel guilty, but then I get disappointed at the same time because I still hope for his support?" In contrast, Jim stated the main issues were "Nutrition – what does Michelle need to eat?" and "Bingeing – how can I provide support?" During the SSFC, the apparent disparity between these needs – one to address the emotional tone and support in the relationship and the other to provide strategies regarding the eating disorder behaviors – was raised and a session agenda negotiated. After identifying these different issues, Michelle and Jim were invited to share more about the effect of the ED problem and what they would like to be different while the other person practiced reflective listening. Intersecting intentions and common aims revealed by these different presenting issues were then summarized by the facilitators. In the course of conducting the SSFC via this non-directive process, a shared concern was able to be identified and reflected back to Michelle and Jim as a tentative formulation of an issue for work: that is, that the ED behaviors had come between them and created distance between the couple that led to uncertainty and unclear expectations. Jim then responded by expressing his concern via over-involvement in Michelle's food choices. They were able to see that they had both unintentionally neglected their relationship and given the ED a central place in their interactions. They both agreed and stated what they wanted was to re-establish their intimacy. Next steps were identified that involved Jim stepping back from his role supervising Michelle's nutrition and instead beginning to plan joint activities that they could enjoy together, such as attending ballet and musical performances. During the follow-up call, Jim required reassurance that Michelle was continuing to attend the treatment program and that the dietitian would be assessing the adequacy of her meal plan. He expressed gratitude for the session and said they had been to some excellent concerts!

Comment: As is often the case with such a dangerous and self-perpetuating cycle as develops in long-term ED problems, the illness symptoms and response had come to dominate interpersonal interactions. Giving Michelle and Jim space to collaboratively identify this and discuss how they actually wanted their relationship to allow an emotional connection to be reasserted and a recognition that their interpersonal relationship was a priority. The SSFC method, although brief, was able to break into the negative cycle that had developed and facilitate a more sustainable and appropriate role for Jim in supporting Michelle in her recovery.

Concluding the SSFC Process

Terri, a 30-year-old teacher with a long history of depression and changing symptoms of unhealthy dieting and binge eating had an SSFC with her partner, Jodie. During the session, Jodie stated she felt there was "too much talk about food and the ED" and "wanted to spend less time and energy worrying about meals." Terri explained how much the issue interfered in her life, stressing "Every mealtime, when I think about food, I struggle with my sense of self … I fear weight gain, fear my negative emotions, shame, disgust, and self-hatred." Terri was able to clarify during the session that her main interpersonal problem was with Jodie's inconsistent reactions and the anxiety and anger this led to for her. She wanted Jodie to provide empathy without advice and was able to identify that Jodie dictating food choices led to resentment. The key worker was able to reflect that this dynamic had also seemed to emerge for Terri with the program staff, especially the dietitian. Jodie stated that there needed to be less pressure on her and that she wasn't sure what level of involvement Terri really wanted from her. A commonly problematic situation for the couple, choosing from a menu at restaurants, was explored to expand on this dynamic, with Terri and Jodie sharing what they had previously tried in this situation and how they would like eating out to be. A range of possible solutions was generated and Terri and Jodie agreed to a planned experiment for Terri to try an online menu check beforehand, observing what their friends ordered, and some conversational strategies during the meal to help with panicky feelings and to slow down eating. The facilitator also suggested the couple build in a review process to check in with how they felt this had worked on the drive home. A written copy of the steps was provided on a take-away sheet. In the follow-up session with her key worker, Terri stated, "After the family meeting I became more committed to recovery and my meal plan. Jodie has also been more supportive. I have noticed my table manners, pace and ability to socialize during meals was better. I'm better able to tolerate uncertainty." On her post-session form, however, Terri identified further questions, including "How can Jodie and I ensure both of our needs are met even when they are conflicting? How do I keep the momentum going when the program ends?" The worker advised that another SSFC could be scheduled but Terri did not request any further family sessions during the remainder of her treatment at the clinic.

Comment: Jodie did not reply to the follow-up phone call. Terri was prematurely discharged from the program as her eating disorder symptoms had only partially improved but her depression had intensified and she was referred to a higher level of care. Although SSFC can be very useful when working with adults with EDs, and a mastery experience over entrenched problems can be experienced via the brief intervention, other treatment issues can take precedence as this group can have additional mental or physical health problems. When this happens, the opportunity for further service support or referral for family members may be lost as contact is contingent on the adult client. (For more on ending an SST, see Hoyt, 2000; Hoyt & Talmon, 2014; and Hoyt & Rosenbaum, 2018.)

Further Considerations Regarding Implementing the SSFC Process

The SSFC process has proved flexible enough to incorporate the variety of presenting psychosocial needs of families and the range of emotional development seen in adults affected by EDs at QuEDS. A recent evaluation of 35 consecutive adult patients who started outpatient therapy at QuEDS revealed that approximately 70% of clients (24/35) took the opportunity to include their family in their treatment via an SSFC. Clients and carers reported that the SSFC process was a safe and accessible way to approach interpersonal problems caused by the ED that may have previously been experienced as overwhelming, conflictual, or were avoided altogether. Utilizing an already existing therapeutic relationship with the client's key worker to introduce the SSFC helped clients accept the idea of family involvement. The one-at-a-time nature of the approach also seemed to assist with this ambivalence. The collaborative agenda setting and co-facilitation of the sessions by a family worker trained in the SSFC method who did not have a prior relationship with either the client or the family members also appeared helpful in encouraging a neutral environment for participants. QuEDS has a large multidisciplinary treatment team and the co-facilitation method also helped to extend clinician exposure to an intervention that was novel to the agency.

The low-intensity nature of the SSFC approach did initially concern some clinicians at the service who suggested that offering only a single session to families would chance "opening Pandora's box," with relational problems being exposed but not able to be fully addressed. Given the difficulty of engaging and retaining clients with EDs in treatment programs in general, and the importance of preserving the therapeutic alliance, this was an understandable concern. Clinicians were able to recognize, however, that family members who were more involved, even briefly, were more likely to encourage their loved one to persist in the treatment program if difficulties arose. Consequently, information and orientation to the model also needed to be provided to clinicians as well as to clients and carers. The evidence base for SSFC with other serious mental illnesses was emphasized and the safe and effective nature of the "as-needed" approach with similar complex issues like drug and alcohol problems was highlighted.

Families can have many roles in the care of an individual affected by an ED: to provide information, investigate help, instigate care, interpret treatment, support identity development, reduce isolation, resource recovery, and instill hope (McDonald, 2018). Clinicians striving to do the same for families of adults with EDs are encouraged to consider expanding their therapeutic practice to include use of single session family consultation.

Note

1 *Editors' note*: Also see Chapter 5.

References

Baucom, D.H., Kirby J.S., Fischer, M.S., Baucom, B.R., Hamer, R., & Bulik, C.M. (2017). Findings from a couple-based open trial for adult anorexia nervosa. *Journal of Family Psychology, 31*(5), 584–591.

Dimitropoulos, G., Landers, A.L., Freeman, V., Novick, J., Garber. A., & Le Grange, D. (2018). Open trial of family-based treatment of anorexia nervosa for transition age youth. *Journal of the Canadian Academy of Child and Adolescent Psychiatry, 27*(1), 50–61.

Fox, J.R., Dean, M., & Whittlesea, A. (2017). The experience of caring for or living with an individual with an eating disorder: A meta-synthesis of qualitative studies. *Clinical Psychology and Psychotherapy, 24*(1), 103–125.

Hampson, R., O'Hanlon, J., Franklin, A., Pentony, M., Fridgant, L., & Heins, T. (1999). The place of single session family consultations: Five years' experience in Canberra. *Australian and New Zealand Journal of Family Therapy, 20*(4), 195–200.

Hodsoll, J., Rhind, C., Micali, N., Hibbs, R., Goddard, E., Nazar, B.P., ... Landau, S. (2017). A pilot, multicentre pragmatic randomised trial to explore the impact of carer skills training on carer and patient behaviours: Testing the cognitive interpersonal model in adolescent anorexia nervosa. *European Eating Disorders Review, 25*(6), 551–561.

Hoyt, M.F. (2000). The last session in brief therapy: Why and how to say "when." In *Some Stories Are Better than Others* (pp. 237–261). Philadelphia, PA: Brunner/Mazel.

Hoyt, M.F., & Rosenbaum, R. (2018). Some ways to end an SST. In M.F. Hoyt, M. Bobele, A. Slive, J. Young, & M. Talmon (Eds), *Single-Session Therapy by Walk-In or Appointment* (pp. 318–323). New York: Routledge.

Hoyt, M.F., & Talmon, M. (2014). The temporal structure of brief therapy: Some questions often associated with different phases of sessions and treatment. In M.F. Hoyt & M. Talmon (Eds.), *Capturing the Moment: Single Session Therapy and Walk-In Services* (pp. 517–522). Bethel, CT: Crown House Publishing.

Magill, N., Rhind, C., Hibbs, R., Goddard, E., Macdonald, P., Arcelus, J., ... Treasure, J. (2016). Two-year follow-up of a pragmatic randomised controlled trial examining the effect of adding a carer's skill training intervention in inpatients with anorexia nervosa. *European Eating Disorders Review, 24*(2), 122–130.

McDonald, J. (2018). Working with parents, partners and other carers. In J. Morris & A. McKinlay (Eds.), *Multidisciplinary Management of Eating Disorders* (pp. 109–121). New York: Springer.

Mottaghipour, Y., & Bickerton, A. (2005). The pyramid of family care: A framework for family involvement with adult mental health services. *Australian e-Journal for the Advancement of Mental Health, 4*(3), 210–217.

National Institute for Health and Care Excellence. (2017). *Eating Disorders: Recognition and Treatment (NICE Guideline NG69)*. London: NICE.

Poon, A.W.C., Harvey, C., Fuzzard, S., & O'Hanlon, B. (2019). Implementing a family-inclusive practice model in youth mental health services in Australia. *Early Intervention in Psychiatry, 13*(3), 461–468.

Runfola, C.D., Kirby, J.S., Baucom, D.H., Fischer, M.S., Baucom, B.R., Matherne, C.E. ... Bulik, C.M. (2018). A pilot open trial of UNITE-BED: A couple-based intervention for binge-eating disorder. *International Journal of Eating Disorders, 51*(9), 1107–1112.

Schmidt, U., Magill, N., Renwick, B., Keyes, A., Kenyon, M., Dejong, H., ... Landau, S. (2015). The Maudsley Outpatient Study of Treatments for Anorexia

Nervosa and Related Conditions (MOSAIC): Comparison of the Maudsley Model of Anorexia Nervosa Treatment for Adults (MANTRA) with specialist supportive clinical management (SSCM) in outpatients with broadly defined anorexia nervosa: A randomized controlled trial. *Journal of Consulting and Clinical Psychology, 83*(4), 796–807.

Schmidt, U., & Treasure, J. (2006). Anorexia nervosa: Valued and visible. A cognitive-interpersonal maintenance model and its implications for research and practice. *British Journal of Clinical Psychology, 45*(3), 343–366.

The Bouverie Centre (2016). *From Individual to Families: A Client-Centred Framework for Involving Families Developed for Mental Health and Alcohol and Other Drug Services.* Melbourne, Australia: The Bouverie Centre: Victoria's Family Institute, La Trobe University.

Treasure, J., Smith, G., & Crane, A. (2016). *Skills-Based Caring for a Loved One with an Eating Disorder: The New Maudsley Method.* New York: Routledge.

Waller, G., Schmidt, U., Treasure, J., Murray, K., Aleyna, J., Emanuelli, F. ... Yeomans, M. (2009). Problems across care pathways in specialist adult eating disorder services. *Psychiatric Bulletin, 33*(1), 26–29. doi: 10.1192/pb.bp.107. 018325.

Whitney, J., & Eisler, I. (2005). Theoretical and empirical models around caring for someone with an eating disorder: The reorganization of family life and inter-personal maintenance factors. *Journal of Mental Health, 14*(6), 575–585.

Wierenga, C.E., Hill, L., Knatz Peck, S., McCray, J., Greathouse, L., Peterson, D., ... Kaye, W.H. (2018). The acceptability, feasibility, and possible benefits of a neurobiologically-informed 5-day multifamily treatment for adults with anorexia nervosa. *International Journal of Eating Disorders, 51*(8), 863–869.

30 Collaborative First Meetings with Young People Who Have Eating Problems and Their Families

Rachel Barbara-May

The Alfred Child and Youth Mental Health Service (CYMHS) is a state hospital run community-based mental health service in the inner southeast of Melbourne, Victoria. For many years we have been trying to design an effective service response for young people with eating problems and their families. This has meant that we have changed our practice many times, adapting and failing, learning and evolving. We're not sure that we have really worked it out for every family, but we have decided that above everything else the first meeting is most important. It presents an opportunity that we believe we may never get again and, if we approach the encounter with the importance of it in mind with each and every family we meet, we can often get started together in a powerful way.

The families we meet in our program have many different stories, experiences and circumstances but at the same time there are things that are much the same. For instance, they all have a young person, a child, or adolescent usually, who is very troubled and often in a life-threatening situation wherein they are no longer able to accept food from their parents or consume it for themselves. They are usually preoccupied by feelings of worthlessness and self-hatred, and often have no other way to cope with overwhelming feelings and the challenges of growing up. For many of these young people, this problem has already greatly interfered with their lives and relationships to the extent that they have been taken out of their family and placed in hospital for medical intervention. Sometimes this has occurred many times before meeting with us. Also similar for all of these families is that their parents and caregivers are experiencing extreme levels of guilt, shame, and blame. They tell us that they feel they have failed as parents and are unequipped to help their child out of this predicament. Although meeting us for the first time, most of these families have had many other encounters with professional teams and clinicians, and as people do, have researched the "problem" and learnt many helpful and sometimes unhelpful things. Their family is in crisis, the people around them who are trying to help are enraged and their young person is feeling unreachable, strange, and alienated. The tasks of the first meeting then are many and supremely important.

With an already flourishing single session family therapy program at the service (Barbara-May et al., 2018; Fry, 2012), clinicians working in the program are highly skilled in and influenced by single session ideas. Also influencing this work is our involvement in developing Open Dialogue practices for young people with psychosis (Haarakangas et al., 2007) in another part of our service. The all-important first meeting and our common factors-informed family approach (Davis & Hsieh, 2019) to helping young people with eating problems and their families occurs with these service cultures and practices as our context.

When developing our response to young people (and their families) with eating problems, we felt it important that it be part of the core business of the child and youth mental health service. To help achieve this, we established the Eating Disorders Consulting Team that functions as a "specialist" team, supporting the work of the treating CYMHS clinicians and the young people and families that they are trying to help. The Eating Disorders Consulting Team is made up of a program co-ordinator/lead clinician, psychiatrist, dietitian, family peer worker, mental health nurse, and mental health clinician. This team "wraps around" the treating clinicians who all have different professional backgrounds and levels of experience, and in addition to helping young people with eating problems, also work with children and young people with various types of behavioral and psychological distress. These case managers are working within three CYMHS clinical teams. We also have a newly developing stream through our headspace[1] primary program where continuing care (for more moderate presentations) is supported through Medicare-funded private providers working in partnership with the CYMHS team.

Program Structure

The structure and different components of the program are illustrated in Figure 30.1.

This program structure means that we are maximizing the capacity of the service to effectively help young people with eating disorders across our system of care. Although we are experiencing increased demand, the young people and families have significantly better access to good-quality care and a system that has a great deal better capacity to respond. Whichever stream the young person continues through, they all start with the collaborative first family meeting, an intensive meeting involving all members of the consulting team. The first meeting has three main elements: (1) to develop a shared understanding of the problem, (2) to build a treatment plan and make collaborative decisions, and (3) to generate a healing dialogue.

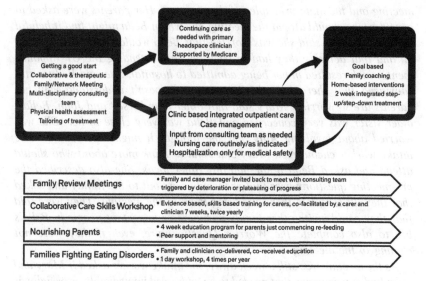

Figure 30.1 The Alfred CYMHS Eating Disorders Program.

Our hopes and beliefs for the program are clear. It should be easy to get in and to get what you need. We should respond early and quickly. The crisis creates energy and opportunity to bring everyone together that can help. The bringing together of important people also creates possibilities for healing, and impactful conversations that may never be possible again. The clinicians who begin with the family stay with the family because relationships are seen to be important, and we want to create a culture with the family that "we are all in this together." However, what works for some doesn't work for all and we adapt and adjust until we find the right way to go on with each young person and their family.

"Bella": Case Illustration with Commentary

Bella is a 16-year-old girl who lives with her parents, John and Mary, older sister Carrie (17), and younger sister Amy (11). Bella was taken to the family general practitioner (GP) by her concerned parents because of intentional weight loss, food aversion, body dysmorphia and preoccupation. These concerns had begun about nine months prior, but in the last three months the parents had become more worried due to significant weight loss. Bella had lost over 10 kg (22 lbs.) in three months and her body was showing signs of malnutrition and medical compromise. The GP arranged a medical admission at hospital where Bella stayed for approximately ten days. She was then referred for follow-up treatment at our service and we quickly organized a family meeting.

The intake worker described to Bella's parents the process of the first meeting and the main principles of the program. Her parents were asked to consider who should attend the meeting and whom Bella might find it helpful to include. Mary said she was worried that Bella wouldn't want to come at all and that actually they had to trick her into attending the GP appointment, which resulted in her being admitted to hospital. She said Bella is still convinced that there is nothing wrong and doesn't understand why her parents are so worried. Mary said that other than herself and John, Bella's older sister was very concerned and Bella was very close to her. She was worried about involving Amy and she thought it might upset Bella. The intake worker encouraged Mary and John to think more about who should attend and asked Bella if she had any other ideas. She also described the pre-meeting questionnaires that she would send out to the family and asked that they all complete them and bring them to the meeting. They were told that they could invite other family members or important people in Bella's life to also complete the Worries Questionnaire, even if they were not coming to the meeting.

As the meeting was still a week away, the intake worker asked if Mary and John had any concerns that needed to be addressed immediately, especially as Bella's weight was low and her body showing signs of becoming unstable. They had a discussion about how, since being discharged from hospital, Mary and John planned to try and limit Bella's exercise and start to create some expectations about food intake. They were encouraged to follow their instincts in regard to these things. They were also asked to contact the service immediately should their worries increase or something change with Bella and we would discuss whether something different should happen.

Getting a good start also requires a quick start. Wherever possible we try to organize the first family meeting quickly after contact is made with our service. In ideal circumstances the young person and family will be invited to meet with us within seven to ten days. Families are encouraged to get in touch with us if their worries increase during that time rather than seeking help elsewhere. This helps us to be able to respond directly to the worries and also avoid an escalation of the worries through the system which in some circumstances might result in premature hospitalization of the young person, or another type of interruption of the healing potential of the first meeting. Also, our intake process tries to prioritize the family's preparedness for the meeting (by focusing on asking about who should be invited, who in the family/network knows about the problem and who could be of helped), over detailed history-taking or gathering extensive information from the family. We try to only get the information needed to get started with the family.

Before the first meeting, we send out questionnaires to the family. The young person with eating troubles is invited to complete our Eating Concerns Questionnaire and her parents are invited to complete our Eating Concerns Questionnaire for Parents. This provides us with much-needed access to multiple perspectives and details about some of the practicalities of the situation, like what happens at mealtimes. We find that these questionnaires can also help families tell us something about their beliefs about change, their explanatory models of eating difficulties, and the real-life effects of these concerns on the family and young person's life. We also send the family the "Worries Questionnaire" (Rober, 2017) and invite all members of the family to complete it. The Worries Questionnaire is not a measuring instrument, it is a conversational tool that is meant to "help the family and the therapist broaden the dialogical space and to talk about things that can't be talked about at home..." and "...focus on worries, rather than on the so-called problem or on the diagnosis of the identified patient" (Rober, 2017, p. 67). We have found that the Worries Questionnaire provides us with insight into the severity of concerns, expectations, and the similarities and differences between family members. It helps us hear the quieter voices in the family, those who might need more help to express their concerns. We hypothesize that the act of completing these questionnaires before coming starts the healing and dialogical process well before the meeting begins.

The young person and their family are always encouraged to invite to the first meeting other important people in their life. The valuing of participation of important people mobilizes support for the family and usually results in them becoming important partners in the healing process. The young person is often a child or adolescent and so our approach is to work with their family and caregivers. We usually encourage all members of the family to participate in the meeting but view the parents and the young person as best placed to determine who should come along. This is particularly true when there are very young children in the family or when a family is split and living across different households. When the young person is a young adult or older adolescent, this approach is broadened, and we try to hold a social network perspective. Informed by the Open Dialogue approach to working with psychosis (Seikkula & Alakare, 2011), the young person in distress is encouraged to consider whom to invite to the first meeting. To help with this, they are usually asked about who else knows about their difficulties, who could be of help and how they should be invited.

At the all-important first meeting special attention is paid to calming the system, getting the young person engaged in thinking about solutions, finding strengths to build on, and creating a reasonable plan of action. Through empathy and with respect and concern for both the young person and the family, we can make thoughtful decisions about what's most important to start working on. We use a collaborative-dialogic process that focuses on the importance of being listened to and together we try to explore some new ideas about the social and relational implications of the situation. We use the family's feedback to create a dialogical space that attends to the process and outcome of the meeting and allows us to reorient and make adjustments along the way. As a common factors-informed approach (Davis & Hsieh, 2019) the meeting emphasizes relationships, relational responding, healing over therapy, and usefulness over truthfulness. Therapists working in the program work hard to locate resources for change in the family and the young person in distress and purposefully and humbly offer expertise and authentic relationships throughout their healing journey.

Our first family meeting is an intensive first encounter with the young person, their family and our multi-disciplinary team. Relinquishing terms like "assessment" and other clinical and diagnostic jargon and adopting the language of the family allows us to begin meeting families and young people in a collaborative way and to adapt to their needs and preferences. Each meeting could be described as a live consultation with a young person and family/network including two therapists and a consulting team, lasting about two hours. The two therapists in the room approach the meeting from a curious, "not-knowing" stance (Anderson & Goolishian, 1992), and bring into the conversation what they have learned from the family through their Worries Questionnaires. The consulting team is positioned behind a one-way mirror listening to the talk with the family, in a similar way to Tom Andersen's (1987) original reflecting teams.

During the first swap over the team talked together about what they had heard the family talking about. They were wondering about what the family might call what is going on? They heard Bella talk about it as a "habit." They noted how quickly everyone had responded to these worries and how it is still really early days. For the next part of the meeting, they wondered if the family could talk about how quickly they want to break the habit, for some it is easier to go quickly, others prefer slowly. Sometimes it works better for Bella to give responsibility to her parents, and they wondered if this might work as it seems that Bella has previously trusted her parents. The dietitian talked about how much food Bella would need and wondered about what support she might need to be able to do that. The nurse was able to provide feedback on Bella's current physical state and provided advice on physical recovery. The family peer worker shared some of her own experience of having a daughter with an eating problem; she resonated with the guilt John and Mary described. She offered some ideas about how her family supported her daughter.

Being client-led and needs-adapted, the therapeutic process and style of the meeting change each time. This includes what is talked about, and how the consulting-reflecting team is utilized throughout the meeting. These adaptations are driven by the family and through the use of the feedback they provide throughout the process. What happens next is also uncertain prior to the meeting and is determined with each family towards the end of the meeting, or afterwards at an agreed follow-up point. All families are provided with a copy of the meeting summary document completed by a member of the consulting team, to take away with them.

Bella and her parents attended a follow-up meeting with their case manager and the dietitian. She and her parents had developed a sound plan for Bella's eating. They were working together to manage her exercise and putting in place lots of alternate strategies to help Bella manage her distress. Bella was continuing to talk to her parents about her fears and struggles and she and her sister Carrie were spending lots of time together. At two weeks from the first meeting, Bella had gained 5 kgs (11 lbs.) and was continuing to work collaboratively with her parents towards her recovery.

Case managers who continue on with the family also join the important first meeting and provide psychological continuity for the family. Operating from the stance of "resources on tap, not on top" most families are seen once or twice with the team, and case managers can invite the team back for a meeting at any time that feels useful or needed.

Conclusion

In the last three years, the number of new cases coming to the service has continued to increase. We have met approximately 100 families this way from January 2019 to June 2020. Many of these families decide to come back only once or twice for some brief follow-up after the first meeting and tell us that they have resolved their worries or are feeling confident to be able to go on. Although we have not yet completed our formal evaluation of the program we also notice, as in Bella's situation, the therapeutic gains achieved in the weeks after the first meeting are significant and such signs of early progress provide us with optimism about the overall outcome for these young people. For those that continue on with us, their involvement is usually of a shorter duration and their lives and relationships restored in ways that are much easier than in our previous way of working. We find that young people who come with their families to meet with us in this way are more able to find a voice in the conversation. By emphasizing the experience of listening to each other and by having the experience of being listened to, family members often feel better understood and are more able to be part of the shared discovery of solutions. Unlike our previous way of working, we work hard to hear the voice of the young person and help those around them hear their voice too. It is our experience that this helps young people be part of the healing process, rather than experiencing others as trying to do it for them. Positioning families and loved ones as partners in the healing process bolsters their existing strengths and restores their confidence in being able to help the young person through the crisis. By believing that the opportunity of the meeting may not happen again and that "all we have is now" we work to find solutions that they can implement together immediately. It is our experience that, informed by ideas about single session thinking and practice, Collaborative First Family Meetings are healing encounters that help young people with eating problems to become engaged in solutions, and to reconnect with those who love them at a time in their lives where they feel troubled, overwhelmed, and un-reachable.

Note

1 *Editors' note*: For more on headspace single session programs, see Fuzzard, Chapter 12 of this volume.

References

Andersen, T. (1987). The reflecting team: Dialogue and meta-dialogue in clinical work. *Family Process*, *26*, 415–428. doi:10.1111/j.15455300.1987.00415.x

Anderson, H., & Goolishian, H. (1992). The client is the expert: A not-knowing approach to therapy. In S. McNamee & K.J. Gergen (Eds.), *Therapy as Social Construction* (pp. 25–39). Newbury Park, CA: SAGE.

Barbara-May, R., Denborough, P., & McGrane, T. (2018). Development of a single-session family program at Child and Youth Mental Health Services, Southern Melbourne. In M.F. Hoyt, M. Bobele, A. Silve, J. Young, & M. Talmon (Eds.), *Single Session Therapy by Walk-In or Appointment: Administrative, Clinical, and Supervisory Aspects of One-at-a-Time Services* (pp. 104–115). New York: Routledge.

Davis, S.D., & Hsieh, A.L. (2019). What does it mean to be a common factors informed family therapist? *Family Process*, *58*, 629–640. doi:10.1111/famp.12477

Fry, D. (2012). Implementing single session family consultation: A reflective team approach. *Australian and New Zealand Journal of Family Therapy*, *33*, 54–69. doi:10.1017/aft.2012.6

Haarakangas, K., Seikkula, J., Alakare, B., & Aaltonen, J. (2007). Open dialogue: An approach to psychotherapeutic treatment of psychosis in northern Finland. In H. Anderson & D. Gehart (Eds.), *Collaborative Therapy: Relationships and Conversations that Make a Difference* (pp. 221–233). New York: Routledge.

Rober, P. (2017). *In Therapy Together: Family Therapy as a Dialogue*. London: Palgrave Macmillan. Retrieved from https://doi.org/ 10.1057/978-1-137-60765-2

Seikkula, J., & Alakare, B. (2011). Open dialogue with psychotic patients and their families. In M. Romme & S. Escher (Eds.), *Psychosis as a Personal Crisis: An Experience-Based Approach* (pp. 178–193). New York: Routledge.

Section VII

Editors' Conclusion

31 Single Session Thinking and Practice – Themes, Lessons, and a Look Toward the Future

Michael F. Hoyt, Jeff Young, and Pam Rycroft

> "Remember then: there is only one time that is important – Now! It is the most important time, because it is the only time when we have any power."
>
> – Leo Tolstoy (1885, *What Men Live By, and Other Tales*)

The preceding chapters have provided a rich array of concepts and methods. In this final section, we will first describe some general themes involved in Single Session Thinking and Practice, highlighting how different authors in the present volume actualize them. We will then turn to several other issues; and will conclude with answers to some Frequently Asked Questions.

Common Themes

Four themes (with variations) inform Single Session Thinking and Practice:

1. *Attitude*, which involves the realization, supported by research, that you may only have one session and hence should make the most of it. As Bob Rosenbaum (in Hoyt, Rosenbaum, & Talmon, 1992, p. 77) wrote: "Training clinicians in SST is more a question of inculcating a certain attitude than it is of passing on a set of techniques." Stephen Appelbaum (1973) noted the operation of "Parkinson's Law in Psychotherapy" – work (and therapy) tends to expand or contract to fit the time allotted. The structure of a *single* session concentrates the mind. Thus, Jay Haley (1977) would often ask, "If we were only going to meet once or a few times, what problem would you want to focus on solving at this point in time?" and Robert and Mary Goulding (1979) would ask, "What are you willing to change today?"

   One of us (PR) recalls a productive conversation in which a father and daughter reflected on their single session. The 15-year-old bubble-gum-chewing girl exclaimed, "I thought there was no point in bullshittin'!" and went on to compare it to her every-week experience with a school counselor where they talked about the week but, as she put it, they "didn't get to any real stuff."

In the present volume, Flavio Cannistrà notes in Chapter 6 that it is the therapist's (and client's) *mindset* that guides the choice of theory and method. Bob Rosenbaum (Chapter 7) explores how the ways that one conceptualizes time may undergird thinking about single session practice, and Rycroft and Young (Chapter 3) invite us to "make time your friend." Martin Söderquist, Malena Cronholm-Nouicer, Lars Dannerup, and Karin Wulff (Chapter 15) describe "taking the leap" to a one-at-a-time (OAAT) mindset.

2. *Accessibility*, which involves responding quickly to take advantage of clients' motivation by not putting any unnecessary barriers in the way of them seeing a therapist when they're ready (sometimes called "Capturing the Moment" – Young & Rycroft, 1997; Hoyt & Talmon, 2014). We endeavor to be "on time in brief therapy" (Hoyt, 1990/ 2017). Although it might be a bit of an exaggeration to say, following Shakespeare (*Hamlet*, Act V, Scene 2), that "the readiness is ALL," whether by appointment or by open access walk-in it is important to "strike while the iron is hot" (Hoyt, 2011, p. xi) in order to capitalize on clients' motivation.

In the present volume, our Editors' Introduction (Chapter 1) reviews some of the advantages of both by-appointment and by walk-in approaches. Monte Bobele and Arnie Slive (Chapter 4) and Nancy McElheran (Chapter 11) cogently highlight the advantages of open access. Good accounts of by-appointment single session services are provided by Rycroft and Young in Chapter 3; by Brendan O'Hanlon and Naomi Rottem in Chapter 5; by Alix Robinson, Grace Harvey, Molly McDonald, and Turi Honegger in Chapter 13; and by Pat Boyhan in Chapter 16.

3. *Action*, which involves the understanding that there is really no time but the present and that the best opportunity to address change is NOW, no matter the diagnosis, severity or complexity of the problem. This entails helping the client to feel empowered and instrumental (not passive or powerless) – which Terry Soo-Hoo (2019) refers to as "client activation" and Karin Schlanger and Esther Krohner (2019) imply in their phrase "Our clients *are* able and strong." James Prochaska (1999) also gets at this when he talks about readiness and the stages of change. Rubin Battino (2006, 2014) highlights the importance of expectation in SST and very brief therapy, the belief that something good is about to occur. Along similar lines, Michael Yapko (1990, p. 191) noted:

What determines whether a client will benefit from brief therapy interventions? I suggest that a principal factor is his or her primary temporal orientation, evident in general life-style as well as in the presenting problem(s). Another factor is the individual's general value regarding 'change.' Is the client more invested in maintaining tradition or in seeking change? A third factor is the client's belief system about what constitutes a complete therapeutic experience.

In *The First Session in Brief Therapy*, Budman, Friedman, and Hoyt (1992, p. 351) observed:

> The brief therapist who is attempting to help his or her patients use treatment in the most productive, time-effective manner possible is advised [... that although] there are widely varied possibilities for the proficient practice of such treatment, the successful clinician "hits the ground running." It is unlikely that treatment that fails to quickly set a tone of active, dynamic intervention and change will lead to celeritous, positive outcomes.

While some clients may stop after one session because they did not find it helpful, others may elect to stop after one – as the chapters in this volume and other publications illustrate – because they came seeking one session and the session provided what they were looking for. Clients want help in a first meeting – and are unlikely to benefit from one session or return for more – if the first encounter is essentially an "intake" procedure in which they are "assessed" but do not come away engaged, encouraged, and with new ideas and skills (see Chow, 2018; Taibbi, 2016). Therapists should be oriented toward and equipped to enhance the possibility of successful SST, and clients should have the choice whether to have one or more than one session.[1]

In the present volume, Hoyt (Chapter 2) emphasizes the importance of inspiring hope, the belief that it is possible to make things better; Sophia Sorensen (Chapter 21) writes of "finding hope in remote places." Client activation and empowerment also are pursued when, in Chapter 3, Rycroft and Young describe how they help their clients focus on what they hope to get from the session, asking what they want to walk away with and checking that the work is on track at different points during the meeting; in Chapter 14, when Windy Dryden explores with his client what are her target issues and specific session goal; in Chapter 20, when Alison Elliott and James Dokona describe making sure that they are honoring clients' goals for the session through deep listening rather than imposing the therapists' ideas of what should be the focus of discussion. Kieran O'Loughlin (Chapter 19) makes explicit the importance, when doing counseling with people having just received an HIV diagnosis, that the single session therapist be knowledgeable in the issues which that particular population is likely to face. The enhanced efficiency of the therapist having both single session training and topical clinical expertise is also demonstrated in the respective reports by Stacey Rabba (Chapter 17, on working with families dealing with autism); by Bonita Cohen, Greta Daley, and Vicky Northe (Chapter 28, on helping individuals and their families affected by problem gambling); by Rosalie Birkin (Chapter 18, on consulting parents concerned about infants); by Martin Söderquist et al. (Chapter 15, on working with couples); and by Carmel Fleming and by Rachel Barbara-May (Chapters 29 and 30, respectively) on assisting individuals and their families dealing with eating disorders.

4. *Alliance*, which involves asking about and honoring what clients want to achieve by the end of the session so that the therapist and client can work collaboratively as allies, in the here and now, to achieve the clients' goals. Mary Goulding and Robert Goulding (1979) referred to the "therapeutic contract"; John Walter and Jane Peller (1994) called this "goaling"; Chris Iveson, Evan George, and Harvey Ratner (2012, p. 1) note that the typical therapeutic process of moving *away* from a problem was reconstructed by Steve de Shazer as a process of moving *towards* a solution; Hoyt (2000/2017, p. 33) used the metaphor of golf and observed that, "It's a long day on the course if you don't know where the hole is." Barry Duncan and Scott Miller (2000) evoke the image of the "heroic client" to be assisted via *client*-directed outcome-oriented therapy, and Miller, Mark Hubble, and Daryl Chow (2020) have developed instruments for Feedback Informed Treatment (FIT) to make sure that the client's goals are being served.

The therapeutic alliance is the soil in which all else may take root.[2] *Alliance* implies being allies, *working on the same team toward a common goal* (Bordin, 1979; Norcross, 2011). There are many illustrations in this volume of how clinicians connect and build rapport, including by showing keen respect for clients' worldviews and goals. As already mentioned, in Chapter 14 Windy Dryden illustrates how he and his client consider and co-create a goal for their session. In the chapters featured in *Section V: Applications in Cross-Cultural/Non-Western Contexts*, all the authors emphasize the importance of being culturally attuned and attending to client-defined goals. In Chapter 20, Alison Elliott and James Dokona in their interview with Henry von Doussa describe how their single session practice with Aboriginal families of carefully listening and actually making it about what the family wants to talk about is a decolonizing approach that is, in itself, therapeutic and healing. Sophia Sorensen (Chapter 21) also notes the importance of allowing Indigenous clients to set the goals and pace of the session; in Chapter 22 about working with Māori clients in *Aotearoa* New Zealand, Bronwyn Dunnachie, Stacey Porter, and Karin Isherwood note that even suggesting a time limit for the single session may be experienced as imposing a Western framework. Consistent with Michael White's (in Hoyt, 2001; also see Andreas, 2014) distinction between "direction and discovery," in Chapter 24, Rafael Núñez and Jorge Abia describe how their single session group hypnotherapy instructions provide a general direction but, in Ericksonian style, invite the clients to fill in the specifics in order to make their own discoveries about what they find calming and healing. In Chapter 25, Tess McGrane and Ron Findlay give charming examples of practice innovations intended to make family SST more friendly and effective.

Sometimes clients return over time for multiple OAAT/SSTs. They may see the same clinician for repeat or serial SSTs; or if sessions occur at an agency where at each visit they see a different clinician, they may form an alliance with the service or organization or with the idea of "therapy" rather than with a particular therapist.[3] In the present volume, examples of *sequential* (Battino, 2014) or *serial* (Bobele et al., 2018) single sessions are provided by Helen Mildred, Lia Hunter, Belinda Goldsworthy, and Peter Brann (Chapter 26) and by Myf Murphy and Denise Fry (Chapter 27).

Different Single Session Theories and Models[4]

The search [is] for a conceptualization that would allow a viable and parsimonious solution. The therapist needs to be versatile, innovative, and pragmatic, asking: "What would help this patient today?" Patients may need to begin a process or complete a process; they may need to take hold or to let go; they may need reassurance or confrontation; they may need to look at something deeply or to shift perspective. [...] Nothing works all the time, but what might work this time? (Hoyt, Rosenbaum, & Talmon, 1992, p. 63)

Writing from his theoretical perspective, Chris Iveson (2019, p. 121; also see Anderson & Goolishian, 1992) said:

My professional world, the world of Solution-Focused Brief Therapy, is a topsy-turvy world where success still depends on trust – but on the therapist trusting the client rather than the other way around [...] Taking the radical position that we cannot know (or prescribe) the "right" way forward for our clients, we have to trust their knowledge and treat them as the only experts in their own lives[5].

Most of the authors in this volume favor SST approaches that align with similar "trust the client – they know what's best" sentiments.[6] Focusing on what the client wants can create a fruitful collaboration between two expertises: the client's lived experience and the practitioner's professional knowledge. Both contribute to the synergy, as Windy Dryden (2020, p. 283) has articulated:

It is a core feature of SST/OAAT therapy that it is client-centered especially where the session's focus and goal are concerned. However, in an attempt to avoid SST/OAAT therapy being highjacked by therapists who operate from the "expert" source of influence, the field has downplayed the contribution of the therapist's expertise ... [T]he expertise of the therapist when allied to the expertise of the client can be a potent force for good in SST/OAAT therapy.

After identifying a client's goals, in one session the therapist could make an interpretation (*à la* David Malan et al.'s 1968 and 1975 psychodynamic studies at the Tavistock Clinic in London); or challenge the client's dysfunctional way of thinking/behaving and perhaps teach a skill (*à la* Albert Ellis and Windy Dryden – see Chapter 14); or see an unsuccessful attempted solution and block it (*à la* MRI; see Hoyt & Bobele, 2019; Vitry, de Scorraille, & Hoyt, in press); or externalize the problem and do narrative therapy (*à la* Karen Young 2018, 2020) or put the problem in another chair and do Gestalt therapy; or give directives to restructure family hierarchies (*à la* Salvador Minuchin or Jay Haley). Our particular theoretical "lenses" (Hoffman, 1990; also see Cannistrà on "mindset," Chapter 6) influence our thinking and practice. Milton Erickson would typically take a hierarchical Therapist-as-Expert position. Erickson also strongly believed, however, in clients' capacities – his *utilization* approach (see Short, 2020; Short, Erickson, & Klein, 2005) was based on his efforts to awaken and engage clients' resources in the service of what the clients want. Of all Erickson's known cases – most of which yielded successful outcomes – one session was the most frequent length of therapy (O'Hanlon & Hexum, 1990; Hoyt, 2000). The developer of Motivational Interviewing, William Miller (2000), has also described positive results in one session.

Some other single session approaches can be seen in this sample of statements from leading practitioners of differing theoretical persuasions:

- "Before each group session I pause and ask myself, 'How can I cure everyone in this room *today*?'" (Eric Berne, founder of Transactional Analysis, quoted by Mary Goulding & Robert Goulding, 1979, p. 4)
- "The idea behind playing as communication is that if we know about regression in the analytic hour, we can meet it immediately and in this way enable certain [...] patients to make the necessary regressions in short phases, perhaps even almost momentarily." (D.W. Winnicott, child psychoanalyst, 1958, p. 261)
- "In a surprising number of cases, people may require no more than an initial interview to precipitate lasting change and achieve profound behavioral readjustment." (Arnold Lazarus, multimodal behavior therapist, 1971, p. 50)
- "From a strategic point of view [...] one can guide the patient to discover new perceptions that determine new reactions to the problem right from the first session. In so doing, we subtlety introduce a chain reaction of changes: knowing through changing [pp. 23–24] [...] By leading the first session this way over the past four years, we found that 69–70% of patients had their symptoms reduced to zero between the first and the second session. These results are reflective of the majority of the psychopathologies treated with this method." (Giorgio Nardone & Alessandro Salvini, 2007/2018, p. 27)
- "I believe that the inpatient group therapist must consider the life of the group to be only a single session." (Irvin Yalom & Molyn Leszcz, 2005, p. 488)
- "In contrast to *Feeling Good* (Burns, 1980), which was all about the cognitive revolution, this book is all about the motivation revolution. It is based on the simple idea that we sometimes get 'stuck' in depression and anxiety because we have mixed feelings about recovery. [...] Through a new approach called TEAM-CBT, you can overcome this resistance and achieve recovery quickly. [p. xv] [...] The entire process took less than an hour and was so joyful. [...] In fact, the final part where she challenged her negative thoughts [...] took less than ten minutes. You *can* change the way you feel, and it *can* happen really fast." [p. 34] (David D. Burns, 2020)
- "I suspect that the most successful outcomes were in the families I only saw once. Forcing the family members to get together and making them think about the family for one hour gave them enough experience to do something about their setup on their own, in their own way, and without ever letting me know about it". (Carl Whitaker, family therapist, 1992, p. 18)

These various examples underscore, as Söderquist et al. (Chapter 15) put it, that "There are many different roads to Rome, as the saying goes, and there are many ways for [...] counselors to make the leap to an OAAT mindset."

What Are Some Single Session Thinking and Practice Ideas to Take with You When You See a Client?

There are many different ways to translate single session thinking into practice (see Talmon & Hoyt, 2014, pp. 473–478). Bloom (1981/1992) offered 15 transtheoretical suggestions:

1. Identify a focal problem
2. Do not underestimate clients' strengths
3. Be prudently active
4. Explore, then present interpretations tentatively
5. Encourage the expression of affect
6. Use the interview to start a problem-solving process
7. Keep track of time
8. Do not be overambitious
9. Keep factual questions to a minimum
10. Do not be overly concerned about the precipitating event
11. Avoid detours
12. Do not overestimate a client's self-awareness (i.e., don't ignore what may seem obvious)
13. Help mobilize social supports
14. Educate when patients appear to lack information
15. Build in a follow-up plan.

Rosenbaum, Hoyt, and Talmon (1990) highlighted:

1. "Seed" change through induction and preparation
2. Develop an alliance by co-creating, with the client, obtainable treatment goals
3. Allow enough time for the session to be a complete process or intervention
4. Look for ways to meet clients in their worldview while, at the same time, offering a new perspective or hope about the possibility of seeing and acting differently
5. Go slowly and look for the client's strengths and resources
6. Focus on "pivot chords," ambiguous situations that can be reframed in therapeutic ways
7. Practice solutions experientially, using the session to help clients rehearse a solution or solutions, thus inspiring hope, readiness for change, and forward movement
8. Consider taking a time-out, break, or pause during the session to think, consult, focus, prepare, and punctuate
9. Allow time for last-minute issues, to help the client have the sense that the session has been complete and satisfactory

10. Give feedback, emphasizing the client's understanding and competency to make changes
11. Leave the door open, follow up, and let the client decide if the session has been sufficiently helpful or if another session (or more) is needed.

Reporting on his experience of providing and directing single session disaster counseling in the wake of Hurricane Katrina, John Miller (2011) recommended:

1. Therapy begins at the first moment of meeting, often focused by the first question: "What is the single most important concern that you have right now?"
2. Seeking client resources, often with questions such as: "What things have you tried?" and "What inner strengths would be useful for us to know about?"
3. Helping clients prioritize problems and goals, as guided by the question: "What will be the smallest change to show you that things are heading in the right direction?"
4. Focusing on pragmatism versus any specific model or intervention, evaluation of results being based on whether the session was able to meet the client's stated goal, not on whether the problem was entirely resolved. Helping clients to adjust to and deal with the range of needs and emotions that emerge from the trauma is primary.
5. Fostering a relationship with the service rather than an individual therapist by informing the client at the end of the session that they can return as needed and desired, and that another worker will be available and would welcome talking with them.

Arnie Slive and Monte Bobele (2011, p. 136) described 11 principles:

1. The session is only one hour
2. Within that hour, we have a whole therapeutic session
3. We narrow the database to the immediate problem
4. We look for common factors
5. The therapist's therapeutic influences are tempered with pragmatism
6. The session involves a consultation with other therapists
7. The therapists focus on what the client wants from the session
8. We seek to understand the client's resources
9. We explore the client's previous attempts at a solution
10. We make use of the client's own motivations
11. We commend the client.

Writing within the context of single session hospital social work, Jill Gibbons and Debbie Plath (2012, p. 52) outlined eight practice guidelines:

1. Manage the immediate situation
2. Explain the system
3. Make an expert assessment
4. Set clear parameters and realistic goals for the session
5. Advocate for the client and negotiate with the system
6. Provide access to practical assistance
7. Provide information that can be accessed in the future....
8. Review goals and resources as part of closure.

Karen Paul and Mark van Ommeran (2013) also provided a valuable primer on the potential application of walk-in SSTs in acute emergency situations. Echoing some of Miller's (2011) suggestions, they advised:

1. Use various evidence-based approaches and techniques that fit your training, skill level, experience, and the client's presenting needs
2. Ensure that the approaches and techniques fit within the culture or context
3. Keep the client focused on what is happening in the moment
4. Recognize that a single session is good for some people, but not for others
5. Allow couples, individuals and small groups to participate in a session together
6. Help clients create a relationship with the service rather than an individual professional
7. Consider how providing single session services can help strengthen the existing mental healthcare delivery system
8. Provide the service in an accessible location where those who need help can access it at the time of need (community halls, schools, information centers, etc.)
9. Ensure cooperation between single session service providers and professionals within the broader mental healthcare and psychosocial support system.

Windy Dryden (2019, 2020), working from an integrated SST/rational emotive behavior therapy approach and offering one-off sessions in a public forum, also articulated the main features of an SST/OAAT mindset:

1. Celebrate the power of "now" and create a realistic expectation for SST/OAAT therapy
2. Ask the client how you may best help them
3. Develop an end-of-session goal
4. Agree on a focus for the session
5. Keep on track

6. Identify and utilize client strengths
7. Encourage the client to use environmental resources
8. Identify and utilize the client's previous attempts to deal with the problem
9. Negotiate a solution
10. Encourage the client to rehearse the solution
11. Encourage the client to reflect on the session, digest what they have learned, act on it, let time pass before seeking further help.

Rycroft and Young (in Chapter 3 and in their online training – see https://events.bouverie.org.au/sst) offer a distillation of 10 core elements:

1. Negotiating a client-led outcome
2. Establishing the client's (or clients') priorities
3. Finding a focus and talking about the most important things ("cutting to the chase")
4. Checking in with the client(s) at regular intervals
5. Interrupting respectfully when necessary (to help clients get what they want)
6. Making time your friend
7. Preparing to end well (reaching closure if not solution or resolution)
8. Sharing your thoughts openly with clients
9. Leaving the door open (an "open door" policy)
10. Listening to client voices (following up, seeking feedback, and utilizing it).

Alistair Campbell (2012, p. 16) noted that:

> SST is not a therapeutic model in itself, and that almost any therapeutic orientation could be adapted to working in a single-session way. The key aspect of the general frame is to ensure that the client walks away from a single session with a plan about how to solve their problem, the confidence that they have the skills and resources available, and the knowledge that they can come back at any time for further work.

We will leave it to the reader to decide what are the essential common elements of these single session practice lists, but the genuine collaboration between therapist and client to address in a focused way what the client wants changed in their life is basic.

Terminology

As we discuss in Hoyt, Young, and Rycroft (2020) and in Chapter 1, to help move the field forward we suggest that the overarching term *Single*

Session Thinking be used to describe the principles highlighted in the previous section; the generic *Single Session Therapy* (*SST*) be used to designate clinical therapeutic models (individual and couple, as well as group and family) that are implemented using single session principles; and that the term *Single Session Work* (*SSW*) be used to refer to other, non-clinical applications. Although Hampson et al. (1999) in Canberra earlier had used the term *Single Session Family Consultation* (*SSFC*) to refer to a single session approach to family therapy, The Bouverie Centre also used the term Single Session Family Consultation when it combined Single Session Thinking with ideas from Family Consultations (Wynne & Wynne, 1986) to assist practitioners working in individually oriented organizations to engage families in a structured way in order to enhance treatment outcomes (see Chapter 5). This practice has spread across Australia and New Zealand, and we suggest that *Single Session Family Consultation* (*SSFC*) be reserved for those times one (or a one-at-a-time) family meeting is held in the course of a client's ongoing individual work.

The Power of Family Contexts

Families (and family therapy) are a "crucible" (Napier & Whitaker, 1978) in which we are formed and can change. As Cathy Renkin, Karen Alexander, and Marianne Wyder (Chapter 8, italics in original) wrote: *"Family is personal for us. It is a source of inspiration, identity and re-lationships. It is also a meaning-making experience we draw on heavily in all our work."* Renkin et al. also note that "family" may be defined to include unpaid carers, relatives, and friends – not just those people who share DNA. In this book, many chapters illustrate aspects of working with families, including the important practice development of sometimes conducting Single Session Family Consultations (SSFC) with the whole family in the course of an individual client's ongoing 1:1 ther-apeutic work.

The Power of Cultural Contexts

Bruce Wampold (2015) noted:

> The contextual model emphasizes that the explanation given for the patient's distress and the therapy actions must be acceptable to the patient. [...] There are many ways to adapt treatments, including those involving language, cultural congruence of therapist and patient, cultural rituals, and explanations adapted to the "myth" of the group.

We need to learn about, from, and with one another (see Lewis & Cheshire, 2007; Miller, 2014). Therapy can be much more effective and efficient if you work within someone's cultural context, and especially if you don't work against their culture. What works in one setting may not translate or fit well in another (Soo-Hoo, 2018; Hoyt, 2019, p. 38), so we expect that there will be increasing attention to the different strengths in different cultures, how they go about it, valuing the diverse belief systems that people embrace.

Richard Fisch (1994, pp. 126–127, emphases in original) observed:

> If one were to take a historic perspective, one might see that, throughout the history of mankind, "therapy" was *always* brief [...] "Therapy" was brief until the advent of psychoanalytic concepts and practices near the turn of this [the 20th] century. "Therapy" changed from a *doing* modality in which the change-agent (oracle, shaman, mesmerist, etc.) either *did* something to the troubled/troublesome person and/or had the person *do* something, to an insight or *understanding* modality, one which required a stylized conversation, mostly one-sided. The "patient" was required to be more active in the conversation, the therapist more passive, often meta-communicating about the "patient's" comments.[7]

Several of the chapters in this book, such as John Miller, Xing Dai, Yaorui Hu, and Yilin Xu's account in Chapter 23 (also see Miller, 2014) of their single session family work in China (and in Cambodia – see Miller, Platt, & Conroy, 2018); Bronwyn Dunnachie, Stacey Porter, and Karin Isherwood's descriptions in Chapter 22 of their work in *Aotearoa* New Zealand; Rafael Núñez and Jorge Abia's report in Chapter 24 of their community interventions with Indigenous people in Mexico; Sophia Sorensen's lovely narrative in Chapter 21 of her work with a remote Indigenous community in Western Canada; and the already mentioned interview with Elliott and Dokona in Chapter 20 all provide readers with fascinating insights about single sessions in settings different from usual Western office practice. Interestingly, we learn that Australian Aboriginal clients find it healing to know how long a session may last but find it NOT helpful to be directed regarding content, and that *Aotearoa* New Zealand Māori may be offended by being told that they are restricted to a specific time frame; but that the Chinese patients seen by Miller et al. want structure and direction by experts! Coming from their different backgrounds, histories, and beliefs, different cultures want different approaches and SST can accommodate them all – but in different ways.

Single session thinking and practice allow more services to be offered to more people, including to disadvantaged populations. In his classic paper, "The Art of Being a Failure as a Therapist," Haley (1969, p. 76) sardonically wrote:

> Perhaps the most important rule is to ignore the real world that patients live in and publicize the vital importance of their infancy,

inner dynamics, and fantasy life. This will effectively prevent either therapists or patients from attempting to make changes in their families, friends, schools, neighborhoods, or treatment milieus. Naturally they cannot recover if their situation does not change, and so one guarantees failure while being paid to listen to interesting fantasies. Talking about dreams is a good way to pass the time, and so is experimenting with responses to different kinds of pills.

In the same paper (1969, p. 76) – perhaps anticipating the utility of SST with disadvantaged populations – Haley also trenchantly advised: "Avoid the poor because they will insist upon results and cannot be distracted with insightful conversations."[8]

The Power of a Global Perspective

A greater awareness of cultural differences goes hand in hand with the growing applications of single session thinking in different parts of the world. It also helps us to realize that the seeking of help in one session is, and has been, a common expectation in many cultures. Recognition of the elemental principles of single session thinking and the global expansion of single session practice is beginning to generate a movement that is connecting diverse practitioners from around the planet, exploring the paradigm shift inherent in making the most of every encounter.

Researchers: Start Your Engines!

In the conclusion of his 2012 SST review, Alistair Campbell (p. 24) wrote: "[T]he next thing is to accept the potential of single sessions as a vehicle for intervention and recognize the opportunity that they pose for clinical research, using them to ask and answer [...] interesting questions." The field of single session thinking and practice is expanding globally, so there are many opportunities for development of new knowledge. The reader can add to the list, but here are a few we'd like to see explored:

- More documentation of the frequency and effectiveness of different SST approaches – in different countries, with different cultures, and with different clinical problems.
- What are the "active ingredients" that make SSTs effective? As Campbell (2012, p. 24) has written: "The circumscribed nature of the single session (lasting an hour or two) would radically reduce the complexity of any process study. It should be quite straightforward to explore a range of specific and nonspecific process factors that can be associated with positive outcomes over both short- and long-term time frames. [...] The really more interesting questions are: What is happening in a single session that is leading to change? Are these

things happening in the first session of multisession therapies? If so, do they lead to change that is not being recognized or tapped? But also: Is the change that happens in a single session modality specific? Does the therapeutic framework matter or does this just provide a structure for a focused change?"

- There has been considerable research on "common (or nonspecific) factors" (see Duncan, Miller, Wampold, & Hubble, 2009), with "client factors" generally being identified as most determining (about 40%) of outcome variance and "relationship factors" accounting for another 30%. In SSTs, do these percentages still obtain? Will the most important factors vary by country/culture, by problem, and/or by some aspects (such as personality dynamics or family structure) of clients – or of therapists? What differences in alliance (or other factors) may there be between those therapies that are "one-and-done" versus those that are OAAT but involve serial single session meetings? When the decision for possible further sessions is made at a phone call following the session, how can the time between session and phone call be used to support and promote client change?

- How might by-appointment versus walk-in SSTs vary? Will one have more appeal to certain socioeconomic or cultural groups and/or people with different problems? What are the economics of walk-in versus by-appointment arrangements? What is the impact of SSTs on other health service utilization? What is the no-show rate for by-appointment single sessions? Are there effective ways to mitigate by-appointment no-shows (e.g., having clients call to confirm appointments)? Does the no-show rate vary by how many days clients wait for the appointment, and what they may be asked to do while they wait? How many walk-ins per shift or per day are needed to make walk-ins cost-effective?

The Need for Training *and* Implementation

Single session thinking and practice require both learning and application. *Training* is the action of teaching and learning a particular attitude, skill or type of behavior. *Implementation* is the process that turns plans and learning into actions in order to accomplish strategic objectives and goals. If implementation is forgotten, innovative initiatives may appear as "good ideas" but they do not come to fruition.

Previously, Young, Weir, and Rycroft (2012) and Young, Rycroft, and Weir (2014) have outlined steps for successfully implementing single session thinking, starting with the identification of a problem that single session practice addresses, articulating that the approaches fit with the strategic directions and values of the organization and its practitioners, and utilizing the supports of training, ongoing consultation, practice champions, and management. In the present volume, the important role of implementation is highlighted especially in Section III. Cathy Renkin, Karen Alexander, and Marianne Ryder in Chapter 8, for example, and Jillian McDonald, Paul Hickey, and Marianne Wyder in Chapter 9 carefully detail various administrative and organizational steps taken to implement SSFC and SST in a public mental health service in the Australian state of Queensland; in Chapter 11 Suzanne Fuzzard lets us see how SSFC came to be embedded in headspace, an Australia-wide national youth mental health service; and in Chapter 13, Alix Robinson and her colleagues take us through the process they implemented for college students to see a counselor for an SST visit at their university counseling center.

Some Frequently Asked Questions

*   *Isn't SST really just a band-aid until real therapy can be provided?*

Although not everything to everyone, SST *is* "real therapy." It has repeatedly been shown to be effective in terms of both therapeutic outcomes (resolving problems) and in terms of satisfying clients. The belief that "one session can't really be therapy" is an ideological position cloaked in theory, not a reflection of the actual abundant research that supports SST. As Slive and Bobele (2019a, p. 16) have noted: "In an era of a well-intentioned focus on evidence-based practices, it is ironic that the evidence that supports SST is unknown to or ignored by many professionals." Indeed, the efficacy of SST requires a high level of therapeutic skill – SST is basically "good practice" (Rycroft & Young, 2014, p. 156) or, as Gibbons and Plath (2012 p. 39) have said, SST is practice "at its highest level of skill" since the clinician must function quickly and with a high level of adeptness.[9] And, by the way, don't knock "band-aids." As Slive and Bobele (2014, p. 85) have noted, a bandage may be just what is needed to allow natural healing to occur.

*   *Haven't some people even contended that a single session can't be real psychotherapy, since one session doesn't allow time for a healing relationship to form?*

Single sessions of therapy have long been established as scientifically supported forms of psychotherapy. A controversy developed, however, in 2019 in Ontario, Canada, when a regulatory board tried to deny SST hours as credits toward psychologist licensure. As Karen Young and Joseph Jebreen (2020) detail, that wrongheaded effort was thoroughly debunked. In their report, Young and Jebreen quoted our colleague, Bob Rosenbaum (2008, p. 4): "Psychotherapy is neither long nor short; to view it as such sets up a false dichotomy." They went on to write (p. 36):

Psychotherapy depends on moments that are 'therapeutic' where something profound or meaningful shifts for a client. This can happen in one or in more than one session. It is not about length; it is about quality and creating impactful moments in the conversation.

They also noted a recent comment by Talmon (2018, p. 149): "The essence of any psychotherapy is the same as that of SST. It is based on the abilities of the therapist and patient to create a therapeutic alliance in the here-and-now of each therapeutic encounter."[10]

The *APA Dictionary* (https://dictionary.apa.org/single-session-therapy; retrieved September 11, 2020) has given the following definition:

> *Single Session Therapy (SST).* Therapy that ends after one session, usually by choice of the client but also as indicated by the type of treatment (e.g., Ericksonian psychotherapy, solution-focused brief therapy). Some clients claim enough success with one hour of therapy to stop treatment, although some therapists believe that this claim represents a flight into health or temporary relief from symptoms. Preparation for the session (e.g., by telephone) increases the likelihood of the single-therapy session being successful.

- *What about the issue of SST/OAAT clients being at risk? Is it safe? Is it ethical?*

This concern would seem to be based on a misunderstanding: a view of a single session approach being limited to a one-only session with no allowance for identifying urgent or emergency risks, incorporating other resources, offering and planning follow-up, or referral to emergency services, etc. In single session practice, risk is managed by responding explicitly to the client's main or immediate concerns and is addressed in the same way as in any ongoing work (e.g., assessment; safety plan; support; additional services, including hospitalization if needed). Further, we would contend that making services more accessible and responsive is a more ethical approach than asking vulnerable and at-risk clients to fall back on their own resources and/or languish on a waitlist.

- *But with all the complexities in people's lives, how could one session (or one session-at-a-time) really get at the underlying truth?*

In his book, *Sapiens: A Brief History of Humankind*, Yuval Noah Harari (2015, p. 259) writes:

> In 1620 Francis Bacon published a scientific manifesto titled *The New*

Instrument. In it he argued that "knowledge is power." The real test of "knowledge" is not whether it is true, but whether it empowers us. Scientists usually assume that no theory is 100 per cent correct. Consequently, truth is a poor test for knowledge. The real test is utility. A theory that enables us to do new things constitutes knowledge.

What we're getting at here is what William James (1907/1987) called "Pragmatism" – is it useful, does it work? Thus, Giorgio Nardone and Paul Watzlawick (2005, pp. 39–40) wrote: "For the clinician, theories must not be irrefutable truths, but hypotheses related to the world, partial points of view, useful for describing and organizing observable data so as to achieve successful therapies or to correct unsuccessful ones." Similarly, Scott Miller (in Hoyt, Miller, Held, & Matthews, 2001, p. 218; also see Amundson, 1996) said: "Ultimately, the meaning of an idea is in its use."

To quote Harari (2015, p. 238) again:

> What is the difference between describing "how" and explaining "why"? To describe "how" means to reconstruct the series of specific events that led from one point to another. To explain "why" means to find causal connection that account for the occurrence of this particular series of events to the exclusion of all others.

As Evan George, Chris Iveson, and Harvey Ratner (2006, p. 34) have explained: "Steve de Shazer was adamant that solution-focused brief therapy [SFBT] is not a theory. Rather, he stated, it is a description of a way of talking with clients."[11] Just as de Shazer asserted that SFBT was not an explanatory theory but, rather, a model, we're not asserting that single session thinking and practice has all the answers. We're saying that many people find it useful in improving their lives. And even more importantly, the research evidence shows that many people themselves are saying that.

• *What are some locations beyond usual office practice where walk-in SSTs could be available?*

Although generally not crisis interventions unless that is what is called for (Hoyt & Talmon, 2014, p. 13; Bobele & Slive, 2015), there are various reports (e.g., Miller, 2011; Paul & van Ommeren, 2013; Dass-Brailsford & Hage Thomley, 2015; Akerele & Yuryev, 2017; Guthrie, 2018) of SST/WIs occurring in tents, the open air, and makeshift shelters during humanitarian emergency situations. In Section V of this volume, Sorensen (Chapter 21) and Núñez and Abia (Chapter 24) describe traveling to Native villages to provide services; in Chapter 22, Bronwyn Dunnachie,

Stacey Porter, and Karin Isherwood describe attending Māori traditional ceremonies as part of their SSFC implementation efforts. There also have been reports published about SST occurring in taxis (Hoyt & Ritterman, 2012; Malm, 2014) and at IKEA furniture stores (Potkewitz, 2015). A walk-in service could be available in a busy neighborhood shopping mall so that someone might drop in to see a counselor while doing their errands or waiting for an appointment elsewhere (see Slive & Bobele, 2018). At the Melbourne symposium, someone suggested having a space and time available in public libraries where someone could walk in to have a therapy session. An employee assistance program (EAP) could have someone available on-site by appointment or drop in at a large factory or office building. There are also a number of services now available on the internet where one can click in for no-wait counseling. There are clinicians available NOW to take your call. As noted in Chapter 1, single session interventions are very common in behavioral medicine, primary care, medical social work, and emergency rooms (e.g., see Gibbons & Plath, 2012; Rosenberg & McDaniel, 2014; Reiter, Dobmeyer, & Hunter, 2018; Luutonen, Santalahti, Makinen, Vahlberg, & Rautava, 2019) – they are efficacious and efficient and thus welcomed by physicians and other frontline workers. The use of SST in these settings can be expected to increase.

• *How would single session thinking and practice apply in clinical supervision?*

Just as in SST and other single session work, *single session supervision* involves structuring each meeting to have a clear beginning, middle, and end. One could think about the parts of the supervision session in various ways. There can be an opening "Exposition" section that introduces themes for the particular meeting, a "Development" section that explores variations, and a last "Recapitulation" section that returns to and resolves the original themes (Rycroft, 2018, p. 349). Hoyt (1991/1995) observed that there is sometimes a parallel process between therapy and supervision, in which phase-specific (beginning, middle, ending of a therapy session) aspects of the client–therapist relationship get repeated in the therapist–supervisor relationship.

Rycroft and Young (2014) describe several exercises used to help supervisees reflect on how they approach SST clients so that they view each contact as complete in itself – including ways to co-create with the client a shared session goal, how to stay on track, and how to end successfully. Other authors (e.g., Bedggood, 2018; Harper-Jaques, 2018) have highlighted different aspects of SST training and supervision. In Chapter 23 in this volume, Miller and his colleagues in Shanghai describe a seven-step protocol in which at each single session family session trainees receive feedback from both the family and their supervisor.

- *What effect(s) do you think the Covid-19 pandemic and the shift toward more online therapy will have on SST?*

We're still early on in this world of the "new normal." Like many places, The Bouverie Centre had to do a very rapid and major reconfiguration of services. As clinicians and clients get used to the technology, we're seeing some very interesting effects. Clients seem to want to get down to the nitty-gritty quickly, so they like the idea of SST. There is also a kind of "virtual" distance (talking to a face on a screen) that allows some folks to open up quickly about personal matters. At the same time, it's a bit like making home visits – you can often see what's behind them in the room (and they can see your space, too!) and get some sense of what their real-life situation is like. Some clients feel more comfortable in their own space and maybe the unspoken power differential of therapist and client levels out a bit. Anxieties about illness and jobs, of course, are especially big right now – but for many people, they quickly move past those and get into the usual topics of family, relationships, and various life difficulties. Doing couple and family work online is interesting – do they all sit in front of one screen or go to their separate spaces and use their individual devices? (In Chapter 25, by the way, Tess McGrane and Ron Findlay suggest sometimes allowing an upset teenager to go to another room to communicate via Facetime or Zoom as a way to modulate family tensions.) There are some additional issues regarding risk management online versus in the office, including if you're doing a session online and the client says something very worrisome, and then goes off-line, to whom do you report it – the local authorities in your community, or theirs? And online, people may be more mobile – they're not physically there in your office with you – hence, it is important to follow online protocols (e.g., see bouverie.org.au) such as setting up risk management processes and gaining contact details before the online therapeutic work begins. Some of these are more general issues, of course, than specific to single session thinking and practice – but in terms of SST, SST online is still SST.

- *Could you also give a couple of single session thinking and practice examples from non-therapy situations?*

Sure. Back in 1982, Kenneth Blanchard and Spencer Johnson published *The One Minute Manager*. Iveson et al. (2012) and Harvey Ratner and Denise Yusuf (2015) have described ways that solution-focused thinking can be used in brief (including one session) coaching. One might consult one time with a cooking instructor, an interior home designer, a computer technologist, or a sports coach (see Giges and Peitpas, 2000; Pitt, Thomas, Lindsay, Hanton, & Bawden, 2015) – they would ascertain what skills you already have and what you're looking for, try to assist you in getting there, and not necessarily expect another session. Visits to the garden nursery or the home improvement center are usually one at a time – they're complete unto themselves, until the next round.

A Look Toward the Future

Single session therapy – and by extension, single session thinking and practice – is not a panacea and should not be oversold, imposed, or forced, but when offered as a choice, many people choose one session and find it helpful (see Cummings, 2000). There should be, and we fully expect that there will be, more SST/OAAT services offered both by-appointment and as walk-ins, both face-to-face and online, and through talk or text. As evidence for the frequency, effectiveness, efficiency, and application of a single session mindset and methods in new contexts continues to expand internationally (see Dryden, 2021; Hoyt & Dryden, 2018; Young & Dryden, 2019; Talmon & Dryden, 2021), there will be more research, more publications, and more training (both in person and online). Clients, providers, families, policymakers, funders, and society will all benefit.

As part of an SST/OAAT mindset, at the end of a meeting – even though it is complete unto itself – thought may be given to next steps and what might occasion another meeting. By parallel process, at the end of the 2019 Melbourne symposium, there was discussion and it was decided that there would be, when the time was ripe, another international symposium. We're not sure yet exactly when, but we hope to see you there … probably in Rome!

Notes

1 Unfortunately, studies of so-called "drop-outs" often do not ask the clients why they had stopped treatment, and there may be no consideration or mention of the possibility of successful one session (or other brief) therapy (see Hoyt et al., 2018, pp. 9–10). If they came for one session and achieved what they sought, they might be designated as "completers" (or "SST graduates") rather than "drop-outs."

2 Although sometimes overlooked or taken for granted in discussions about SST (or other brief therapies), the therapeutic alliance has been the focus of several recent qualitative studies. Nozomo Ozaki (2017) conducted a conversational analysis of therapist–client patterns in an SST, highlighting moment-to-moment collaborative interactions; a report by Catalina Perdomo (2017) described using a single session narrative approach to help a client re-author trauma; Kristin Matthews (2018) examined the integration of emotion-focused therapy (EFT) within SST, noting the importance of a strong therapeutic alliance; a conversational analysis by Chrystal Fullen (2020) of an SST depicted how therapist and client co-construct the therapeutic alliance; another conversational analytic study by Jesse Henneberry (2021) illustrated how in one session therapist and client co-construct the client's identity.

3 This has sometimes been called *institutional transference* (Reider, 1953). Miller (2011), in his report about using single session principles after the Hurricane

Katrina disaster, advised fostering a relationship with the service rather than an individual therapist by informing the client at the end of the session that they could return as needed and desired, and that another worker would be available and would welcome talking with them.

4 Single session thinking is not a particular model of therapy but rather an overarching philosophy of practice and, as suggested by Young (2018), a way of delivering services. It lends itself to many therapeutic models.

5 From a 1994 interview with Steve de Shazer and John Weakland (Hoyt 1994/ 2001, p. 21): *Hoyt*: What I'm getting from what you're saying is that it's best to accept that what the patient is communicating about is accurate. *Weakland*: That's an interesting way of putting it, rather than converting them. *de Shazer*: I'm not sure about the last part [...] just, "it's accurate."

6 See Figure 2.4.

7 And thus, James Hillman and Michael Ventura (1992, p. 17) commented: "If you're out of your mind in another culture or quite disturbed or impotent or anorexic, you look at what you've been eating, who's been casting spells on you, what taboo you've crossed, what you haven't done right, when you last missed reference to the gods or didn't take part in the dance, broke some tribal custom. Whatever. It could be thousands of other things—the plants, the water, the curses, the demons, the gods, being out of touch with the great spirit. It would never, never be what happened to you with your mother and your father 40 years ago. Only our culture uses that model, that myth."

8 Haley (1990 pp. 14–15) also opined that the most important decision in the history of therapy was to charge for therapy by the hour: "Historians will someday reveal who thought of this idea. The ideology and practice of therapy was largely determined when therapists chose to sit with a client and be paid for durations of time rather than by results."

9 Yet, as Slive and Bobele (2019a, p. 16) commented, "Most graduate programs do not teach brief therapy approaches, let alone single session therapy." The present volume is intended to help rectify that oversight.

10 Young and Jabreen (2020, p. 33) also importantly noted: "Increasing accessibility and affordability is a social justice issue" and went on (p. 33) to quote Hoyt and Talmon (2018, p. iv): "Recognizing the potential of single-session therapy is especially important nowadays as so many more people would benefit from mental-health services if they were affordable and did not carry the daunting stigma of seemingly endless dependency. Resources are limited, and SST has a valuable ecological function: it preserves time and money. More is not better; *better* is better (Hoyt, 1995, p. 327) – and *better* can sometimes be achieved here and now, even in one visit."

11 Simon and Nelson (2007, p. 7) elaborate: "The Solution-Focused Brief Practice approach is, above all, an approach, a stance, a perspective. It is not a Theory of how people develop, how people change, or how therapy should be conducted. One could say, we suppose, that 'one theory' (note the small *t*) is that a solution-focused approach in therapy helps clients to make the changes they wish to make because they focus on what they want rather than on what they do not want."

References

Akerele, E., & Yuryev, A. (2017). Single session psychotherapy for humanitarian missions. *International Journal of Mental Health, 46*(2), 133–138.

Amundson, J. (1996). Why pragmatics is probably enough for now. *Family Process*, *35*(4), 473–486.

Anderson, H., & Goolishian, H.A. (1992). The client is the expert: A not-knowing approach to therapy. In S. McNamee & K.J. Gergen (Eds.), *Therapy as Social Construction* (pp. 25–39). Newbury Park, CA: SAGE.

Andreas, S. (2014). SST with NLP: Rapid transformations using content-free instructions. In M.F. Hoyt & M. Talmon (Eds.), *Capturing the Moment: Single Session Therapy and Walk-In Services* (pp. 277–298). Bethel, CT: Crown House Publishing.

Appelbaum, S. (1973). Parkinson's law in psychotherapy. *International Journal of Psychoanalytic Psychotherapy*, *4*, 426–436.

Battino, R. (2006). *Expectation: The Very Brief Therapy Book*. Bethel, CT: Crown House Publishing.

Battino, R. (2014). Expectation: The essence of very brief therapy. In M.F. Hoyt & M. Talmon (Eds.), *Capturing the Moment: Single Session Therapy and Walk-In Services* (pp. 393–406). Bethel, CT: Crown House Publishing.

Bedggood, J. (2018). The first time: Teaching skills that prepare interns and new therapists for walk-in counseling. In M.F. Hoyt, M. Bobele, A. Slive, J. Young, & M. Talmon (Eds.), *Single-Session Therapy by Walk-In or Appointment: Administrative, Clinical, and Supervisory Aspects of One-at-a-Time Services* (pp. 327–333). New York: Routledge.

Bloom, B.L. (1981). Focused single-session therapy: Initial development and evaluation. In S.H. Budman (Ed.), *Forms of Brief Therapy*, (pp. 167–216). New York: Guilford Press. A revised and extended version ("Bloom's focused single-session therapy") appeared in B.L. Bloom, Planned Short-Term Psychotherapy: A Clinical Handbook (2nd ed., pp. 97-121). Boston: Allyn & Bacon, 1992.

Bobele, M., Fullen, C., Houston, B., Martinez, A.M., Moffat, L., & Santos, J. (2018). Westside stories: Walk-in and single-session therapy in San Antonio. In M.F. Hoyt, M. Bobele, A. Slive, J. Young, & M. Talmon (Eds.), *Single-Session Therapy by Walk-In or Appointment: Administrative, Clinical, and Supervisory Aspects of One-at-a-Time Services* (pp. 221–250). New York: Routledge.

Bobele, M., & Slive, A. (2015). Walk-in psychotherapy: A new paradigm. *The Milton H. Erickson Foundation Newsletter*, *35*(2), 9.

Blanchard, K., & Johnson, S. (1982). *The One Minute Manager*. New York: William Morrow.

Bordin, E.S. (1979). The generalizability of the psychoanalytic concept of the working alliance. *Psychotherapy: Theory, Research & Practice*, *16*(3), 252–260.

Budman, S.H., Friedman, S., Hoyt, M.F. (1992). Last words on first sessions. In S.H. Budman, M.F. Hoyt, & S. Friedman (Eds.), *The First Session in Brief Therapy*, (pp. 345–358). New York: Guilford Press.

Burns, D.D. (1980). *Feeling Good: The New Mood Therapy*. New York: William Morrow.

Burns, D.D. (2020). *Feeling Great: The Revolutionary New Treatment for Depression and Anxiety*. Eau Claire, WI: PESI Publishing & Media.

Campbell, A. (2012). Single-session approaches to therapy: A time to review. *Australian and New Zealand Journal of Family Therapy*, *33*(1), 15–26.

Chow, D. (2018). *The First Kiss: Undoing the Intake Model and Igniting the First Sessions in Psychotherapy*. Correlate Press.

Cummings, N.A. (2000). The single-session misunderstanding. In *The Collected Papers of Nicholas A. Cummings. Vol. 1: The Value of Psychological Treatment* (p. 77). Phoenix, AZ: Zeig, Tucker, & Theisen.

Dass-Brailsford, P., & Hage Thomley, R.S. (2015). Using walk-in counseling services after Hurricane Katrina: A program evaluation. *Journal of Aggression, Maltreatment, and Trauma, 24*(4), 419–432.

Dryden, W. (2019). *Single-Session One-at-a-Time Therapy: A Rational Emotive Behavior Therapy Approach*. Abinsdon, Oxon, UK: Routledge.

Dryden, W. (2020). Single-session one-at-a-time therapy: A personal approach. *Australian and New Zealand Journal of Family Therapy, 41*(3), 283–301.

Dryden, W. (2021). *Single-Session Therapy and Its Future: What SST Leaders Think*. Abingdon, Oxon, UK: Routledge.

Duncan, B.L., & Miller, S.D. (2000). *The Heroic Client: Doing Client-Directed, Outcome-Oriented Therapy*. San Francisco: Jossey-Bass.

Duncan, B.L., Miller, S.D., Wampold, B.E., & Hubble, M.A. (2009). *The Heart and Soul of Change: Delivering What Works in Therapy* (2nd ed.). Washington, DC: APA Books.

Fisch, R. (1994). Basic elements in the brief therapies. In M.F. Hoyt (Ed.), *Constructive Therapies* (pp. 126–139). New York: Guilford Press.

Fullen, C.T. (2020). The therapeutic alliance in a single session: A conversation analysis. *Journal of Systemic Therapies, 38*(4), 45–61.

George, E., Iveson, C., & Ratner, H. (2006). *BRIEFER: A Solution-Focused Manual*. London: Brief Therapy Press.

Gibbons, J., & Plath, D. (2012). Single session work in hospitals. *Australian and New Zealand Journal of Family Therapy, 33*(1), 39–53.

Giges, B., & Peitpas, A. (2000). Brief contact interventions in sport psychology. *The Sport Psychologist, 14*, 176–187.

Goulding, M.M., & Goulding, R.L. (1979) *Changing Lives Through Redecision Therapy*. New York: Grove Press.

Guthrie, B. (2018). Reflections on providing single-session therapy in post-disaster Haiti. In M.F. Hoyt, M. Bobele, A. Slive, J. Young, & M. Talmon (Eds.), *Single-Session Therapy by Walk-In or Appointment: Administrative, Clinical, and Supervisory Aspects of One-at-a-Time Services* (pp. 303–317). New York: Routledge.

Haley, J. (1969). The art of being a failure as a therapist. In *The Power Tactics of Jesus Christ and Other Essays* (pp. 69–78). New York: Avon.

Haley, J. (1977). *Problem-Solving Therapy: New Strategies for Effective Family Therapy*. San Francisco: Jossey-Bass.

Haley, J. (1990). Why not long-term therapy? In J.K. Zeig & S.G. Gilligan (Eds.), *Brief Therapy: Myths, Methods, and Metaphors* (pp. 3–17). New York: Brunner/Mazel.

Hampson, R., O'Hanlon, J., Franklin, A., Petony, M., Fridgant, L., & Heins, T. (1999). The place of single-session family consultations: Five years' experience in Canberra. *Australian and New Zealand Journal of Family Therapy, 20*(4), 195–200.

Harari, Y.N. (2015). *Sapiens: A Brief History of Humankind*. New York: Harper Perennial.

Harper-Jaques, S. (2018). Supervision and the single-session therapist: Learnings from ten years of practice. In M.F. Hoyt, M. Bobele, A. Slive, J. Young, & M. Talmon (Eds.), *Single-Session Therapy by Walk-In or Appointment: Administrative, Clinical, and Supervisory Aspects of One-at-a-Time Services* (pp. 334–346). New York: Rutledge.

Henneberry, J. (2021). *A Foucauldian Discourse Analysis of the Co-Construction of Client Identity within a Single-Session Therapy*. Unpublished doctoral dissertation, Ottawa, ONT, Canada: University of Ottawa.

Hillman, J., & Ventura, J. (1992). *We've Had a Hundred Years of Psychotherapy – and the World's Getting Worse*. San Francisco, CA: HarperSanFrancisco.

Hoffman, L. (1990). Constructing realities: An art of lenses. *Family Process, 29*, 1–12.

Hoyt, M.F. (1991). Teaching and learning short-term psychotherapy within an HMO. In C.S. Austad & W.H. Berman (Eds.), *Psychotherapy in Managed Health Care: The Optimal Use of Time and Resources* (pp. 98–108). Washington, DC: American Psychological Association. Reprinted in M.F. Hoyt, *Brief Therapy and Managed Care* (pp. 63–68). San Francisco: Jossey-Bass, 1995.

Hoyt, M.F. (1995). *Brief Therapy and Managed Care: Readings for Contemporary Practice*. San Francisco: Jossey-Bass.

Hoyt, M.F. (1994). On the importance of keeping it simple and taking the patient seriously: A conversation with Steve de Shazer and John Weakland. In M.F. Hoyt (Ed.), *Constructive Therapies*. (pp. 11–40). New York: Guilford Press. Reprinted in M.F. Hoyt, *Interviews with Brief Therapy Experts* (pp. 1–33). New York: Brunner/Routledge, 2001.

Hoyt, M.F. (2000). What can we learn from Milton Erickson's therapeutic failures? In *Some Stories Are Better than Others* (pp. 189–194). Philadelphia, PA: Brunner-Mazel.

Hoyt, M.F. (2001). Direction and discovery: A conversation about power and politics in narrative therapy with Michael White and Jeff Zimmerman. In *Interviews with Brief Therapy Experts* (pp. 265–293). New York: Brunner-Routledge.

Hoyt, M.F. (2011). Foreword. In A. Slive & M. Bobele (Eds.), *When One Hour is All You Have: Effective Therapy for Walk-In Clients* (pp. ix–xv). Phoenix, AZ: Zeig, Tucker, & Theisen.

Hoyt, M.F. (2017). *Brief Therapy and Beyond: Stories, Language, Love, Hope, and Time*. New York: Routledge.

Hoyt, M.F. (2019). Strategic therapies: Roots and branches. *Journal of Systemic Therapies, 38*(1), 30–43.

Hoyt, M.F., & Bobele, M. (Eds.). (2019). *Creative Therapy in Challenging Situations: Unusual Interventions to Help People*. New York: Routledge.

Hoyt, M.F., Bobele, M., Slive, A., Young, J. & Talmon, M. (Eds.). (2018). *Single-Session Therapy by Walk-In or Appointment: Administrative, Clinical, and Supervisory Aspects of One-at-a-Time Services*. New York: Routledge.

Hoyt, M.F., & Dryden, W. (2018). Toward the future of single-session therapy: An interview. *Journal of Systemic Therapies, 37*(1), 79–90. Reprinted in

W. Dryden, *Single Session Therapy and Its Future: What SST Leaders Think* (pp. 31–45). New York: Routledge, 2021.

Hoyt, M.F., Miller, S.D., Held, B., & Matthews, W. (2001). About constructivism (or, if four colleagues talked in New York, would anyone hear it?): A conversation with Scott Miller, Barbara Held, and William Matthews. In M.F. Hoyt (Ed.), *Interviews with Brief Therapy Experts* (pp. 206–225). New York: Brunner-Routledge.

Hoyt, M.F., & Ritterman, M. (2012). Brief therapy in a taxi. *The Milton H. Erickson Foundation Newsletter, 32*(2), 7.

Hoyt, M.F., Rosenbaum, R., & Talmon, M. (1992). Planned single-session psychotherapy. In S.H. Budman, M.F. Hoyt, & S. Friedman (Eds.), *The First Session in Brief Therapy* (pp. 59–86). New York: Guilford Press.

Hoyt, M.F., & Talmon, M. (Eds.) (2014). *Capturing the Moment: Single-Session Therapy and Walk-In Services*. Bethel, CT: Crown House Publishing.

Hoyt, M.F., & Talmon, M. (2018). *Prefazione* [Preface]. In F. Cannistrà & F. Piccirilli (Eds.), *Terapia a Seduta Singola: Principi e Pratche* (pp. ix–xiv). Florence, Italy: Giunti. (In Italian: translated as *Single-Session Therapy: Principles and Practices*.)

Hoyt, M.F., Young, J., & Rycroft, P. (2020). Single Session Thinking 2020. *Australian and New Zealand Journal of Family Therapy, 41*(3), 218–230.

Iveson, C. (2019). However great the question, it's the answer that makes a difference. In M.F. Hoyt & M. Bobele (Eds.), *Creative Therapy in Challenging Situations: Unusual Interventions to Help Clients* (pp. 121–133). New York: Routledge.

Iveson, C., George, E., & Ratner, H. (2012). *Brief Coaching: A Solution Focused Approach*. New York: Routledge.

James, W. (1987). *William James: Writings 1902–1910: The Varieties of Religious Experience/Pragmatism/A Pluralistic Universe/The Meaning of Truth/Some Problems of Philosophy/Essays*. (B. Kluklick, Ed.). New York: Library of America. (*Pragmatism* originally published 1907).

Lazarus, A.A. (1971). *Behavior Therapy and Beyond*. New York: McGraw Hill.

Lewis, D., & Cheshire, A. (2007). *Te whakaakona*: Teaching and learning as one. *Journal of Systemic Therapies, 26*(3), 43–56.

Luutonen, S., Santalahti, A., Makinen, M., Vahlberg, T., & Rautava, P. (2019). One-session cognitive behavior treatment for long-term frequent attenders in primary care: Randomized controlled trial. *Scandanavian Journal of Primary Health Care, 37*(1), 98–104. doi: 10.1080/02813432.2019.1569371.

Malan, D.H., Bacal, H.A., Heath, E.S., & Balfour, F.H.G. (1968). A study of psychodynamic changes in untreated neurotic patients: Improvements that are questionable on dynamic criteria. *British Journal of Psychiatry, 114*, 525–551.

Malan, D.H., Heath, E.S., Bacal, H.A., & Balfour, F.H.G. (1975). Psychodynamic changes in untreated neurotic patients. II. Apparently genuine improvements. *Archives of General Psychiatry, 32*, 110–126.

Malm, S. (2014). The taxis in which the passengers get tips! Cab firm puts therapists in back of its cars to counsel lonely Swedes. Retrieved from www.dailymail.co.uk/news/article-2812359.

Matthews, K.M. (2018). The integration of emotion-focused therapy within single-session therapy. *Journal of Systemic Therapies, 37*(4), 15–28.

Miller, J.K. (2011). Single-session intervention in the wake of Hurricane Katrina: Strategies for disaster mental health counseling. In A. Slive & M. Bobele (Eds.), *When One Session is All You Have: Effective Therapy for Walk-In Clients* (pp. 185–202). Phoenix, AZ: Zeig, Tucker, & Theisen.

Miller, J.K. (2014). Single session therapy in China. In M.F. Hoyt & M. Talmon (Eds.), *Capturing the Moment: Single Session Therapy and Walk-In Services* (pp. 195–214). Bethel, CT: Crown House Publishing.

Miller, J.K., Platt, J.J., & Conroy, K.M. (2018). Single-session therapy in the majority world: Addressing the challenge of service delivery in Cambodia and the implications for other global contexts. In M.F. Hoyt, M. Bobele, A. Slive, J. Young, & M. Talmon (Eds.), *Single-Session Therapy by Walk-In or Appointment: Administrative, Clinical, and Supervisory Aspects of One-at-a-Time Services* (pp. 116–134). New York: Routledge.

Miller, S.D., Hubble, M.A., & Chow, D. (2020). *Better Results: Using Deliberate Practice to Improve Therapeutic Effectiveness.* Washington, DC: APA Books.

Miller, W.R. (2000). Rediscovering fire: Small interventions, large effects. *Psychology of Addictive Behaviors, 14*(1), 6–18.

Napier, A.Y., & Whitaker, C.A. (1978). *The Family Crucible.* New York: Harper & Row.

Nardone, G., & Salvini, A. (2018). *The Strategic Dialogue: Rendering the Diagnostic Interview a Real Therapeutic Intervention.* New York: Routledge. (Work originally published in 2007).

Nardone, G., & Watzlawick, P. (2005). *Brief Strategic Therapy: Philosophy, Techniques, and Research.* New York: Jason Aronson.

Norcross, J.C. (Ed.) (2011). *Psychotherapy Relationships that Work: Therapist Contributions and Responsiveness to Patients* (2nd ed.). New York: Oxford University Press.

O'Hanlon, & Hexum (1990). *An Uncommon Casebook: The Complete Clinical Work of Milton H. Erickson, M.D.* New York: Norton.

Ozaki, N. (2017). *A Conversation Analysis of Therapist-Client Interactional Patterns in Single Session Therapy: A Researcher's Interpretation.* Doctoral dissertation. Fort Lauderdale, FL: Nova Southeastern University. Retrieved from https://nsuworks.nova.edu/shss_dft_etd/45.

Paul, K.E., & van Ommeren, M. (2013). A primer on single session therapy and its potential application in humanitarian situations. *Intervention: Journal of Mental-Health and Psychosocial Support in Conflict-Affected Areas, 11*(1), 8–23.

Perdomo, C. (2017). Undocumented and deportable: Re-authoring trauma within the context of immigration in a narrative informed single session. *Journal of Systemic Therapies, 36*(4), 3–15.

Pitt, T., Thomas, O., Lindsay, P., Hanton, S., & Bawden, M. (2015). Doing sports psychology briefly? A critical review of single session therapeutic approaches and their relevance to sport psychology. *International Review of Sport and Exercise Psychology.* doi: 10.1080/1750984X.2015.1027719.

Potkewitz, H. (2015). Can your relationship handle a trip to IKEA? *Wall Street Journal.* Retrieved from www.wsj.com/articles/can-your-relationship-handle-a-trip-to-ikea-1429724227.

Prochaska, J.O. (1999). How do people change and how can we change to help many more people? In M.A. Hubble, B.L. Duncan, & S.D. Miller (Eds.),

The Heart and Soul of Change: What Works in Therapy (pp. 227–255). Washington, DC: APA Books.

Ratner, H., & Yusuf, D. (2015). *Brief Coaching with Children and Young People.* New York: Routledge.

Reider, N. (1953). A type of transference to institutions. *Journal of Hillside Hospital, 2,* 23–29.

Reiter, J.T., Dobmeyer, A.C., & Hunter, C.L. (2018). The primary care behavioral health (PCBH) model: An overview and operational definition. *Journal of Clinical Psychology in Medical Settings, 25,* 109–126.

Rosenbaum, R. (2008). Psychotherapy is not short or long. *APA Monitor on Psychology, 39*(7), 4, 8.

Rosenbaum, R., Hoyt, M.F., & Talmon, M. (1990). The challenge of single-session therapies: Creating pivotal moments. In R.A. Wells & V.J. Giannetti (Eds.), *Handbook of the Brief Psychotherapies* (pp. 165–189). New York: Plenum Press. Reprinted in M.F. Hoyt, *Brief Therapy and Managed Care* (pp. 105–139). San Francisco: Jossey-Bass, 1995.

Rosenberg, T., & McDaniel, S. (2014). Single-session medical family therapy and the patient-centered medical home. In M.F. Hoyt & M. Talmon (Eds.), *Capturing the Moment* (pp. 349–362). Bethel, CT: Crown House.

Rycroft, P. (2018). Capturing the moment in supervision. In M.F. Hoyt, M. Bobele, A. Slive, J. Young, & M. Talmon (Eds.), *Single-Session Therapy by Walk-In or Appointment: Administrative, Clinical, and Supervisory Aspects of One-at-a-Time Services* (pp. 347–365). New York: Routledge.

Rycroft, P., & Young, J. (2014). SST in Australia: Learning from teaching. In M.F. Hoyt & M. Talmon (Eds.), *Capturing the Moment: Single Session Therapy and Walk-In Services* (pp. 141–156). Bethel, CT: Crown House Publishing.

Schlanger, K., & Krohner, E. (2019). Our clients *are* able and strong: MRI problem-solving brief therapy in action. In M.F. Hoyt & M. Bobele (Eds.), *Creative Therapy in Challenging Situations: Unusual Interventions to Help Clients* (pp. 172–182). New York: Routledge.

Short, D. (2020). *From William James to Milton Erickson: The Care of Human Consciousness.* Bloomington, IN: Archway Publishing.

Short, D., Erickson, B.A., & Klein, R.E. (2005). *Hope and Resiliency: Understanding the Psychotherapeutic Strategies of Milton H. Erickson, M.D.* Bethel, CT: Crown House Publishing.

Simon, J.K., & Nelson, T.S. (2007). *I Am More than My Label: Solution-Focused Brief Practice with Long-Term Users of Mental Health Services.* New York: Haworth Press.

Slive, A., & Bobele, M. (2011). *When One Hour is All You Have: Effective Therapy for Walk-In Clients.* Phoenix, AZ: Zeig, Tucker, & Theisen.

Slive, A., & Bobele, M. (2014). Walk-in single session therapy: Accessible mental health services. In M.F. Hoyt & M. Talmon (Eds.), *Capturing the Moment: Single Session Therapy and Walk-In Services* (pp. 73–94). Bethel CT: Crown House.

Slive, A., & Bobele, M. (2018). The three top reasons why walk-in/single-sessions make perfect sense. In M.F. Hoyt, M. Bobele, A. Slive, J. Young, & M. Talmon (Eds.), *Single-Session Therapy by Walk-In or Appointment:*

Administrative, Clinical, and Supervisory Aspects of One-at-a-Time Services (pp. 27–39). New York: Routledge.

Slive, A., & Bobele, M. (2019a). Introduction to the special section: What's so scary about single-session therapy? *Journal of Systemic Therapies, 38*(4), 15–16.

Slive, A., & Bobele, M. (2019b). Ideas for addressing doubts about walk-in/single-session therapy. *Journal of Systemic Therapies, 38*(4), 17–30.

Soo-Hoo, T. (2018). Working within the client's cultural context in single-session therapy. In M.F. Hoyt, M. Bobele, A. Slive, J. Young, & M. Talmon (Eds.), *Single-Session Therapy by Walk-In or Appointment: Administrative, Clinical, and Supervisory Aspects of One-at-a-Time Services* (pp. 186–201). New York: Routledge.

Soo-Hoo, T. (2019). Beyond reason and insight: The 180-degree turn in therapeutic interventions. In M.F. Hoyt & M. Bobele (Eds.), *Creative Therapy in Challenging Situations: Unusual Interventions to Help Clients* (pp. 193–208). New York: Routledge.

Taibbi, R. (2016). *The Art of the First Session: Making Psychotherapy Count from the Start.* New York: Norton.

Talmon, M. (2018). The eternal now: On becoming and being a single-session therapist. In (Eds.), *Single-Session Therapy by Walk-In or Appointment: Administrative, Clinical, and Supervisory Aspects of One-at-a-Time Services* (pp. 149–154). New York: Routledge. M.F. Hoyt, M. Bobele, A. Slive, J. Young, M. Talmon

Talmon, M., & Dryden, W. (2021). The future of single-session therapy. In Dryden W. (Ed.), *Single-Session Therapy and Its Future: What SST Leaders Think* (pp. 26–30). Abingdon, Oxon, U.K.: Routledge.

Talmon, M., & Hoyt, M.F. (2014). Moments are forever: SST and walk-in services now and in the future. In M.F. Hoyt & M. Talmon (Eds.), *Capturing the Moment: Single Session Therapy and Walk-In Services* (pp. 463–485). Bethel, CT: Crown House Publishing.

Vitry, G., de Scorraille, C., & Hoyt, M.F. (in press). Redundant attempted solutions: 50 years of theory, evolution, and new supporting data. *Australian and New Zealand Journal of Family Therapy,* forthcoming.

Walter, J., & Peller, J. (1994). "On track" in solution-focused brief therapy. In M.F. Hoyt (Ed.), *Constructive Therapies* (pp. 111–125). New York: Guilford Press.

Wampold, B.E. (2015, October). How important are the common factors in psychotherapy? An update. *World Psychiatry, 14*(3), 270–277.

Whitaker, C.A. (1992). Symbolic experiential family therapy: Model and methodology. In J.K. Zeig (Ed.), *The Evolution of Psychotherapy: The Second Conference* (pp. 13–20). New York: Brunner/Mazel.

Winnicott, D.W. (1958). *Through Paediatrics to Psychoanalysis.* New York: Basic Books.

Wynne, A.R., & Wynne, L.C. (1986). At the center of the cyclone: Family therapists as consultants with family and divorce courts. In Lynne L.C., McDaniel S.H., & Weber T.T. (Eds.), *Systems Consultation: A New Perspective for Family Therapy* (pp. 300–319). New York: Guilford Press.

Yalom, I., & Leszcz, M. (2005). *The Theory and Practice of Group Psychotherapy* (5th ed.). New York: Basic Books.

Yapko, M.D. (1990). Brief therapy tactics in longer-term psychotherapies. In J.K. Zeig & S.G. Gilligan (Eds.), *Brief Therapy: Myths, Methods, and Metaphors* (pp. 183–202). New York: Brunner/Mazel.

Young, J. (2018). Single session therapy: The gift that keeps on giving. In M.F. Hoyt, M. Bobele, A. Slive, J. Young, & M. Talmon (Eds.), *Single-Session Therapy by Walk-In or Appointment: Clinical, Supervisory, and Administrative Aspects* (pp. 40–58). New York: Routledge.

Young, J. (2020). Putting single session therapy to work the Bouverie way: Conceptual, practical, training and implementation ideas. *Australian and New Zealand Journal of Family Therapy*, *41*(3), 231–248.

Young, J., & Dryden, W. (2019). Single-session therapy – Past and future: An interview. *British Journal of Guidance and Counseling*, *47*(5), 645–654. Reprinted in W. Dryden, *Single Session Therapy and Its Future: What SST Leaders Think* (pp. 46–63) New York: Routledge, 2021.

Young, J., & Rycroft, P. (1997). Single-session therapy: Capturing the moment. *Psychotherapy in Australia*, *4*, 18–23.

Young, J., Rycroft, P., & Weir, S. (2014). Implementing single session therapy: Practical wisdoms from Down Under. In M.F. Hoyt, & M. Talmon (Eds.), *Capturing the Moment: Single Session Therapy and Walk-In Services* (pp. 121–140). Bethel, CT: Crown House Publishing.

Young, J., Weir, S., & Rycroft, P. (2012). Implementing single session therapy. *Australian and New Zealand Journal of Family Therapy*, *33*(1), 84–97.

Young, K. (2018). Change in the winds: The growth of walk-in therapy clinics in Ontario, Canada. In M.F. Hoyt, M. Bobele, A. Slive, J. Young, & M. Talmon (Eds.), *Single-Session Therapy by Walk-In or Appointment: Administrative, Clinical, and Supervisory Aspects of One-at-a-Time Services* (pp. 59–71). New York: Routledge.

Young, K. (2020). Multi-story listening: Using narrative practices at walk-in clinics. *Journal of Systemic Therapies*, *39*(3), 34–45.

Young, K., & Jebreen, J. (2020). Recognizing single-session therapy as psychotherapy. *Journal of Systemic Therapies*, *38*(4), 31–44.

Index

haiku 34, 37
Haley, Jay vii, 4, 37, 337, 346
Harari, Yuval Noah 341–342
Harwood, Gwen 337
headspace 133–138, 267
health center staff 230
health funding, limited resources 107
  competing priorities 107
history of single session therapy 5–6
homework 33
hope 29–41, 215, 222
Houston Galveston Institute (HGI) 8,
  10, 223–224
Huineng 89
human immunodeficiency virus (HIV)
  202–208
  acquired immune deficiency
  syndrome (AIDS) 202
  antiretroviral therapies 202–203
  community-based counseling service
  204–208
  cross-cultural/non-western contexts
  211–264
  diagnosis 202–210
  test, discussions 203–208
  testing 202–203
hypnotherapy 255–264
  Erickson, Milton 255
  Ericksonian strategic model 256–258
  Esdaile, James 255
  family single session practice
  265–322
  group hypnotherapy 258–261
  Mesmer, Franz Anton 255

identifying intervention 105
identifying need 143
identifying solution 158
implementation and training 339
implementation challenges 112–113
implementation science 104–108
improvement of families' lives 184–185
increased staff, lobbying for 105
Indigenous communities 18, 223–233
  availability of counseling 230
  challenges 230
  collaborative relationship 227–228
  community context 229–230
  cultural healers 230
  First Nation Communities 225–227
  First Nations Health Authority 225
  Health Centre staff 230
  hope 231–232

informal conversations, therapeutic
  value 230
  leadership, connect with 226
  mistrust 230
  Nuu-Chah-Nulth community
  227–229
  reflexive responses 230
  Royal Canadian Mounted
  Police 226
  thinking 228–229
  traditional ceremonies, participation
  in 230
Indigenous populations 18, 213, 231
infants 192–201
  alliance with family 199
  alliance with professionals 198
  clinical example 198–200
  collaborative single session model
  194, 197–198
  engagement in process 199–200
  framework 199
  review 200
  structure of collaborative 195–197
  types of sessions 193–194
informal conversations, therapeutic
  value 230
inquiry interview with family 249–250
intake 44
integrating with existing structures 144
inter-session 148–149
internal states 93
  emotions 93
international conferences 7–9, 345
intervention characteristics
  framework 107
  SSFC framework 107
invitations 169
issue selection 156, 160
Italian Center for Single Session
  Therapy 6
Iveson, Chris 329

James, William 341
jealousy 155
joy 29–41

Kaimahi 237
Kaiser Permanente xxvii, 5

lack of control 155
language 217
large numbers of consumers 107
Lao Tzu 3